ADVANCES IN
Pediatrics

VOLUMES 1 THROUGH 56 (OUT OF PRINT)

VOLUME 57

The GH/IGF-1 Axis in Growth and Development: New Insights Derived from Animal Models, *by Dara Cannata, Archana Vijayakumar, Yvonne Fierz, and Derek LeRoith*

Fetal Surgery: Progress and Perspectives, *by Miho Watanabe and Alan W. Flake*

Advances in the Surgical Management of Gastroesophageal Reflux, *by John A. Sandoval and David A. Partrick*

Vice President, Continuity Publishing: Kimberly Murphy
Editor: Jessica McCool

Editorial Office:
Elsevier
1600 John F. Kennedy Blvd,
Suite 1800
Philadelphia, PA 19103-2899

International Standard Serial Number: 0065-3101
International Standard Book Number: 13: 978-0-323-08405-5

Printed and bound by CPI Group (UK) Ltd, Croydon, CR0 4YY

Transferred to Digital Print 2011

ADVANCES IN
Pediatrics

CONTRIBUTORS

ERAKA BATH, MD, Director, Child Forensic Services, Assistant Professor, University of California, Los Angeles, Department of Psychiatry, University of California, Los Angeles Neuropsychiatric Institute, David Geffen School of Medicine at University of California, Los Angeles, Los Angeles, California

TERI BOOK, RN, MSN, CPNP, Pediatric Nurse Practitioner, For OC Kids Neurodevelopmental Center, Orange, California

JANE D. CARVER, PhD, MS, MPH, Department of Pediatrics, College of Medicine, University of South Florida, Tampa, Florida

KEVIN CHAN, MD, MPH, Division of Pediatric Emergency Medicine, Department of Pediatrics, Hospital for Sick Children; Fellow, Munk Centre for Global Studies, University of Toronto, Toronto, Ontario, Canada

AGNES H. CHEN, MD, Assistant Clinical Professor of Pediatrics and Neurology, Division of Pediatric Neurology, Los Angeles County-Harbor-University of California, Los Angeles Medical Center, David Geffen School of Medicine at University of California, Los Angeles, Torrance, California

DAI H. CHUNG, MD, Departments of Pediatric Surgery and Cancer Biology, Vanderbilt University Medical Center, Nashville, Tennessee

NADJA C. COLON, MD, Department of Pediatric Surgery, Vanderbilt University Medical Center, Nashville, Tennessee

JEFFREY J. DEHMER, MD, Department of Surgery, University of North Carolina at Chapel Hill, Chapel Hill, North Carolina

SUSAN B. EDELSTEIN, LCSW, Adjunct Assistant Director, University of California, Los Angeles, Department of Pediatrics, Executive Director, University of California, Los Angeles TIES for Families, Los Angeles, California

STEVEN G. FEDERICO, MD, Medical Director, School-Based Health Centers, Denver Health, Denver; Associate Professor of Pediatrics, University of Colorado School of Medicine, Aurora, Colorado

VINCENT A. FULGINITI, MD, Chancellor Emeritus, University of Colorado Health Sciences Center, Denver; Professor Emeritus at Universities of Colorado and Arizona (Pediatrics), Tucson, Arizona

MEGAN K. FULLER, MD, Department of Surgery, University of North Carolina at Chapel Hill, Chapel Hill, North Carolina

FRANK R. GREER, MD, Professor of Pediatrics, Wisconsin Perinatal Center, Meriter Hospital, University of Wisconsin School of Medicine and Public Health, Madison, Wisconsin

MICHAEL A. HELMRATH, MD, Division of Pediatric Surgery, Cincinnati Children's Hospital Medical Center, Cincinnati, Ohio

PAUL KAPLOWITZ, MD, PhD, Chief of Endocrinology, Professor of Pediatrics, Division of Endocrinology, Children's National Medical Center, George Washington University School of Medicine and the Health Sciences, Washington, DC

MICHAEL S. KAPPY, MD, PhD, FAAP, University of Colorado Health Sciences Center, The Children's Hospital, Aurora, Colorado

RUSSELL S. KIRBY, PhD, MS, FACE, Department of Pediatrics, College of Medicine; Department of Community and Family Health, College of Public Health, University of South Florida, Tampa, Florida

CAROLINE M. LEE, MA, CCC-SLP, University of California, Los Angeles Senior Speech-Language Pathologist, Speech and Language Consultant, University of California, Los Angeles TIES for Families, Los Angeles, California

WANDA MARSHALL, MS, CPNP, Program Manager, School-Based Health Centers, Denver Health, Denver, Colorado

PAUL MELINKOVICH, MD, Professor of Pediatrics, University of Colorado School of Medicine, Aurora; Director of Community Health, Denver Health, Denver, Colorado

BRADLEY S. MILLER, MD, PhD, Assistant Professor, Division of Endocrinology, Department of Pediatrics, University of Minnesota Amplatz Children's Hospital, Minneapolis, Minnesota

AYESHA MIRZA, MD, FAAP, Assistant Professor, Department of Pediatrics, University of Florida, Jacksonville, Florida

JUDITH D. RANELLS, MD, Department of Pediatrics, College of Medicine, University of South Florida, Tampa, Florida

MOBEEN H. RATHORE, MD, CPE, FAAP, FIDSA, FACPE, Professor and Associate Chairman, Department of Pediatrics, University of Florida; Chief, Section of Infectious Diseases and Immunology, Wolfson Children's Hospital, Jacksonville, Florida

KENNETH B. ROBERTS, MD, Professor Emeritus of Pediatrics, University of North Carolina School of Medicine, Chapel Hill; Moses Cone Health System, Greensboro, North Carolina

JOSÉ R. ROMERO, MD, FAAP, Professor of Pediatrics, Horace C. Cabe Chair in Infectious Diseases; Director, Pediatric Infectious Diseases Section, Arkansas Children's Hospital, University of Arkansas for Medical Sciences, Little Rock, Arkansas

RANGARAJ SELVARANGAN, BVSc, PhD, Associate Professor, Children's Mercy Hospital, University of Missouri-School of Medicine, Kansas City, Missouri

ROBIN STEINBERG-EPSTEIN, MD, Associate Clinical Professor of Pediatrics, Division of Developmental-Behavioral Pediatrics, University of California, Irvine School of Medicine; Attending Physician, For OC Kids Neurodevelopmental Center, Orange, California

LORI WALDINGER, MA, Rehabilitation Specialist, University of California, Los Angeles TIES for Families, Educational Consultant–General and Special Education, Los Angeles, California

CLAUDIA WANG, MD, Clinical Professor of Pediatrics, University of California, Los Angeles Department of Pediatrics; Medical Director, University of California, Los Angeles Suspected Child Abuse and Neglect (SCAN) Team; Pediatric Consultant, University of California, Los Angeles TIES for Families, Mattel Children's Hospital at University of California, Los Angeles, David Geffen School of Medicine at University of California,Los Angeles, California

SHARON B. WIGAL, PhD, Clinical Professor of Pediatrics, Department of Pediatrics, Child Development Center, University of California, Irvine, California

PATRICIA J. YOON, MD, Associate Professor, Department of Otolaryngology–Head and Neck Surgery, University of Colorado School of Medicine; Associate Medical Director, The Bill Daniels Center for Children's Hearing, The Children's Hospital, Aurora, Colorado

CONTENTS VOLUME 58 • 2011

Immunization Update III

By Ayesha Mirza and Mobeen H. Rathore

The Human Parechoviruses: An Overview

By José R. Romero and Rangaraj Selvarangan

Care of the Foster Child: A Primer for the Pediatrician

By Claudia Wang, Susan B. Edelstein, Lori Waldinger, Caroline M. Lee, and Eraka Bath

School-Based Health Centers: A Model for the Provision of Adolescent Primary Care

By Steven G. Federico, Wanda Marshall, and Paul Melinkovich

The Past Decade in Pediatric Education: Progress, Concerns, and Questions

By Kenneth B. Roberts

rhGH Safety and Efficacy Update
By Bradley S. Miller

Update on Precocious Puberty: Girls are Showing Signs of Puberty Earlier, but Most Do Not Require Treatment
By Paul Kaplowitz

Update on Pediatric Epilepsy
By Agnes H. Chen

Hearing Loss and Cochlear Implantation in Children
By Patricia J. Yoon

Neuroblastoma
By Nadja C. Colon and Dai H. Chung

Advances in Pediatrics 58 (2011) xxi

ADVANCES IN PEDIATRICS

Introduction

Michael S. Kappy, MD, PhD

The editors present volume 58 of *Advances in Pediatrics*. In keeping with our tradition of honoring those who contributed greatly to pediatrics, we feature Waldo Nelson, MD, a giant in our field, as our annual honoree in the "Foundations of Pediatrics" segment of this issue. The article by Chan is in keeping with our recent addition of articles on international health. As with the past issues, a variety of topics related to general pediatric care are presented, as well as topics related to infectious disease, endocrinology, surgery, pharmacology, and others. We welcome suggestions for topics to be included in future volumes of *Advances in Pediatrics*, and these may be communicated to us at: kappy.michael@tchden.org.

Michael S. Kappy, MD, PhD
Department of Pediatrics
University of Colorado Health Sciences Center
The Children's Hospital
13123 East 16th Avenue
B-265, Aurora, CO 80045, USA

E-mail address: kappy.michael@tchden.org

0065-3101/11/$ – see front matter
doi:10.1016/j.yapd.2011.03.016

Advances in Pediatrics 58 (2011) 1–10

ADVANCES IN PEDIATRICS

Waldo E. Nelson, MD (1898–1997) Giant of Pediatrics

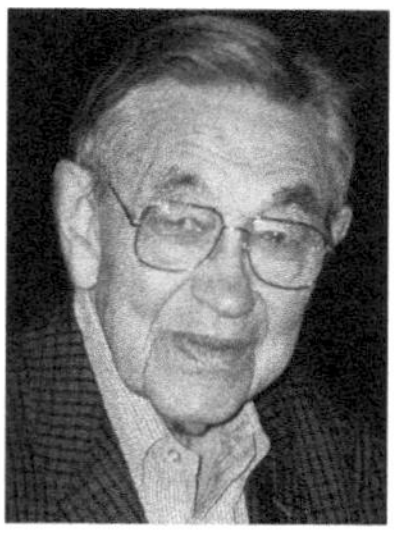

Vincent A. Fulginiti, MD

University of Colorado Health Sciences Center, 4260 North Osage Drive, Tucson AZ 85718, USA

How to describe a man who was mentor to many, editor supreme, taskmaster, husband, father, grandfather, great grandfather, and overall a powerful influence on pediatric education and clinical care in the world? One could simply recite his biography and accomplishments but that would simply be the facts; underlying them is a force in pediatrics felt even today by his disciples throughout the world and continual publication of his seminal text and the journal he devoted his expertise to for many years. Perhaps the best way to start is to discuss this influence and force and then give the so-called backstory of his personal and professional life.

If one looks at current pediatric education and practice, one must consider what influences the educational process and the professionals in this discipline. Today, most learners in medical schools use the *Nelson Textbook of Pediatrics* as the *Green Bible* for comprehensive coverage of available knowledge. Most of us who were educators used this text as the basis for our students to learn about the art and science of pediatrics. For Dr Nelson, it was a labor of both love and dedication. Dr Nelson described its genesis in a note to his grandson, Ted, son of Jane Nelson Beatty. After describing his mentor and prior editor of the *Textbook of Pediatrics*, A. Graeme Mitchell, he goes on to state the reasons he should not be the editor, "1. I did not feel competent, 2. I had just assumed the chairmanship of the Department of Pediatrics at Temple and did not have the time, and 3. Not the least, that having come from a department where the textbook was published, I felt I would lose the respect of those in the pediatric world,

E-mail address: vfulginiti@comcast.net

0065-3101/11/$ – see front matter
doi:10.1016/j.yapd.2011.03.014

whose friendship I valued, if I accepted such an offer." Most of us who knew Dr Nelson do not believe any of these reasons. He was competent, he always did what was required and found the time, and taking on the task of upgrading and modernizing that text gained him more respect and friendship than he could even imagine. To the great delight of the pediatric world, he was urged to overcome his objections and to accept the assignment. He further states, "...I had the advantage of being solely responsible for the reorganization of the book. On this basis I started anew and selected contributors for those sections I did not feel comfortable in handling myself." The rest of the story is known to all of us in pediatrics. He did change the nature of textbooks by insisting on multiple authorships by experts in a given area, in contrast to the previous efforts that had been a single authorship modified only by consultation with experts. He also made clear that although the content was the author's area of expertise, "...material would be edited in order to maintain throughout the book a similarity in style of writing." Those of us who participated learned what that meant. I can recall one submission of mine that I thought contained prose for the ages. When returned to me there were more words in the editing than I had written. The effect was enormous; the text caught on and became the sole authoritative source for thousands upon thousands of students of pediatrics the world over. Even today, many decades after his last editorial efforts, and 23 years after his death, students and practitioners refer to it for clear, concise, and lucid expression of almost all aspects of pediatrics.

Not to be forgotten was his family's influence in making the book the ideal that it was. His wife Margery contributed mightily to the editing process; she was an accomplished grammarian and stylist and was the behind-the-scenes editor along with her husband. All of the family was involved. Dr Nelson said, "It was a hot Sunday in late summer of 1953. The long aluminum table had been set up in the living room and I faced 'the three gals,' Jane, Ann, and (Margery), with page proof in hand." This scene was duplicated with each edition, with manuscripts strewn throughout the house, not just on the table. In the inscription for the fifth edition, he wrote, "Recognizing that children, like adults, prosper under the stimulus and responsibility of a task to be done, WE ACKNOWLEDGE the contributions that this book has made to JANE, ANN, AND BILL in providing them such privileges and the satisfaction in family living which has come from group activity." Dr Nelson indicated that his role was "to edit for content, manner of presentation, and style." Then Margery took over and determined if he had altered the author's intent, edited his editing, and constantly searched for brevity in expression. It was truly a partnership of successful editing.

The success of the text is remarkable. It is used worldwide, has been translated into multiple languages, even obscure ones, and is read avidly by students. It is also used as a reference manual by experienced practitioners who seek complete, authoritative information about a given condition. I personally have used it that way more times than I can count.

Dr Nelson also gave credit to all those who contributed, including his family and his colleagues at St Christopher's. In fact, that was a consistent trait; he always acknowledged other's contributions in any arena in which he was involved. He was a tough taskmaster, some might even call him a martinet, but all who were associated with him came to appreciate that discipline and it often forged spine in their own activities and a sense of integrity, hard work, and dedicated purpose. Dr Nelson was a mentor to many throughout the world. He gathered a remarkable faculty at Temple/St Christopher's Hospital for Children: men and women who were dedicated teachers, experienced clinicians, and avid researchers in bedside medicine and in the burgeoning laboratory emphasis on research in the 1960s and beyond. My own experience was in this early period as a student at Temple, a resident at St Christopher's, and a colleague thereafter as I moved through my own career. I was asked to give a talk on the occasion of being selected as a St Geme awardee by the Federation of Pediatric Societies. My theme was mentoring and here is what I said about Dr Nelson:

> Bill Nelson offered a model of unselfish, dedicated service to the profession, service that was totally child oriented. To all of his students, he stressed the appropriate application of skills, our duty to respond, and other aspects of pediatric care. He left those he mentored with inspiration to apply their best efforts always, without regard to self, and with an intense energy devoted to their professional responsibilities.

By those words, I was attempting to characterize the complex relationship Dr Nelson had with those he mentored. When one considers the persons who came in contact with him as students, residents and faculty, one can see the positive results of his influence. For example, he mentored several individuals who became department heads, deans, and academic educators and administrators, carrying the messages learned with him into another realm of those mentored. This mentoring put the stamp of Dr Nelson's influence on an even greater range of health care workers than by his own direct contact. Angelo DiGeorge, one of Dr Nelson's faculty and lifelong, dedicated friend, presented the introduction to the Howland Award of the American Pediatric Society and said this of his boss: "To work for him was like joining a monastic order, one took vows of poverty, dedication and self-denial. As a consequence the perceptive medical student's sobriquets for the hospital became St Waldo's." Dr DiGeorge went on to say, "inculcating his staff and students in his values has far outweighed the pain of self-denial."

A word about his personality: I have alluded to his strict taskmaster attitude toward the work of pediatrics. All of us have felt his stern admonitions and can relate anecdotes about such encounters. He appeared emotionless to many and his sharp assessments sometimes stung. But as I have looked at those who eulogized him and recounted this characteristic, all have pointed out that his treatment of them, harsh as it seemed at the time, was not only justified, but led to a better performance than might have occurred otherwise. His daughter, Jane, also indicates that this characteristic did not end with his professional associations but extended to his family as well. One must understand that Dr Nelson's critique was always based on love, respect and a desire for those he interacted with to be the best they could be. His stimulation of their efforts sometimes seemed harsh and martinetlike, but he always lauded their talents, skills, and accomplishments, both of his own family and the St Chris family. I can personally attest to this as, at each junction of my academic life, he sent me a message of both approbation and a stern note to do my best, better than I had done before.

His editing style was also severe, as I have alluded to earlier. His role was not just as a text editor but as the Editor of the Journal of Pediatrics. He assumed this position in 1959 and continued until 1977, often with the able help of one that he had mentored, Joe Garfunkel, who succeeded him as editor. The journal rapidly rose in prominence under his editorship. Prior to his taking this position, the journal received only 200 manuscripts annually; it soon reached 1600 and the quality of submissions and publications improved dramatically. He ultimately worked 50 to 60 hours a week on editing and other necessary duties of his position. Dr Garfunkel wrote an editorial upon Dr Nelson's death and said, "Within a few years the journal was receiving more manuscripts than any other pediatric publication, and both circulation and readership had grown steadily." He also noted that Dr Nelson's editorial style contributed to the clarity and expression in the published articles. Even after his retirement he continued to contribute to the journal as emeriti and defined the definition of emeritus as "no one pays any attention to you anymore." Dr Garfunkel indicates he attended every board meeting and offered advice and occasional editing during the 18 years Dr Garfunkel was editor.

NOW FOR THE BACKSTORY

Dr Nelson was born in 1898 in McClure, Ohio, a town of 600. His father was a pharmacist, general store keeper, and postmaster. His mother fed and kept track of 7 sons and initiated and ran the only movie theater in town. He was named after Ralph Waldo Emerson but as with many children he did not like fancy names, so he insisted on being called Bill, which stuck for his lifetime. (Note: Most of us who were associated with him could not call him Bill even after he insisted and we had achieved mature status; it just seemed wrong, so we always called him Dr Nelson). After high school he wanted to go into finance; he applied to the Wharton School, was accepted, but could not attend for lack of financial resources. So he went to work as a mail clerk and office boy at the Willys-Overland plant in Toledo, Ohio. He sold peaches and insurance subsequently and the *Saturday Evening Post* and the *Country Gentleman.* He won a prize for selling the most Curtis Publications in Northern Ohio. As an accomplished salesman he sold fender braces, ordered from a Chicago mail order house, installed them on a car and asked for $1 for them (he paid $0.33 for each). In college at Wittenberg he became a steward at his fraternity and helped it climb out of a financial hole.

In 1917 he enlisted in the army and the next year entered the Student Army Training Corps at Wittenberg College. On his first night there he met another student, Marge Harris, whom he married after a 7-year engagement. When he finally married Marge she was teaching high school math in Illinois and he was beginning his final year of residency. His daughter Jane reports that he always wondered if they should have married earlier in the relationship. Marriage to Marge was eventful in later life as she was a professional helper in editing, as already pointed out, but also took advantage of Dr Nelson's many invitations to visit former students and admirers across the world. They traveled extensively with Marge researching each trip's possibilities. She was born in India to Lutheran missionaries and this may in part account for her wanderlust. Their travels included Europe, Japan, India, China, Iran, Greece, Turkey, Egypt, Spain, Argentina, Brazil, Hawaii, and many other places. Often his host was a former resident at St Christopher's; Dr Nelson insisted on having excellent foreign students each year and they were integrated into the St Christopher's family along with US trained residents. Upon leaving St Christopher's and returning home, they would invite him to visit and speak. Hence, the many sites around the world that the couple visited. When traveling abroad they took time to write detailed letters back to their children and some to the faculty at St Christopher's.

Dr Nelson attended medical school at Cincinnati College of Medicine graduating in 1926. He then became an intern and resident at Cincinnati General Hospital and the new Cincinnati Children's Hospital. He came under the preceptorship of A. Graeme Mitchell, then a giant in pediatrics and author of the text that was to become Dr Nelson's hallmark later. In a few years he became a member of the faculty and participated in the growth of the department into a major force in American pediatrics. There was a new model for academicians, the combination of teaching, clinical care, and research, which Dr Mitchell pioneered and in which Dr Nelson was his right hand man. Dr Nelson became interested in tuberculosis, diabetes, and nephritis. He developed clinical activities for each of these diseases and conducted clinical research, publishing a series of articles on each in the pediatric literature. The identification of diabetes and how to manage it, particularly with one patient, became a highlight for Dr Nelson. The child was Billy Talbert, who was encouraged by Dr Nelson to take up tennis, and who became captain of the United States Davis Cup Team and excelled as a tennis player for many years despite his diabetes. Dr Nelson often referred to this early patient association in his lectures to us as students at Temple, and later as an example of the kind of total patient care that gave children a chance at an active, productive life.

In 1940 Nelson was invited to become the Professor of Pediatrics and to head the department at Temple University Medical School. By his own accounts this decision was not an easy one; he had decided to go into more active research in diabetes. But Dr Mitchell encouraged him to consider the offer and after much hesitation and indecision, he did so. At Temple, by Dr Nelson's own account, he found no pediatric residency, and he had only one full-time faculty, Dr Nina Anderson, a neonatologist who came with him from Cincinnati. He relied on volunteer pediatricians to staff the clinical and educational services and began to build a faculty, including John Bartram (also from Cincinnati), Walter Cohn, and Bob High. In sequence he developed a residency program, further developed the volunteer faculty staff, attempted to get an integrated program with the 5 Philadelphia area medical schools (failed), and decided to affiliate with St Christopher's Hospital for Children, then a private hospital. This activity was both controversial and risky by his own account. However, he quickly completed the affiliation agreement, including a separate board for the hospital, and incorporation of the visiting clinicians. He built a full-time faculty representing the developing specialty fields in pediatrics; recognized the talent in his resident staff, and nurtured some of them into the full-time faculty after their training; built a 150-bed specialty pediatric hospital; found a way to finance the venture and developed a first-class, respected department with the combination of Temple and St Christopher's. Dr Nelson often referred to the financial difficulties of managing this arrangement. He spent a great deal of time encouraging philanthropy and blending funds from Temple University, local and state grants, and federal support, wherever he could find it. As faculty joined him he encouraged them to assist in generating funding for the various academic programs and for clinical care. Many faculty commented on the low pay at St Christopher's compared to other institutions. These comments were often heard after faculty attended national meetings and compared notes. Remarkably this was not a deterrent to most and long-term relationships grew with the St Christopher's family. In a few instances, the rather meager offers led to promising individuals leaving for more lucrative positions, but these were few.

I have indicated the major accomplishments outside of St Christopher's but it would be incomplete if I did not provide insight into the remarkable teaching/clinical care atmosphere there. Residents were recruited from promising students at Temple and from referrals to those who had gone elsewhere in pursuit of specialty training. The resident staff was tightly bound together in purpose. As co-chief resident with Ray Helfer, I found a spirit of cooperation that I learned later was unique to St Christopher's. Residents helped each other constantly, substituted for each other when circumstances dictated an absence, and participated in teaching of medical students to a degree that they were often cited at Temple for their excellence in medical student education. But beyond the bonding among the residents, there was an intimate teaching relationship with faculty. I can recount numerous instances but will only cite a few from my own experience. In my first year I encountered a seriously ill young child and was puzzled as to why she was in shock. Because of my inexperience and because as a team we suspected that she possibly had an adrenal crisis, I asked Dr Angelo DiGeorge to come in from home. He did so in the middle of the night and we not only successfully cared for the child but had an entire session of the endocrinologic underpinning of the diagnosis and treatment of her condition, all at 3:00 AM. I have been in other settings where that simply would not have happened.

In another instance, I was caring for a child with a distended abdomen, high fever, and near unconsciousness. After examining him I thought he had an abdominal crisis and obtained a radiograph examination of his abdomen. John Kirkpatrick was head of pediatric radiology and I was startled to have him appear on the ward with a stethoscope. He handed it to me and said, "examine his chest now and carefully." I did so and discovered lack of breath sounds low in his chest. Dr Kirkpatrick then explained that in the margins of the abdominal radiograph he saw obliteration of the costophrenic angles bilaterally and thought the child had empyema, which he had. His cultures grew *Staphylococcus aureus*, then epidemic in our community. Finally, there were many times when we all gathered in Dr Jim Arey's pathology department for examination of either microscopic or autopsy evidence of the conditions our patients had experienced.

The St Christopher's spirit was often cited by those involved in pediatric care there and among colleagues who went elsewhere. The spirit involved all members of the St Christopher's family, nurses, administrators, hospital staff, and all those involved in patient care, regardless of their specific role. This concept that we were one group all striving to give the best care possible in a congenial atmosphere permeated the institution and inspired those of us who left to imitate it in our new settings.

I cite these examples as a few among many that profile the close working relationships that faculty, residents, and the entire health care team had and continued to have under Dr Nelson's leadership and mentorship. We cherished the time we spent at St Christopher's and carried many of the attitudes we perceived into our subsequent roles in academic medicine and clinical practice.

Finally, there is an anecdote that has been recounted numerous times that irked Dr Nelson sometimes, and caused him some paternal pride at other times. It is the famous "for the birds" insertion in his textbook's index. He often said that this one incident had more impact than any other in his professional career. Although there are many versions, I am reporting his own account of what he called the consecration to the birds as follows: "Certainly no feature brought the book as much attention from the lay population and perhaps even the medical one." After recounting the steps that led up to having the sixth edition in preparation for final editing of the index, he tells of each child having index cards with a single entry for each index point. By midafternoon on a hot Sunday he had exhausted his slaves and proposed a swim. Jane and Ann, his daughters, disappeared quickly, relieved that the task was over, but Ann returned, took a single index card and wrote "birds, for the" with the pagination for the entire book. The entry was caught and never made the index then. For the seventh edition, some 4 years later, Ann, now married to Dick Behrman, who would become a future editor of the textbook, returned for a visit and Dr Nelson put her to work. (Ann died in 2005.) The suggestion was made that the "birds, for the" be again entertained for the index. What happened subsequently is not as clear as the previous account. Somehow the entry made it into galleys, and even though crossed out, was inserted into the seventh edition's index. When published, it created a sensation in the lay press, garnered publicity for Saunders, who published the textbook, and was widely discussed in medical circles, despite Dr Nelson claiming a lesser focus in that arena. The humor intrinsic to the insertion offered relief to students who used the text and smiles to those of us who appreciated the fact that his daughter, overtaxed by the taskmaster, saw the humor in such an insertion and perhaps a commentary on the impact on her life and participation. Dr Nelson did not like the insertion and often expressed his dissatisfaction to me and others. But in his letter to his grandson he also relates some of the humorous side to the incident. For example, he was occasionally introduced by allusion to the "birds," and twice, in Rio and Atlanta, was introduced by a slide showing birds in flight. He cited Cleveland's *THE PLAIN DEALER* comment: "They simply liked a light touch in high places." As Dr Nelson often said, enough of the birds!

Dr Nelson received many official awards and numerous unofficial ones as he was invited to speak around the world. When I became head of the department of pediatrics at the University of Arizona, I asked him to become a visiting professor, as did many of his former students, residents, and faculty. He gave a wonderful talk on the need for town-gown integration and his activities in Philadelphia to bring that about. Two humorous incidents occurred during his visit. He was in his 90s at the time and an avid golfer. In our department, Grant Morrow was an expert golfer who had been almost professional in Philadelphia before choosing a medical career. Dr Nelson wanted to play golf and I asked Grant to arrange a foursome, which he did. Dr Nelson came back and told me that he enjoyed the course but that Grant was more avid than he. Dr Nelson had landed one shot in a tire track and thought that he could lift the ball onto a better surface, but Grant insisted that he hit it from where it lay. Dr Nelson was not amused.

We had placed him at the wonderful Arizona Inn, a local hostelry famed for its history, ambiance, and food. Speaking the next day he recounted two incidents that amused him. Upon awakening he saw snow on the threshold and thought that he had escaped that by coming to Tucson. It was one of the rare times that we had snow in the 20 years we lived there. Further, he complained publicly that the furniture in the Inn was older than his grandmother's. It is true because in the interest of southwestern flavor many of the rooms have antique furniture with drawers that do not quite fit, and closet doors that are akimbo somewhat. His room was one of those.

Dr Nelson has received the highest recognition pediatric organizations and others can give. He was the recipient of the Abraham Jacobi Award of the American Academy of Pediatrics; the Howland Award of the American

Pediatric Society; the Order of Mayo by the Government of Argentina; Honorary Professorships from Santos Tomas, Philippines and the University of Santo Domingo; Doctor of Humane Letters of Temple University; Honorary Member of the Latin American Society of Research; Doctor of Medical Science from the Medical College of Pennsylvania; Gold Medal Award of the Children's Hospital of Philadelphia; and the University of Cincinnati's College of Medicine's Daniel Drake Award. He was interviewed at 97 years old for the Columbia University Oral History Research Office for hours. This project was an oral history project for the American Academy of Pediatrics.

This remarkable man did not end his career when he retired from the department chair at Temple, the editorship of the textbook, from the *Journal of Pediatrics*, and from other official titles and positions. Instead he began a quest for collaboration between town and gown. He gathered pediatric leaders in Philadelphia to promote the concept, preparing a missive indicating the steps that might be taken. He lectured on the concept and established a fund at St Christopher's to promote the idea. He continued such an active life that he complained to his daughter that he did not have enough free time at 93 years old.

In short, Dr Waldo E. (Bill) Nelson was a major force in pediatrics by promoting education through his editorial efforts, by his development of a child-oriented clinical entity at St Christopher's Hospital for Children, and by mentoring a myriad of professionals who carried his message of integrity, dedication, attention to the written word, hard work and focus on the health and well being of children. His reach went beyond Philadelphia to the entire country and to the world with his disciples spreading his philosophy and attitudes. He was an amazing, active, intelligent man who was and is an inspiration to students of pediatrics at all levels. One final note: If Dr Nelson were alive, he would edit this manuscript mercilessly and then suggest that it be ripped to pieces, never to see the light of day.

Acknowledgments

I am deeply indebted to Jane Nelson Beatty who provided me with many private papers of Dr Nelson's from which some of the quotes in this narrative are taken. I am grateful for her careful review of the manuscript. Her editorial suggestions indicate that DNA transmits more than physical genes; she has her father and mother's editorial skills and instincts!

Further Readings

DiGeorge AM. Presentation of the Howland Award to Waldo E. Nelson. Pediatr Res 1972;6: 843–7.

DiGeorge AM. Reflections on Waldo E. Nelson M.D. (1898–1997) Temple University Medical Alumni. Newsletter 1999;11–2.

Garfunkel J. In Memoriam, Waldo E. Nelson, 1898–1997. J Pediatr 1997;130:849.

Gerhardt W. Octogenarian visits "Home", Bulletin Alumni Association College of Medicine. Cincinnatti (OH): University of Cincinnati; 1987.

Historical Archives Advisory Committee. Committee report: American pediatrics: milestones at the millennium. Pediatrics 2001;107:1482–91.
Nelson MD Waldo E. Main line life. Ardmore (PA): Penn; 1997.
Obituary Nelson Waldo. Author of Pediatric Text, New York Times, March 9, 1997. Waldo Nelson, 'father of pediatrics', dead at 98. Available at: http://aapnews.aapublications.org. Accessed March 9, 1997.

Advances in Pediatrics 58 (2011) 11–26

ADVANCES IN PEDIATRICS

Developing Leadership in Global Child Health

Kevin Chan, MD, MPH[a,b,*]

[a]Division of Pediatric Emergency Medicine, Department of Pediatrics, Hospital for Sick Children, University of Toronto, 555 University Avenue, Toronto, Ontario, Canada M5G 1X8
[b]Munk Centre for Global Studies, University of Toronto, Toronto, Ontario, Canada

Twenty years ago, when I (the author, K.C.) was a young medical student, a little girl asked the group of us who were working in rural Malawi, "Why can you who have so much not help us who have so little?" Twenty years ago, the challenge was identifying health as an issue. I remember speaking at a meeting of leaders in Malawi in the late 1990s about the specter of HIV/AIDS affecting both men and women, and was told that the disease was something seen only in Western countries.

Around the world, we have seen a large transformation occurring in the attitudes toward health, with a significant push made by governments and leading philanthropic organizations, such as the Bill and Melinda Gates Foundation and the One Foundation, led by the rock star Bono. These visible leaders have put global health into the conversation of important priorities, especially in developing countries.

Yet despite a 30% decline in childhood deaths around the world from 1990 to 2009, the United Nations Children's Emergency Fund (UNICEF) still reports 8.1 million deaths in children under the age of 5 in 2009 [1]. Approximately 70% of these deaths are preventable by available knowledge and technology [2]. Therefore, 5.5 million deaths in children can be prevented by what we know and have available to us. These simple questions still exist: Why do these deaths occur when we know how to prevent them? How can we reduce the gap between our knowledge base and our actions leading to these poor health outcomes?

Obviously there is a large gap between what is known and what is done to improve global child health. One of the issues is how do we make these solutions, visible, viable, and acted upon? The challenge is not just to review the

There are no disclosures of relevance to this study.

*Corresponding author. Division of Pediatric Emergency Medicine, Department of Pediatrics, Hospital for Sick Children, University of Toronto, 555 University Avenue, Toronto, Ontario, Canada M5G 1X8. *E-mail address*: kevinjchan@aol.com

0065-3101/11/$ – see front matter
doi:10.1016/j.yapd.2011.03.015

state of where global child health is, but to provide fresh, new insight into possible solutions. The missing gap is something that is not discussed in many medical or public health schools, but something we find in business and management schools: leadership. My belief is that the major weakness is a lack of global child health leadership globally, nationally, and locally that prohibits faster improvements in morbidity and mortality.

What is known about global child health leadership? The unfortunate answer is: not very much.

This article looks at the realm of global child health leadership and examines prior attempts to reduce mortality and morbidity. The philosophy and outlook at building global child health leadership currently being developed between sub-Saharan Africa and the Hospital for Sick Children in Toronto is highlighted. Examples are provided of concrete programs and efforts being worked upon to develop this global child health leadership capacity. The author hopes to inspire more participation in building global child health leadership.

First, a brief survey is given of global child health programs: Primary Health Care, the Integrated Management of Childhood Illnesses, and Millennium Development Goal #4.

PRIMARY HEALTH CARE

In 1978, Primary Health Care (PHC) was launched at Alma Ata with the slogan "Health for All by the Year 2000" [3]. PHC aimed to create national health systems, based on the economic abilities of each country [4]. The type of health care employees would be dependent on each country's goals and resources available.

The specific Alma Ata declaration aimed to increase the participation of community members in the development of health care, and aimed to decentralize health care to individuals at a local level [3].

The key principles can be summarized as follows: (1) PHC aimed to promote equity within health care; (2) community participation was paramount at all decision-making points; (3) prevention was highlighted over cure; (4) available technology should be used; (5) other sectors should be involved in health care (such as education, agriculture and housing); (6) decentralization of decision-making was important; and (7) leadership was needed to achieve the goals of PHC [5].

Therefore, as far back as 1978 it was clear that global health leadership was a basic requirement to achieving health for all people. However, although there were programs to "train" health leaders, there was little systematic development that targeted national or local leaders effectively.

THE INTEGRATED MANAGEMENT OF CHILDHOOD ILLNESSES

In the mid 1990s, the World Health Organization (WHO) and UNICEF adopted the Integrated Management of Childhood Illnesses (IMCI). IMCI builds on the concept of PHC, using the community health worker (CHW) as the cornerstone of assessing a child's well-being. If a sick child presents to the CHW, the CHW decides how to best treat a child, using a color-coded system with red (danger), yellow (caution), or green (safe) to determine whether a child should be managed at home or in hospital.

IMCI has other foci including improving the training of CHWs, strengthening preventive health care measures, and upgrading existing health care services. It provides a first-line approach to treating child health problems. Although IMCI has been a standard of care, its proper adoption has been a challenge.

THE MILLENNIUM DEVELOPMENT GOAL #4: REDUCING CHILD MORTALITY

The fourth Millennium Development Goal (MDG #4) is to reduce the under-5 mortality rate by two-thirds from 1990 to 2015 [6]. We have seen the number of children dying from developing countries decrease from 100 (1990) to 72 (2008) deaths per 1000 live births, with only 10 of 67 countries with high child mortality on track to meet the MDG target [7]. The continuing challenge, however, has been the slow decline in childhood deaths in sub-Saharan Africa, with high fertility rates and a slow reduction in under-5 mortality rates (Fig. 1).

Other associated MDG #4 objectives include reducing the infant mortality rate, and increasing the proportion of 1-year-old children immunized against measles (Fig. 2).

There are obvious trends downward in the number of childhood deaths. There have been large falls in under-5 mortality rates across all areas of the world, but because of high fertility rates, there has been little progress in overall numbers of childhood deaths in sub-Saharan Africa [7].

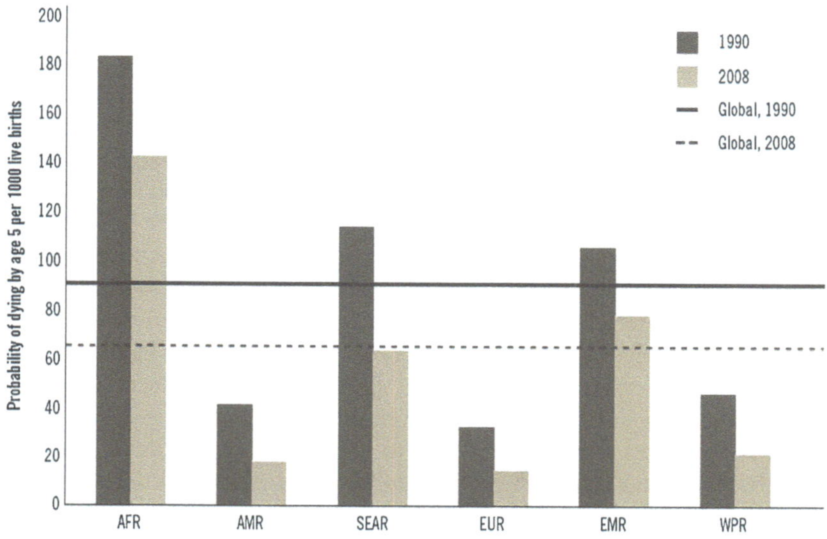

Fig. 1. Mortality rate in children younger than 5 years by WHO region. (*Reprinted from* www.who.int/whosis/whostat/EN_WHS10_Part1.pdf, p. 13; copyright The World Health Organization; with permission.)

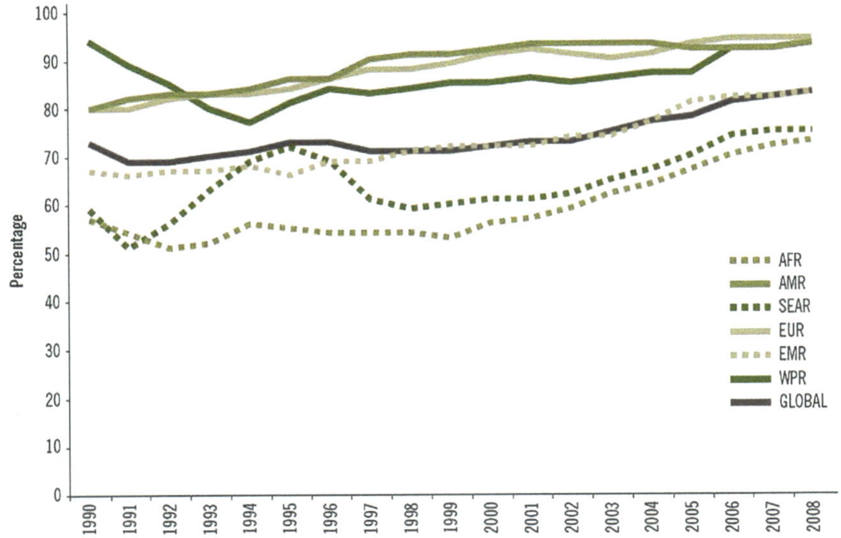

Fig. 2. Measles immunization coverage among 1-year-olds by WHO region. (*Reprinted from* www.who.int/whosis/whostat/EN_WHS10_Part1.pdf, p. 14; copyright The World Health Organization; with permission.)

WHY ARE WE FAILING TO REDUCE CHILD DEATHS FASTER?

As far back as David Morley's classic textbook on global child health, *Paediatric Priorities in the Developing World,* there was widespread recognition that improvements in children's health were not strictly rooted in medical answers [8]. The challenge is that many of the underlying root causes of child deaths are not simple and straightforward medical causes that health professionals tackle on a daily basis. For example, poverty, poor female education, and poor water and sanitation remain barriers to successfully reducing childhood mortality.

The challenge in children's health is but one small portion of a government's list of competing priorities. Child health competes with adult health; health competes with other departments, such as defense, industry, education, transportation, and agriculture for limited government resources. Improving children's health requires both technological improvements in tackling children's diseases, and providing enough funding and resources to deliver proper services.

Regarding the solution to global child health mortality, the technical aspects are not the problem as much as access to health care. For example, one area where there has been little reduction in global child mortality in the past decade has been on perinatal mortality. The challenge remains in identifying mothers who will run into trouble, getting access to the right level of care, and ensuring the quality of care once they arrive at the facility [9].

Our current global child health leaders continue to face a combination of economic, policy and political challenges to improve health systems and health outcomes for children. In particular, a cadre of child health leaders who can advocate for children and policy change should be developed in the existing health care system. Leveraging existing collaborative networks, such as the Program for Global Pediatric Research, can bring together child health leaders from Africa and around the world to forward the global child health agenda [10].

It is with this in mind that the author now looks at leadership as an integral part of developing global child health programs.

WHAT IS LEADERSHIP?

There is great difficulty in defining what leadership is. Is it experience? Is it logic? Is it vision? Pulitzer Prize winner James MacGregor Burns, in his influential book *Transforming Leadership,* aptly states: "I have come to see leadership not only as a field of study but as a master discipline that illuminates some of the toughest problems of human needs and social change" [11]. The reality is that leadership occurs at various levels, both from positions of power and from individuals at the grassroots level.

Leaders such as Gandhi in India, Mao Tse-Tung in China, and Alexander the Great are well-known leaders who helped transform countries and societies. The question is whether the intrinsic characteristics of an individual, the "Great Man" theory proposed by Sidney Hook, "creates" leadership through the natural intellect and strength of character [12]. Countervailing ideas suggest that leadership may be a product of time and circumstances, and by decisions made at opportune times. This idea was championed by Karl Marx [13] and later by the philosopher, Herbert Spencer [14]. In particular, Spencer championed the concept that complex influences were what created the conditions by which leaders, through a Darwinian process, would succeed through the creation of wealth and power. So the concept of a great leader was hypothesized either to be intrinsic to the leader oneself, or a concept dependent on the circumstances and the situation. Thus, leadership can also occur at local levels around specific issues that lead to direct activism, such as protecting women from being sexually exploited or by protecting a local park or forest from being harmed.

The development of the program for global child health leadership comes from a perspective that leadership qualities, characteristics, and traits can be maximized, and specific situational opportunities identified to improve global child health.

Leadership begins with "vision": what is the purpose and goal we seek? Leadership provides purpose to an idea or goal. However, vision is insufficient. Leadership should bring components such as logic and pragmatic approaches that can be performed in a systematic fashion. There are also some basic characteristics that are important for a leader to bring to the fore, such as integrity, adherence to principles and values, humility and respect for others, communication, and the ability to persuade people and demonstrate commitment to the vision. Experience often helps in leadership, but it may act as a barrier if preconceived notions limit the capacity to invoke change.

WHAT DOES LEADERSHIP IN GLOBAL CHILD HEALTH MEAN?

Before 2000, global child health leadership was provided internationally by UNICEF and the WHO. There were many local champions of child health, but little systematic training of these leaders.

There are 3 fundamental components of global child health leadership. First, there must be recognition that children have increased morbidity and mortality around the world. Second, it is important to work out how to make the problem a priority issue, facilitating resources and funding. Finally, it is important to identify the means and methods to address problems and resolve issues, and communicate how to effectively promote constructive change.

There are cross-cutting themes that exist no matter what level of health care provider and leader is sought. These themes include: identification of problems and issues; setting policy priorities and agendas; communication; team building; managing conflict and change; understanding and interacting with the political system; building health capacity; and conducting health system planning at the district, national, and international levels.

The goal of training global child health leaders is to develop a cadre of individuals who can effect positive change and help shape policy within the existing and future health care systems. Leveraging on large-scale collaborative networks around the world can help advance the skills and agendas of global child health leaders. The aim is to create agents of change and advocates for children's health issues.

WHAT DO WE KNOW ABOUT HEALTH LEADERSHIP IN DEVELOPING COUNTRIES?

Although there is a broad recognition of the need to develop health leadership, there is very little information on systematic training for health leadership. A review of PubMed and a Google search revealed the several global child health leadership programs (Table 1) and global health leadership programs (Table 2).

There is a surprising paucity of concrete leadership training programs that help train global child health leaders. Most programs do not present an organized approach to training leaders.

The hospital for sick children and developing a leadership program in global child health

In 2009, The Hospital for Sick Children was given a grant by the Canadian International Development Agency (CIDA) to develop a leadership program in global child health. The grant was to help developed leadership programs in global child health in 3 countries, namely Ghana, Ethiopia, and Tanzania, with very different leadership requirements. Ghana's leadership program focuses on pediatric nursing leaders; Ethiopia's program focuses on building academic leaders; and Tanzania's leadership program focuses on developing maternal and child health community leaders.

With these varying requirements, there exists a large challenge in finding a core set of values, skills, and principles to teach leaders.

Table 1
Global child health leadership programs

Organization	Program Name	Description	Internet Address
African Medical and Research Foundation (AMREF)	Child Health	A self-contained 16-unit course on how to take a sick child's history, perform physical examinations, and ensure the proper management of a sick child	www.amref.org/info-centre/amref-courses-training-programmes/distance-education-programme
Johns Hopkins University	Maternal and Child Health	A set of training modules designed for small group to explore different leadership concepts in a Maternal Child Health (MCH) context	www.jhsph.edu/wchpc/MCHLDS/index.html
Tanzanian Training Center for International Health (TTCIH)	Integrated Management of Childhood Illnesses (IMCI)	This is an innovative software application to support IMCI. It is meant as a tool to adopt with IMCI guidelines at the national and subnational levels	www.healthtraining.org/schools/ifakara.php#Crs4
USAID	Global Health eLearning Center	The eLearning Center provides Internet-based courses on a variety of health topics	www.globalhealthlearning.org/learnmore.cfm

Table 2
Global health leadership programs

Organization	Program Name	Description	Internet Address
Higher Education Alliance for Leadership Through Health (HEALTH) Alliance	Leadership Initiative for Public Health in East Africa (LIPHEA) Projects	Aims to strengthen the capacity of the Makerere School of Public Health (Uganda) and Muhimbili University College of Health Sciences (Tanzania) through effective public health leadership training	www.liphea.org
International Council of Nurses (ICN)	Leadership for Change	Program assists senior nurses to influence health policy and decisions and to be effective leaders and managers	www.icn.ch/pillarsprograms/leadership-for-change
McGill University	International Masters for Health Leadership	Designed to act as a catalyst for developing an integrated and sustainable approach to health	www.mcgill.ca/desautels/imhl
Open University	The HEAT (Health Education and Training) Program	Work-based training initiative with Web-based health education resources	www.open-ac.uk/africa/HEAT_project.shtm
African Medical and Research Foundation (AMREF)	Executive Healthcare Management Program	Trainees will develop skill sets and leadership qualities to create high-performing health care organizations	sbs.ac.ke/index.php/programs/executive-programs/advanced-healthcare-management-program
Synergos Institute	African Public Health Leadership & System Innovation Initiative	Increases leadership effectiveness in a health care environment by cultivating managerial skills and addressing the attitudes, values, and relationships that drive behavior	www.synergos.org/partnerships/publichealthnamibia.htm
Johnson&Johnson	Management Development Institute (MDI)	Designed to enhance the management and leadership skills of healthcare leaders in families with HIV/AIDS	www.jnj.com/connect/caring/corporate-giving/healthcare-leadership/doctor-training
Management Science for Health (MSH)	Leadership Management System and Sustainability Programs (LMS)	The program is intended to develop leaders and managers in family planning, reproductive health, HIV/AIDS, and health service delivery	www.msh.org/projects/lms
Management Science for Health (MSH)	Virtual Leadership Development Program (VLDP)	A combination of a general leadership program with CD-ROMs and workbooks with on-site team meetings	www1.msh.org/projects/lms/ProgramAndTools/LeadingAndManaging/VLDP.cfm
Tanzania Training Centre for International Health	Best Practices for Maternal Survival in Sub-Saharan Africa	This course is to strengthen nonphysician clinicians including midwives to help reduce maternal mortality	www.healthtraining.org/schools/ifakara.php/Crs#4

This section highlights some thought processes in developing a leadership program in global child health. Although some steps seem basic, the combination of these steps will help develop and enhance the skills of leaders to forward the child health agenda. The basic modules in global child health are highlighted.

Identifying the scope of the problem

One of the first aspects of the training program is the need to develop basic concepts and understanding of epidemiologic conditions on health, including the understanding of how to survey and collect data on health conditions for an area. Although the scope of the course does not outline the details of how to survey and collect mortality and morbidity data, the aim is to outline basic epidemiologic concepts for child health, including verbal autopsies to identify causes of death; create and understand neonatal, infant, and under-5 mortality rates; identify disease outbreaks, including proper water and sanitation sources; highlight health care access points to identify where populations can get primary, secondary, and tertiary levels of health care, including basic health practices such as immunization and maternal and perinatal health care; and identify the population's health care knowledge, understanding, and practices. The goal for the trainee is not necessarily to conduct all of these surveys, but to understand how to gather, organize, and understand information collected from the field, and to recognize gaps in knowledge and understanding in child health.

Identify personalities, motivations, and skills

The second module assesses a participant's personality, sources of motivation, natural skills, and areas that may require development. The concept comes from the Meyer Briggs personality test, which is a standard assessment tool for many leadership training courses [15]. The module aims to make participants appreciate different personality types, how to work and communicate with different personality types, and how to use their natural skills and minimize potential conflicts.

1. Approach to People and Participation in Activities. Some people are quite extroverted, whereas others are introverted. Descriptions of extroverted people include being active, open, outward-focused, sociable, expressive, breadth, and liking variety; they enjoy acting with other people in the world. Descriptions of introverted people include being reflective, private, inward-focused, reserved, quiet, depth, and focused on tasks at hand; they tend to require "private" time to feel refreshed.
2. Approach to Processing Information. There are two major personality types: sensing and intuitive individuals. "Sensors" are individuals who are detail-oriented, practical, precise in directions, and focused on the present situation. These people trust what they perceive with their senses to be the truth and thus tend to be "reality"-based. The second group looks at the gestalt or bigger picture to find patterns, using hunches and imagination, and tend to be forward-looking. These individuals also tend to look at a myriad of possibilities to try and find the optimal future.
3. Approach to Making Judgments and Decisions. The two major categories are thinking and feeling. Thinkers tend to be objective, logical, analytical, and evaluate cause and effect; they operate from core principles and apply

logic in a formal, critical manner to come up with conclusions. Feelers tend to be subjective empathizers who stress personal relationships and values; they tend to enjoy harmony and avoid conflict.

4. Approach to Getting Things Done. The two major categories are judging and perceiving. Judgers tend to like things in an organized, structured fashion, and like to make deliberate, decisive, controlled plans. Perceivers like to adapt to things as they experience them; they like to be spontaneous and wait for things to occur, and can manage ambiguity more easily.

Creating vision

In the first 2 modules the importance is established of collecting baseline information and understanding the situational context in developing programs by identifying the scope of the problem, and providing an evaluation of the people who will be working in the process. In this third module, the aim is to teach how to create vision.

Vision is looking at the larger picture and imagining what can be achieved in the future through enabling possibilities, and enlisting others to participate in their own dreams through shared goals and aspirations. However, it is insufficient to create vision without a means to achieving these aims.

Vision should take into account the aspirations and goals of each stakeholder to ensure that each stakeholder's wishes are achieved, or to minimize opposition to a project or proposal. It should also take into account reasonable short-, medium-, or long-term frames to meet each stakeholder's goals and clarify who is responsible for achieving each goal.

Vision should also stretch the goals of individual members, to take them out of comfort zones and push their capabilities.

In the context of global child health, the aim may be to develop a global child health program, to strengthen the overall health system to deliver a package of goods, or to promote collective advocacy to highlight a shortfall (such as perinatal care) at the global level. Successful vision development, however, allows as many stakeholders as possible to participate in the engagement process, and involves as many parties as possible in a concrete, focused objective that is measurable and achievable.

Communication

One of the most important skills to develop is the ability to communicate effectively with other team members, stakeholders, clients, and the public. There are various methods of communication including reflective listening, verbal communication through the media and press, and presentations such as video, social media, and Powerpoint. There are also important nonverbal communication clues to observe and act upon.

It is important that roles are clearly defined, yet sufficiently flexible to adapt to changing circumstances. It is also important that the environment created enables members to maximize their potential and to come up with new and creative ideas.

Communication should allow honest views, opinions, and feelings. In many cultures this may not be the norm, and may take time to develop. However, there should be means by which team members can communicate their feelings if open forums do not allow their opinions to be heard.

The other important aspect of communication is providing feedback. The key in providing feedback is to be as objective as possible, and to be positive and constructive. Often feedback is seen as being highly critical; however, when provided in a positive, constructive way, it may help enhance and energize fellow team members.

Team building

Leadership requires followers to help deliver the message and to perform the tasks that help make the vision reality [16].

To build a successful team, several things are important. The values and vision should be aligned for all team members, so that they can work together effectively. Roles should be clearly defined and a supportive environment created. Meetings and gatherings should be focused, with clear implementation and outcome goals. Decisions should be discussed and agreed upon by the members of the team, allowing for dissention, but ultimately agreeing on a common pathway to achieve the vision. There should be a clear timeline and pathway for deliverables, with focused, measurable achievements. Individual goals should challenge each individual team member to achieve to the best of their ability.

One of the other important aspects is for constant feedback and examination of ways to improve how effectively the team works together. There should also be an analysis by which team members look at how their working relationship interacts with their fellow team members and with other people that may be involved with their organization (including patients, clients, suppliers, and the public).

Some characteristics of successful teams include strong individual initiative, including team members making suggestions, and volunteering to solve problems; finding creative ways to resolve disputes, and developing consensus on complex issues; open communication between team members, including anticipating and communicating about potential problems; allowing members to lead at different times depending on the task to be completed; frequent social exchange and little hesitation in expressing concerns; maintaining calm even in the face of significant problems; and positive constructive encouragement and honest feedback throughout the process.

Edgar Schein highlighted how leaders convey to their teams, their beliefs, values, and assumptions through 6 primary mechanisms [17]:

1. What they pay attention to, measure, and control on a regular basis
2. How they react to critical incidents and organizational crises
3. How resources are allocated
4. By role modeling, teaching, and coaching
5. How they provide reward and status
6. How recruitment, selection, promotion, or removal of team members occurs.

Team building is one of the most difficult aspects to implement, especially in hierarchical societies, but it is helpful to build consensus and sustainability in projects. Without broader buy-in, projects can build up and dissipate relatively quickly; however, with buy-in, people get broader-based ownership of an idea and sustain a program over time.

Managing conflict and change

Edgar Schein, one of the great management thinkers of the twentieth century, in his influential book *Organizational Culture and Leadership*, highlighted the intrinsic biases that leaders bring to their organizations by imposing their beliefs, values, and assumptions on other members of the group [17].

Conflict occurs in all manners of leadership. One of the key aspects in addressing conflict is to effectively listen to the problem at hand before attempting to find a resolution to the problem. If the problem is between team members, open communication is necessary between both sides to resolve any conflict. If the problem is between leaders and their team it is necessary to clearly identify the problem, seek resolution, or to find amicable ways to part.

Change is an inevitable part of organizations. Change occurs through various stages: (1) introduction and growth; (2) maturity; and (3) decline. During each of these stages, organizations may face different types of challenges to change and adopt different approaches.

Often change cannot be anticipated, especially by external outside forces [18]. However, if change is anticipated, one should try to be proactive and fix things ahead of time. Positive change can occur when recognition of opportunities occur. To recognize these opportunities, it is important to look at resource capabilities but also to interact with customers, suppliers, team members, and the public to increase awareness of existing opportunities. Change should happen incrementally and be clearly understood by all key stakeholders. It does not have to be quick and sweeping. Rapid changes can lead to confusion, and a lack of clarity of mission and purpose. Change should also attempt to provide the best outcomes for any given resources, and should focus on the present situation and not only look to the future. If change fails to address current issues, change is unlikely to be sustainable.

The politics of health

Health and health care remain one of the most contentious areas of any government. The first part of this module focuses on recognizing how health competes with other sectors of government for priority standing. This approach includes both financial and public policy support at the various government levels and how this translates into both fiscal and nonfiscal resources developed by health.

The second part focuses on how to practically make a local vision sustainable, and how to broaden the vision to a state, national, regional, or international level. For example, malaria bed netting was tested in the 1990s in Tanzania. After research showed its benefits, it was publicized nationally and internationally, and local companies began producing malaria bed nets for use through East Africa. The international accolades played an important role in influencing and adopting malaria bed nets in Africa.

Building health capacity and health system planning
So how do we tie this all together for global child health leadership? The first module focuses on obtaining an understanding of the diseases, problems, and underlying health conditions of the area that is being served. The module focuses on acquiring facts that can help shape decisions and provide information to the leader in question. It does not focus on the "how to," but on what to do to try and elicit information and what to do once information is available.

The second module focuses on looking at the actors in the program. What are their underlying characteristics and motivations? The module focuses on how to engage different individuals, and listen, shape, and change their thoughts and motivations to make them align with the leader's goals and objectives. Understanding individuals and what shapes their desires is important in getting them to buy into the vision.

The third module focuses on the development of the vision. Using the best available information and recognizing the players involved in the situation, how can we create a collective vision congruent with a leader's personal vision, and recognize potential barriers and harms that may make the vision unachievable? For example, Bill Clinton's health care vision to provide health care to every American was a wonderful vision, but ended up having significant barriers because of the opposition from health care associations, Health Maintenance Organizations, businesses, and leaders from the pharmaceutical industry. Failing to recognize how the different actors would react led to its general downfall.

More successfully, the Campaign for Access to Essential Medicines, led by Médecins Sans Frontières, brought together HIV/AIDS organizations and health leaders of developing countries, and with public health pressure forced governments and drug companies to allow cheaper generic drugs to replace more expensive developed-country drugs. Vision, when combined with a focused message, clear goals, and simple steps to achieving outcomes, works best.

The fourth module focuses on communication needs. Communication occurs at many different levels, within and outside the organization. There are verbal, written, and nonverbal communication skills essential for any leader. Establishing clear lines of communication and being aware of backchannel talking is important to being an effective leader.

The fifth module looks at the concept of the team, and building teams to work effectively to turn vision into reality. It emphasizes that successful teams have great communication, various expertise, and different people who can effectively lead at different times. The role of the "leader" in effective teams is to act as a role model, and can help shape and determine the behavior of individual team members. At the same time, effective team leaders listen to their members and facilitate open discussion of novel approaches to address problems.

The sixth module focuses on the times when things are not going well or when change is happening. This time of conflict and change creates problems within team dynamics and may question the capacity and role of the leader itself. The module focuses on getting leaders to address issues of conflict directly and to look at change from a positive fashion, focusing on concrete, incremental changes, rather than bold changes without clear focus.

The seventh module looks at the importance of putting health into a political context. Politics occurs at all levels–regional, national, state, and local. Understanding the different political actors, their agenda, and their perceptions are important in making improvements in global child health a reality.

The final module ties in all the modules looking at the broader vision and looking at the global child health sector, to figure out how this can be integrated in the bigger picture. How do we build capacity in global child health? Although this could be seen as a "what do we want in the future" exercise, the constant challenge is, given our current and future resources and our current skill level and expertise, how can we best use it to obtain the "best" health outcomes?

The concept is to create health planning, by looking at trade-offs between areas that can potentially grow quickly to improve health, or be eliminated if there is little evidence of health impact. The aim is to improve health conditions over time. The module looks at the alignment between current personnel and health delivery, services, and outcomes, and identifies areas of weaknesses and gaps in knowledge and the means to address them. It compares the potential impact of financing health directly versus collaborating with other political entities, such as improving maternal education through the Ministry of Education, or improving roads through the Ministry of Planning or Infrastructure. Finally, it emphasizes the use of different tools, including using political pressure, media, and developing collaborations with other organizations, to translate the underlying vision into reality.

The goal of this module is to strengthen health planning and health capacity building, by emphasizing creative vision-building to promote global child health by all means possible.

How do we turn the training into the global child health reality?

The Leadership Training Program in Global Child Health aims to provide each trainee with the following skills.

The ability to collect and understand epidemiologic data in global child health

At the most basic level, the leader should develop the means, techniques, and understanding of how to gather the best information available, and interpret the meaning of these data.

Formulate a plan to address priority areas

Leaders will be expected to have the capability of forming teams, identifying people's strengths, create common goals and vision, and articulate a clear plan to address priority areas. Part of the process must be the ability to communicate not only internally but externally, the wanted and desired goals, and the road map to achieve them. Furthermore, the ability to anticipate and adapt to challenges is important.

Create a sustainable plan

A successful program will sustain itself through financial and nonfinancial means. There will be a combination of human resource planning, resource acquisition and development, and continued public awareness. The organization will clearly have succession plans, and promote knowledge dissemination to other organizations, government agencies, and international neighbors, if the program is seen to be successful.

Evaluation and measurement

The global child health leader will constantly evaluate and collect new information, reevaluate goals, values, and vision, and create new sustainable plans with teams and stakeholders alike.

SUMMARY

In an era of vast knowledge, when we know what to do to improve children's health, there is still a massive global failure in preventing mortality and morbidity in millions of children around the world. The author argues that this failure is because we have not developed a cadre of global health leaders that puts child health at the forefront of political agendas nationally and globally.

Unfortunately, we have failed to find, develop, and champion enough of these global child health leaders at the local, national, regional, and global levels. The Sick Kids Global Child Health Leadership program aims to change that, by providing a leadership component combined with global child health care knowledge and understanding. By promoting leadership, we aim to develop champions who can evaluate health care conditions and the quality of personnel, and bring them together to achieve a common goal and vision to improve child health. Only then can we achieve "Health Care for All."

Acknowledgments

The author gratefully acknowledges Katie Johnson and Leticia Rebello for their work on Tables 1 and 2.

References

[1] Inter-agency group for child mortality estimation. CME info. Available at: www.childmortality.org. Accessed November 6, 2010.

[2] Jones G, Steketee RW, Black RE, et al. How many child deaths can we prevent this year? Lancet 2003;362:65–71.

[3] WHO. Primary health care: report of the international conference on primary health care, Alma-Ata, USSR, 6-12 September, 1978. Available at: www.who.int/hpr/NPH/docs/declaration_almaata.pdf. Accessed December 1, 2010.

[4] Bender DE, Pitkin K. Bridging the gap: the village health worker as the cornerstone of the primary health care model. Soc Sci Med 1987;24:515–28.

[5] Hillman D, Hillman E, Mukelebai K. The primary health care manual for East Africa. New York: UNICEF; 1996.

[6] Millennium development goal #4: reduce child mortality. Available at: www.un.org/millenniumgoals/cldhealth.shtml. Accessed December 1, 2010.

[7] Murray CJL, Laakso T, Shibuya K, et al. "Can we achieve Millennium Development Goal 4 (reduce under-five mortality by two-thirds?). New analysis of country trends and forecasts of under-5 mortality to 2015." Lancet 2007;370:1040–54.
[8] Morley David. Paediatric priorities in the developing world. London: Butterworths Publishing; 1973.
[9] WHO. Integrated management of pregnancy and antenatal complications. Available at: www.who.int/making_pregnancy_safer/about/impac/en/index.html. Accessed March 15, 2011.
[10] Programme for global paediatric research. Available at: www.sickkids.ca/PGPR/index.html. Accessed March 15, 2011.
[11] Burns James MacGregor. Transforming leadership. New York: Grove Press; 2003. p. 9.
[12] Hook Sidney. The hero in history: a study in limitation and possibility. Boston: John Day Company; 1943.
[13] Marx Karl. In: Fernbach David, editor. Marx's political writings: the revolutions of 1848, surveys from exile, the first international and after, vol. 1–3 (Marx's political writings). New York: Verso Publishers; 2011.
[14] Spencer Herbert. Illustration of universal progress: a series of discussions. Charleston: Nabu Press; 2010.
[15] Meyer Briggs personality test. Available at: www.personalitypathways.com/type_inventory.html. Accessed March 1, 2011.
[16] Edersheim Elizabeth Haas. McKinsey's Marvin Bower: vision, leadership & the creation of management consulting. Hoboken (NJ): John Wiley & Sons Inc; 2004.
[17] Schein Edgar H. Organization culture and leadership. 3rd edition. San Francisco (CA): Jossey-Bass; 2004.
[18] Drucker Peter F. The essential Drucker. New York: Harper Business; 2004.

Advances in Pediatrics 58 (2011) 27–39
ADVANCES IN PEDIATRICS

Update on Nutritional Recommendations for the Pediatric Patient

Frank R. Greer, MD
Wisconsin Perinatal Center, Meriter Hospital, University of Wisconsin School of Medicine and Public Health, 202 S Park Street, Madison, WI 53715, USA

In the last several years there have been several reports with new nutritional recommendations for infants and children. These reports have included new ideas on how to prevent the development of atopic disease that suggest that the established practices of restricting the introduction of complementary foods to infants may promote atopic disease [1]. There are new recommendations for iron supplementation for infants and toddlers that point out the importance of introducing iron-rich complementary foods much earlier in the diet of infants, particularly if they are exclusively breastfed [2]. There are also new recommendations for increased supplements of vitamin D for infants, children, and adolescents [3,4]. In addition, there are new recommended nutritional guidelines for children at risk for overweight hypercholesterolemia [5], and a new American Academy of Pediatrics (AAP) statement that questions the benefits of the addition of probiotics and prebiotics to the diet of healthy children [6]. These new recommendations are reviewed in this article for pediatric health care providers.

PREVENTION OF ATOPIC DISEASE WITH NUTRITIONAL INTERVENTIONS EARLY IN LIFE

In the past 30 years, the incidence of atopic diseases such as asthma, atopic dermatitis, and food allergies have increased dramatically [1]. The incidence of peanut allergy has increased threefold and the incidence of asthma has increased 160%. It has long been believed that the diet in early childhood has been important in the development of atopic disease, including the diet of the mother during pregnancy and lactation. The AAP has previously recommended that lactating mothers with infants at high risk for developing allergy avoid peanuts, cow milk, and fish in their diets while lactating [7].

However, studies have not supported a protective effect of a maternal exclusion diet during pregnancy or lactation on the development of atopic disease

E-mail address: frgreer@pediatrics.wisc.edu

0065-3101/11/$ – see front matter
doi:10.1016/j.yapd.2011.03.010

in infants [1]. Even though dietary food allergens can be detected in breast milk, it cannot be concluded from published studies to date that the exclusion of eggs, cow milk, fish, or peanuts from the diet of lactating women prevents atopic disease in the infant [1].

Breastfeeding has long been believed to prevent atopic disease in children. Although there is evidence that exclusive breastfeeding protects against wheezing in early life (generally believed to be related to infection and airway size), evidence that exclusive breastfeeding prevents asthma in children older than 6 years is unconvincing [1]. There is evidence that mothers with asthma who exclusively breastfeed increase the risk of asthma in their children [1]. For breastfeeding, the most convincing evidence to date is for the prevention of atopic dermatitis. For infants at high risk of developing atopic disease (parent or sibling with allergic disease) there is evidence that exclusive breastfeeding for at least 4 months, compared with feeding intact cow milk protein formula, decreases the incidence of atopic dermatitis and cow milk allergy during the first 2 years of life. However, there is not enough evidence to conclude that exclusive breastfeeding for at least 4 months prevents the development of food allergy (discussed later) [1].

The role of special infant formulas in preventing atopic disease has also been reviewed by the AAP and other groups [1]. There is no convincing evidence that the use of soy-based formula prevents allergy [1,8], and the use of amino acid–based formulas for the prevention of atopic disease has not been studied [1].

The role of hydrolyzed formula is less clear and most of the studies have been done in infants at high risk of developing allergy. No studies have compared completely or partially hydrolyzed formula with exclusive breastfeeding, so there is no evidence that the use of these formulas is any better than human milk in the prevention of atopic disease [1]. One of the largest studies, the German Infant Nutritional Intervention Program, showed the complexity of comparing various hydrolysate formulas [9]. This study included 945 infants who were at high risk for allergy and who were initially breastfed. The study compared a cow milk formula with 1 of 3 other formulas: partially hydrolyzed whey-based formula, an extensively hydrolyzed whey-based formula, and an extensively hydrolyzed casein-based formula. These formulas were started with weaning or when breast milk was not available. This study showed that different hydrolysates have different effects on atopic disease in infants who were initially breastfed and at high risk for the development of atopic disease. The best results for prevention of atopic disease (atopic dermatitis, urticaria, food allergy) were found for the extensively hydrolyzed casein-based formula compared with cow milk formula (odds ratio [OR] 0.51; 95% CI 0.28–0.92; $P<.025$). Lesser effects were seen with the partially hydrolyzed whey-based formula (OR 0.65; 95% CI 0.38–1.1) and extensively hydrolyzed whey-based formula (OR 0.86; 95% CI 0.52–1.4), compared with cow milk formula [9]. Why extensively hydrolyzed whey-based formula was less effective than partially hydrolyzed whey-based formula was not answered in this study. Follow-up of these infants has shown that the preventive effect of hydrolyzed infant formulas persists to a lesser degree until 6 years of age [10]. However, the higher cost of the hydrolyzed formulas must be considered in any decision-making process for their use. The most convincing data supporting their use are only for children at high risk for atopic disease who were initially receiving breast milk.

Although there have been many studies of the duration of exclusive breastfeeding and its effect on atopic disease, fewer studies have examined the timing of the introduction of complementary foods as an independent risk factor in breastfed or formula-fed infants. Most groups have recommended exclusive breastfeeding for between 4 and 6 months. However, there is no current convincing evidence that delaying the introduction of complementary food beyond this period has a significant protective effect on the development of atopic disease, regardless of whether infants are fed cow milk protein formula or human milk [1]. However, there is evidence that the early introduction of some complementary foods between 4 and 6 months may prevent food allergy [1,11], including foods that are highly allergic, such as wheat/gluten, fish, eggs, and foods containing peanut protein [1,11–19]. For instance, introducing cereal grains before 6 months of age (compared with later introduction) has been shown to be protective against wheat-specific immunoglobulin E [14,15]. With gluten allergy, there is similar evidence that introducing gluten between 4 and 6 months of age prevents celiac disease [11,17]. There is also evidence that introducing highly allergic foods while still breastfeeding may be protective against food allergy. Thus, celiac disease can be prevented in children less than the 2 years of age if they are still breastfeeding at the time of introduction of dietary gluten (OR 0.59; 95% CI 0.42–0.83), and even further decreased by continuing to breastfeed after introducing gluten (OR 0.36; 95% CI 0.26–0.51) [11]. Again, earlier introduction of egg in the first year of life affects allergic sensitization to eggs [12,13]. Introducing eggs at between 4 and 6 months compared with 7 to 9 months increases the risk for egg allergy (OR 1.4; 95% CI 1.2–3.0), and introducing egg between 10 and 12 months increases the risk for egg allergy even more (OR 6.5; 95% CI 3.6–11.6) [13].

A major concern remains the impact of early introduction of peanut-containing products and the effect on peanut allergy [16,18,19]. A recent epidemiology study from Israel found that the prevalence of peanut allergy was tenfold lower in Jewish people living in Israel, where peanut butter is used in the weaning food Bamba, compared with London-based Jewish families with much less exposure to peanut-containing products [18]. At present, there are 2 ongoing studies looking at the effect of peanut exposure early in life on the development of peanut allergy at 3 to 6 years, and the results of these are eagerly awaited [16].

IRON

The AAP recently published its first official report on the diagnosis and prevention of iron deficiency (ID) and iron deficiency anemia (IDA) in infants and toddlers [2]. In the United States there has been a decline in prevalence of IDA, but it still accounts for about 20% of all anemias (hemoglobin [Hb]<11.0 g/dL) in young children between 12 and 35 months of age, with a prevalence of 2.1% [2] (Table 1). However, the prevalence of ID in young children between the ages of 12 and 35 months is much higher. It affects 9.2% of children between 12 and 35 months of age in the general US population and up to 15% of Mexican Americans of the same age group (see Table 1) [2].

IDA represents the severe form of iron deficiency and is associated with irreversible neurodevelopmental delay [2]. Given the likelihood that ID also has some effect on long-term neurodevelopment and behavior that may be irreversible, ID also remains a serious concern [2]. Because iron is prioritized to red cells more than other body tissues, its role in the transport of oxygen in the red blood

Table 1
Iron deficiency, IDA, and anemia in NHANES 1999 to 2002, children aged 12 to 35 months[a]

Population Sampled (n)	US Toddler Population, % (se)[b]	Iron Deficiency, % (se)	Iron Deficiency Anemia, % (se)	All Anemia, % (se)
General US population (672)		9.2 (1.3)	2.1 (0.6)	5.1 (0.8)
Above poverty line (355)[c]	66.4 (2.9)	8.9 (1.7)	2.2 (0.8)[e]	4.6 (1.1)
Below poverty line (268)	33.6 (2.9)	8.6 (1.6)	2.3 (1.2)[e]	6.2 (1.3)
Enrolled in WIC (360)[d]	44.4 (3.2)	10.7 (2.1)	3.1 (1.2)[e]	6.6 (1.4)
Non-Hispanic white (196)	58.0 (3.8)	7.3 (1.9)	2.0 (0.8)[e]	4.6 (1.2)
Non-Hispanic black (173)	14.1 (2.1)	6.6 (1.8)	1.6 (0.9)[e]	8.3 (1.9)
Mexican American (231)	15.0 (2.2)	13.9 (3.1)	0.9 (0.7)[e]	3.2 (1.2)[e]
Other ethnicity (72)	13.0 (2.7)	15.2 (4.7)[e]	4.4 (2.7)[e]	5.5 (2.7)[e]

Anemia defined as hemoglobin <11.0 g/dL.
Iron deficiency defined as an abnormal value for at least 2 of 3 indicators: serum ferritin (abnormal cutoff <10 μg/dL), zinc protoporphyrin (>1.42 μmol/L red blood cells), and transferrin saturation (<10%).
IDA defined as anemia plus iron deficiency.

Abbreviations: se, standard error; WIC, Special Supplemental Nutrition Program for Women, Infants, and Children.

[a]Unweighted n's and weighted %'s and standard errors (se) for all children with complete data for hemoglobin, serum ferritin, transferrin saturation, and zinc protoporphyrin.

[b]Proportion of row descriptor out of all children in analytical sample (n = 672).

[c]Children with income data, n = 623.

[d]Any member of household received benefits from the Special Supplemental Nutrition Program for Women, Infants, and Children in the past 12 months. Children with food security data, n = 668.

[e]Estimate is statistically unreliable. Relative standard error (standard error of estimate/estimate ×100) ≥30%.

From Baker RD, Greer FR. Diagnosis and prevention of iron deficiency and iron deficiency anemia in infants and young children (0–3 years). American Academy of Pediatrics, Committee on Nutrition. Pediatrics 2010;126(5):1042; with permission.

cells is clearly its most critical function. This prioritization of iron for red cells, even more than the brain, would account for the adverse neurodevelopmental effects of iron deficiency with or without anemia in the infant. Iron is essential for neuronal proliferation, myelination, energy metabolism, neurotransmission, and various enzyme systems in the central nervous system [20].

The iron supplied in breast milk (averaging 0.27 mg/d assuming a breast milk intake of 0.78 L/d) coupled with the iron stores at birth in the healthy term infant, meets the iron needs only until the infant doubles its birth weight and thus doubles its blood volume, usually by 4 months of age. Between 4 and 6 months of age, there is a dramatic increase in the iron requirement, to 11 mg/d, for the remainder of the first year of life [2]. Thus, because of concerns about ID, the AAP has recommended that breastfed infants be supplemented with 1 mg/kg/d of oral iron beginning at 4 months of age until appropriate iron-containing complementary foods (including iron-fortified cereals) are introduced into the diet [2]. The best source of iron is heme iron found in red meat. Because breast milk contains no heme iron, the early introduction of complementary foods containing meat is advised. It is acknowledged that this would require a significant paradigm shift in the way complementary foods are generally introduced in the diets of infants by pediatric health care providers in the United States. For formula-fed infants, the iron needs for the first 12 months of life can be met by a standard infant formula (iron content 10–12 mg/L) and with the introduction of iron-rich complementary foods after 4 to 6 months of age [2]. Whole milk should not be used before 12 completed months of age.

For toddlers from 1 to 3 years of age, the AAP recommends an iron intake of 7 mg/d [2]. Again, this is best delivered by eating red meats, whole-grain cereals fortified with iron, vegetables that contain iron (ie, legumes), and fruits with vitamin C, which augments iron absorption. An alternative source of iron is liquid iron supplements up to 36 months of age, after which time chewable multivitamins can be used.

Because 80% of iron stores are accumulated during the last trimester of pregnancy, preterm infants need an iron intake of 2 mg/kg/d through 12 months of age, which can be supplied by iron-fortified formulas [2,21]. If fed human milk, these infants should receive an iron supplement of 2 mg/kg/d by 1 month of age and this should be continued until the infant is weaned to iron-fortified formula or eats enough complementary foods to supply 2 mg/kg/d of iron. An exception to this practice would be the preterm infant who has received an iron load from multiple packed red blood cell transfusions.

The AAP has also recommended universal screening for IDA and ID at 12 months of age, with a determination of Hb concentration and an assessment of risk factors associated with ID/IDA [2]. These risk factors include low socioeconomic status (especially in infants of Mexican American descent), a history of prematurity or low birth weight, exposure to lead, exclusive breastfeeding beyond 4 months of age without supplemental iron, and weaning to whole milk or complementary foods that do not include iron-fortified cereals or food naturally rich in iron. Other risk factors are feeding problems, poor growth, and the inadequate nutrition typically seen in infants with special health care needs. If, as a result of this screen, the Hb is less than 11.0 g/dL, then further work-up is required to establish the cause of anemia [2]. Regardless of the Hb, if there is a high risk of dietary ID, then further testing should be performed, given the potential adverse effects of ID on neurodevelopmental outcomes.

The AAP recognized that it was desirable to use the fewest tests that will accurately reflect iron status, and that, at the present time, there is no ideal test to screen for ID/IDA in the pediatric age group. The gold standard for determination of iron stores has been a measurement of bone marrow iron. However, serum ferritin (SF) is recognized as a sensitive parameter for the assessment of iron stores in healthy children. SF of 1 μg/L corresponds to 8 to 10 mg of available storage iron, and a cutoff of 10 μg/L has been recommended in children [2]. However, SF is an acute-phase reactant, and its concentration is increased in the presence of inflammation/infection, malignancy, and liver disease. A simultaneous C-reactive protein (CRP) is always required to rule out inflammation or infection. However, reticulocyte hemoglobin concentration (CHr), a test that is not familiar to most pediatric health care providers, is not affected by inflammation/infection or malignancy, and is a much more desirable biomarker for iron deficiency [22,23]. The CHr assay makes use of flow cytometry, and 2 of the 4 automated hematology analyzers commonly used in the United States have the capability to measure CHr [23]. It provides a measure of the iron available to cells recently released from the bone marrow. A low CHr concentration has been shown to be the strongest predictor of ID in children [22,23]. Therefore, the following screening tests have been recommended by the AAP for ID/IDA along with a screen for Hb when there is a risk for ID:

Serum ferritin and CRP levels; or
Reticulocyte hemoglobin concentration (CHr)

In the AAP report, serum transferring receptor concentration (TfR1) was acknowledged as a potential marker for the iron status of infants and children, and it has been promoted by the World Health Organization as a screening test for ID [24]. It is a measure of iron status and detects ID at the cellular level. TfR1 is found on cell membranes and facilitates transfer of iron into the cell. When iron supply is inadequate, there is upregulation of TfR1 to enable the cell to compete more effectively for iron, and subsequently more circulating TfR1 is found in serum. However, the TfR1 assay is not widely available and standard values for infants and children have not been established, so it cannot be recommended as a screening test at this time [2].

There have been some concerns about harmful effects of iron supplements on infants. In general, no ill effects have been reported in infants given formula with up to 12 mg/L of iron during the first year of life, which have been used for more than 30 years in the United States [2]. Evidence is insufficient to associate iron-containing formulas with gastrointestinal symptoms. No studies have convincingly documented decreased linear growth in iron-replete infants given medicinal iron [2]. In addition, data on the effect on iron on infection has been contradictory, and a systematic review has concluded that iron supplementation has no impact on infections in children [25].

In summary, there is evidence that both IDA and ID have adverse effects on cognitive and behavioral development in many studies [26–32]. Iron is essential for normal neurodevelopment in several animal models. Therefore it is important to minimize IDA and ID in infants and toddlers even if unequivocal evidence is not yet available [33,34].

VITAMIN D

Vitamin D continues to be in the forefront of human nutrition. Both the AAP and Institute of Medicine have recently recommended increased intakes of vitamin D for children [3,4]. For infants in the first 12 months of life, the recommended vitamin D intake has been increased from 200 to 400 IU/d. For children/adolescents 1 year to 18 years of age, the recommendation has been increased from 200 IU to 600 IU a day for vitamin D. These recommendations are based on the intake of vitamin D to maintain serum levels of at least 50 nmol/L (20 ng/mL), a level that benefits 97.5% all of the US population based on the present evidence [4].

Because human milk contains minimal amounts of vitamin D, cases of rickets in infants secondary to inadequate vitamin D intake and decreased exposure to sunlight continue to be reported in the United States [35–38], which represents an extreme degree of deficiency of the vitamin. Most of these cases have been reported in infants who are exclusively breastfed without supplemental vitamin D, because the vitamin D content of human milk is minimal [39]. Infants with rickets often have increased skin pigmentation and a history of decreased sunshine exposure, but, in many areas of the United States sunshine exposure during the winter months is not effective for the cutaneous synthesis of vitamin D [3,4,40]. Vitamin D deficiency can be prevented in breast feeding infants with a vitamin D supplement of 400 IU/d or until they are receiving adequate amounts of vitamin D from vitamin D–fortified formula or dairy products [3,4].

In understanding the growing importance of vitamin D beyond rickets and skeletal health, it must be realized that vitamin D is not a vitamin but a hormone or a prohormone. Like all hormones in the steroid family, its synthesis begins with cholesterol. In the case of vitamin D, 7-dehydrocholesterol in the skin is converted to the parent compound vitamin D_3 (cholecalciferol) with exposure to sunlight (ultraviolet-B radiation). The parent compound is then hydroxylated in the liver to form 25-hydroxy vitamin D_3 (calcidiol) and hydroxylated again in the kidney to form 1,25-hydroxy vitamin D_3 (calcitriol). Though 1,25-$(OH)_2$ vitamin D_3 is the true hormone that effects gene transcription at the cellular level, the most plentiful form of the vitamin in circulation (by a factor of 10) is 25-OH vitamin D_3. It is believed to be the best marker for vitamin D status, again with an ideal level greater than or equal to 50 nmol/L (20 ng/mL) set by the Institute of Medicine (IOM) [4]. However, for the classic endocrine function of vitamin D, it is 1,25-$(OH)_2$ vitamin D_3 that acts in concert with parathyroid hormone to tightly regulate calcium metabolism and maintain the skeletal system [41,42].

The hormone 1,25-$(OH)_2$ vitamin D_3 promotes gene transcription through its interaction with genomic (nuclear) vitamin D receptors (VDRs) present in many types of cells [42]. It is these genomic VDRs, found in many different cells in the body, that have led to the association of vitamin D deficiency with many chronic diseases including hypertension, atherosclerosis/myocardial infarction, type 1 and 2 diabetes, obesity, colorectal cancer, prostate cancer, breast cancer, ovarian cancer, multiple sclerosis, rheumatoid arthritis, inflammatory bowel disease, and even wheezing in early childhood [3,4,41,43]. There is some plausibility for these nonendocrine functions of vitamin D, given new in vitro evidence that 25-OH vitamin D can be taken up by cells other than those in the kidney and hydroxylated at the 1 position to synthesize 1,25-dihydroxyvitamin D locally, where it has autocrine (within the cell) or paracrine (nearby cells) effects [42]. This process has been best shown in the immune system where VDRs are found in the nuclei of monocytes, macrophages, dendritic dells, natural killer cells, T cells, and B cells [44]. In cell culture, 1,25-dihydroxy vitamin D can be shown to alter cytokine secretion patterns, suppress T-cell activation, affect maturation and migration of dendritic cells, enhance phagocytic activity of macrophages, as well as increase the phagocytic activity of killer cells. However, these potential nonendocrine, nonskeletal outcomes of vitamin D deficiency have not been supported by adequate clinical trials showing that vitamin D is casually related to the disease process [3,4].

One of the most frequently cited studies in pediatrics is a Finnish study showing a relationship between the incidence of type 1 diabetes and vitamin D intake during childhood [45]. This study was done in Lapland, whose population has the highest known incidence of type 1 diabetes. That vitamin D may play a role is supported by the observation that it is far more common in northern latitudes where sunshine exposure is decreased and serum 25-OH D levels are low in winter. In animal and cell culture models, vitamin D also seems to stimulate insulin release and insulin receptor expression [46]. As noted earlier, vitamin D may play a role in immune function, and type 1 diabetes is known to be an autoimmune process directed against the β cells of the pancreas [46]. However, the Finnish study was a retrospective birth cohort study in children born in 1966, during a time period when the recommended vitamin D intake for children in this part of Finland was 2000 IU of vitamin D per day [45]. Though serum 25-OH vitamin D levels are known to be low in northern Finland, no 25-OH vitamin D levels were measured in these subjects, and the vitamin D intake was estimated from retrospective chart reviews of medical records. Again, although the epidemiologic association seems to be strong, this paper does not shed light on vitamin D and the causality of type 1 diabetes, which also has a strong genetic component.

The recent IOM report has concluded that the data do not provide compelling evidence that vitamin D is related to extraskeletal health outcomes and advises against the large intakes of vitamin D recommended by some vitamin D advocates [4]. In addition, though the measurement of 25-OH vitamin D level in children and adolescents indicates vitamin D exposure and status, the information available is not adequate to use 25-hydroxy vitamin D as a biomarker for an intermediate health endpoint (eg, blood pressure) or disease (eg, rickets, or osteoporosis) [4]. It is not recommended at this time to measure serum 25-OH vitamin D concentrations in children as a routine screening tool for vitamin D deficiency [3,4].

LIPID SCREENING AND THE USE OF LOW-FAT DAIRY PRODUCTS

The AAP recommended new guidelines for lipid screening and cardiovascular health in children in 2008 [5]. It recommended a population approach to a healthful diet for all children older than 2 years that was in accordance with the Dietary Guidelines for Americans [47]. This recommendation included the use of low-fat dairy products for all children more than 2 years of age. However, a little-noticed recommendation from the AAP report was that, for children between the ages of 12 months and 2 years for whom overweight (body mass index [BMI] $\geq$85% but <95%) or obesity (BMI$\geq$95%) is a concern, or who have a family history of obesity, dyslipidemia, or cardiovascular disease (CVD), the use of reduced-fat milk would be appropriate [5]. Previously, the AAP had recommended the use of whole milk until 24 months of completed age [48]. The new recommendation was largely based on the increasing risk for overweight in young children and results of the ongoing Special Turku Risk Intervention Program [49]. This program was a randomized dietary intervention study beginning at approximately 7 months of age with weaning from breast milk. Children in the intervention group were maintained on a diet with total fat equal to less than 30% of calories, saturated fat less than 10% of calories, and cholesterol intake of less than 200 mg/d, using 1.5% cow milk after 12 months of age. Outcomes in the study included both growth and neurologic function. No adverse effects of the intervention diet were observed on growth or neurologic and cognitive outcomes through 5 years of age [50]. Other significant observations included lowering the low-density lipoprotein concentrations in boys and decreasing the prevalence of obesity in girls in the intervention group, compared with the controls. The study concluded that there was no effect of introducing reduced-fat milk in children beginning at 12 months of age. However, the new Special Supplemental Nutrition Program for Women, Infants, and Children (WIC) food programs instituted in the United States in October of 2009 have specifically excluded any low-fat or reduced-fat milk for children before 24 months completed age. Before this time, some WIC programs had dispensed low-fat milk after the first year of life to toddlers who were overweight or at risk for overweight (Frank R. Greer, MD, personal observations, 2009).

The AAP report also recommended targeting lipid screening for children sometime after 2 years of age but no later than 10 years of age [5]. Children and adolescents who are targeted for a fasting lipid profile are those with a positive family history of dyslipidemia or premature CVD ($\leq$55 years of age for men and $\leq$65 years of age for women). Screening with a fasting lipid profile is also recommended for pediatric patients for whom family history is unknown, or for those with CVD risk factors such as overweight, obesity, hypertension (blood pressure $\geq$95 percentile), cigarette smoking, or diabetes mellitus [5].

New guidelines for lipid screening and cardiovascular health from the National Heart, Lung and Blood Institute are expected in late in 2011, and some changes for the pediatric population are anticipated.

PROBIOTICS AND PREBIOTICS

The AAP recently published a clinical report on the use of probiotics and prebiotics in pediatrics [6]. Probiotics are dietary supplements or foods (including infant formula) that contain viable microorganisms that cause alterations of the microflora of the host. Typically these microorganisms are members of the genera *Lactobacillus*, *Bifidobacterium*, and *Streptococcus*. These organisms are fermentative, obligatory, or facultative anaerobic organisms typically found in the digestive tract, where they predominate and prevail over potential pathogenic microorganisms. Probiotic bacteria are believed to exert positive effects on the development of the mucosal immune system [51–53].

Prebiotics are usually in the form of oligosaccharides that may occur naturally but are now added as dietary supplements to foods, beverages, and infant formula. Although indigestible by humans, their presence in the digestive system selectively enhances proliferation of certain probiotic bacteria in the colon, especially *Bifidobacterium* species. Commercially available prebiotics include fructooligosaccharides (FOSs), galactooligosaccharides (GOSs), soybean oligosaccharides, and inulin. Inulin is a composite oligosaccharide that contains several FOS molecules. Human milk contains hundreds of identifiable prebiotic oligosaccharides and the identification of the most significant forms is the goal of ongoing research. These prebiotics have a significant influence on the preponderance of naturally occurring probiotic bacteria in the digestive system of breastfed infants [6].

Probiotics and prebiotics are added to many food products marketed to children and adolescents, including infant formula. When marketed as dietary supplements (not for treatment or prevention of a disease), they do not require premarket review and approval by the US Food and Drug Administration (FDA) [6]. Probiotics and prebiotics are also available as over-the-counter dietary supplements.

The AAP concluded in its report that the benefits of probiotics or prebiotics to healthy children and adolescents are largely of unproven benefit, including those added to food products marketed to children. However, there is no evidence that they are of any harm to healthy children and adolescents, although long-term effects, including those on the gut microflora, are unknown. Probiotics should not be given to children who are seriously or chronically ill until the safety of their administration to this population has been established [6].

The AAP has also noted that the addition of probiotics to powdered infant formula (they cannot be added to liquid formula, which is sterile) has not been shown to be harmful to healthy term infants. However, evidence of clinical efficacy for their addition is insufficient to recommend the routine use of these formulas at this time [6]. Furthermore, no randomized trials have directly compared the health benefits of feeding human milk versus infant formulas supplemented with probiotics. It also noted that, although prebiotics may prove to be beneficial in reducing common infections and atopy in otherwise healthy infants, confirmatory evidence in infants fed formula that is not also partially hydrolyzed is needed before any recommendations can be made [6].

The prebiotics and probiotics that are now being added to commercially available infant formulas are classified as generally regarded as safe (GRAS) as long as they are used in accordance with the food-additive regulations of the FDA. However, there is no cost-benefit information on their addition, particularly to infant formula. As dietary supplements in food products marketed for infants and children, they are not known to be harmful to healthy subjects. However, probiotics should not be given to children who are seriously or chronically ill until the safety of administration has been established [6].

References

[1] Greer FR, Sicherer SH, Burks AW. Effects of early nutritional interventions on the development of atopic disease in infants and children: the role of maternal dietary restriction, breastfeeding, timing of introduction of complementary foods, and hydrolyzed formulas. American Academy of Pediatrics, Committee on Nutrition and Section on Allergy and Immunology. Pediatrics 2008;121:183–99.

[2] Baker RD, Greer FR. Diagnosis and prevention of iron deficiency and iron deficiency anemia in infants and young children (0–3 years). American Academy of Pediatrics, Committee on Nutrition. Pediatrics 2010;126(5):1040–50.

[3] Wagner CL, Greer FR. Prevention of rickets and vitamin D deficiency in infants, children, and adolescents. American Academy of Pediatrics, Committee on Nutrition, Section on Breastfeeding. Pediatrics 2008;122:1142–52.

[4] Ross AC, Taylor CL, Yaktine AL, et al. Dietary reference intakes for calcium vitamin D. Committee to Review Dietary Reference Intake for Vitamin D and Calcium, Food and Nutrition Board, Institute of Medicine. Washington, DC: The National Academies Press; 2011.

[5] Daniels R, Greer FR. Lipid screening and cardiovascular health in childhood. Pediatrics 2008;122:198–208.

[6] Thomas DW, Greer FR. Probiotics and prebiotics in pediatrics. Clinical report. American Academy of Pediatrics, Committee on Nutrition, and Section on Gastroenterology and Nutrition. Pediatrics 2010;126:1217–31.

[7] American Academy of Pediatrics. Committee on Nutrition. Hypoallergenic infant formulas. Pediatrics 2000;106:346–9.

[8] Bhatia J, Greer FR. The use of soy protein-base formulas in infant feeding. American Academy of Pediatrics, Committee on Nutrition, clinical report. Pediatrics 2008;121:1062–8.

[9] Von Berg A, Koletzko S, Gurbl A, et al. The effect of hydrolyzed cow's milk formula for allergy prevention in the first year of life: the German Infant Nutritional Interventions Study, a randomized double-blind trial. J Allergy Clin Immunol 2003;111:533–40.

[10] Von Berg A, Filipiak-Pittroff B, Kramer U, et al. Preventative effect of hydrolyzed infant formulas persists until age 6 years: long-term results from the German Infant Nutritional Intervention Study (GINI). J Allergy Clin Immunol 2008;121:1442–7.

[11] Agostoni C, Decsi T, Fewtrell M, et al. Complementary feeding: a commentary by the ESPGHAN Committee on Nutrition. J Pediatr Gastroenterol Nutr 2008;46:99–110.
[12] Nwaru BI, Erkkola M, Ahonen S, et al. Age at the introduction of solid foods during the first year and allergic sensitization at age 5 years. Pediatrics 2010;125:50–9.
[13] Koplin JJ, Osborne NJ, Wake M, et al. Can early introduction of egg prevent egg allergy in infants? A population-based study. J Allergy Clin Immunol 2010;126:807–13.
[14] Poole JA, Barriga K, Hoffman M, et al. Timing of initial exposure to cereal grains and the risk of wheat allergy. Pediatrics 2006;117:2175–82.
[15] Zutavern A, Brockow I, Schaaf B, et al. Timing of initial exposure to cereal grains and the risk of wheat allergy. Pediatrics 2008;117:2175–82.
[16] McLean S, Sheikh A. Does avoidance of peanuts in early life reduce the risk of peanut allergy? BMJ 2010;340:c424.
[17] Carlsson A, Agardh D, Borulf S, et al. Prevalence of celiac disease: before and after a national change in feeding recommendations. Scand J Gastroenterol 2006;41:553–8.
[18] Tuit Du, Katz Y, Sasieni P, et al. Early consumption of peanuts in infancy is associated with a low prevalence of peanut allergy. J Allergy Clin Immunol 2008;122:984–91.
[19] Thompson RL, Miles LM, Lunn J, et al. Peanut sensitization and allergy: influence of early life exposure to peanuts. Br J Nutr 2010;103:1278–86.
[20] Andrews NC. Iron deficiency and related disorders. In: Greer JP, Foerster J, Lukens JN, editors. Wintrobe's clinical hematology. 11th edition. Philadelphia: Lippincott Williams & Wilkins; 2004. p. 979–1009.
[21] Raghavendra R, Georgieff M. Microminerals. In: Tsang RC, Uauy R, Koletzko B, et al, editors. Nutrition of the preterm infant: scientific basis and practical guidelines. Cincinnati (OH): Digital Educational Publishing; 2005. p. 277–310.
[22] Ulrich C, Wu A, Armsby C, et al. Screening healthy infants for iron deficiency using reticulocyte hemoglobin content. JAMA 2005;294(8):924–30.
[23] Brugnara C, Schiller B, Moran J. Reticulocyte hemoglobin equivalent (Ret He) and assessment of iron-deficient states. Clin Lab Haematol 2006;28(5):303–8.
[24] World Health Organization. Assessing the iron status of populations: report of a joint World Health Organization/Centers for Disease and Control and Prevention technical consultation on the assessment of iron status at the population level. Geneva (Switzerland): World Health Organization; April 6–8, 2004. Available at: http://whqlibdoc.who.int/publications/2004/9241593156_eng.pdf. Accessed April 13, 2011.
[25] Gera T, Sachdev HP. Effect of iron supplementation on incidence of infectious illness in children: a systematic review. BMJ 2002;325(7373):1142.
[26] Friel JK, Andrews WL, Aziz K, et al. A randomized trail of two levels of iron supplementation and developmental outcome in low birth weight infants. J Pediatr 2001;139:254–60.
[27] Lozoff B, Jimenez E, Wolf AW. Long-term developmental outcome of infants with iron deficiency. N Engl J Med 1991;325(10):687–94.
[28] Idjradinata P, Pollitt E. Reversal of developmental delays in iron-deficient anaemic infants treated with iron. Lancet 1993;341:1–4.
[29] Armony-Sivan R, Eidelman AI, Lanir A, et al. Iron status and neurobehavioral development of premature infants. J Perinatol 2004;24(12):757–62.
[30] Lozoff B, Jimenez E, Hagen J, et al. Poorer behavioral and developmental outcome more than 10 years after treatment for iron deficiency in infancy. Pediatrics 2000;105:E51.
[31] McCann JC, Ames BN. An overview of evidence for a causal relation between iron deficiency during development and deficits in cognitive or behavioral function. Am J Clin Nutr 2007;85(4):931–45.
[32] Martins S, Logan S, Gilbert R. Iron therapy for improving psychomotor development and cognitive function in children under the age of three with iron deficiency anaemia. Cochrane Database Syst Rev 2001;2:CD001444.
[33] Carlson ES, Tkac I, Magid R, et al. Iron is essential for neuron development and memory function in mouse hippocampus. J Nutr 2009;139(4):672–9.

[34] Tran PV, Fretham SJ, Carlson ES, et al. Long-term reduction of hippocampal brain-derived neurotrophic factor activity after fetal-neonatal iron deficiency in adult rats. Pediatr Res 2009;65(5):493–8.
[35] Kreiter SR, Schwartz RP, Kirkman HN Jr, et al. Nutritional rickets in African American breast-fed infants. J Pediatr 2000;137:153–7.
[36] Pugliese MT, Blumberg DL, Hludzinski J, et al. Nutritional rickets in suburbia. J Am Coll Nutr 1998;17(6):637–41.
[37] Ward LM. Vitamin D deficiency in the 21st century: a persistent problem among Canadian infants and mothers. CMAJ 2005;172:769–70.
[38] Weisberg P, Scanlon KS, Li R, et al. Nutritional rickets among children in the United States: review of cases reported between 1986–2003. Am J Clin Nutr 2004;80: 1697S–705S.
[39] Lamin-Keefe CJ. Vitamin D and E in human milk. In: Jensen RD, editor. Handbook of milk composition. San Diego (CA): Academic Press; 1995. p. 706–17.
[40] Webb AR, Kline L, Hollick MF. Influence of season and latitude on the cutaneous synthesis of vitamin D_3: exposure to winter sunlight in Boston and Edmonton will not promote vitamin D_3 synthesis in human skin. J Clin Endocrinol Metab 1988;67(2):373–8.
[41] Holick MF, Chen TC. Vitamin D deficiency: a worldwide problem with health consequences. Am J Clin Nutr 2008;87(Suppl):1080S–6S.
[42] Norman AW. From vitamin D to hormone D: fundamentals of the vitamin D endocrine system for good health. Am J Clin Nutr 2008;88(Suppl):419S–99S.
[43] Misra M, Pacaud D, Petryk A, et al. Vitamin D deficiency in children and its management: review of current knowledge and recommendations. Pediatrics 2008;122:398–417.
[44] Hewison M. Vitamin D and the immune system: new perspectives on an old theme. Endocrinol Metab Clin North Am 2010;39(2):365–79.
[45] Hypponen E, Laara E, Reunanen A, et al. Intake of vitamin D and risk of type 1 diabetes: a birth-cohort study. Lancet 2001;358(9292):1500–3.
[46] Mathieu C, Badenhoop K. Vitamin D and type 1 diabetes mellitus: state of the art. Trends Endocrinol Metab 2005;16(6):261–6.
[47] US Department of Health and Human Services. Dietary Guidelines for Americans 2010. Available at: http://www.health.gov/dietaryguidelines/. Accessed February 15, 2011.
[48] American Academy of Pediatrics. National Cholesterol Education Program: report of the expert panel on blood cholesterol levels in children and adolescents. Pediatrics 1999;89:525–84.
[49] Salo P, Viikari J, Hamalainen M, et al. Serum cholesterol ester fatty acids in 7- and 13-month children in prospective randomized trial of a low-saturated fat, low-cholesterol diet: the STRIP baby project. Special Turku Coronary risk factor intervention project for children. Acta Paediatr 1999;88:505–12.
[50] Rask-Nissila L, Jokinen E, Ronnemaa T, et al. Prospective, randomized, infancy-onset trial of the effects of a low-saturated-fat, low-cholesterol diet on serum lipids and lipoproteins before school age: the Special Turku coronary risk factor intervention project (STRIP). Circulation 2000;102:1477–83.
[51] Corthesy B, Gaskins HR, Mercenier A. Cross-talk between probiotic bacteria and the host immune system. J Nutr 2007;137(3 Suppl 2):781S–90S.
[52] Matsuzaki T, Takagi A, Ikemura H, et al. Intestinal microflora: probiotics and autoimmunity. J Nutr 2007;137(3 Suppl 2):798S–802S.
[53] Yuan Q, Walker WA. Innate immunity of the gut: mucosal defense in health and disease. J Pediatr Gastroenterol Nutr 2004;38(5):463–73.

Advances in Pediatrics 58 (2011) 41–64
ADVANCES IN PEDIATRICS

Immunization Update III

Ayesha Mirza, MD[a], Mobeen H. Rathore, MD, CPE, FIDA[a,b,*]
[a]Department of Pediatrics, University of Florida, 653-1 West 8th Street, Mail Box L-13, Jacksonville, FL 32209, USA
[b]Wolfson Children's Hospital, 800 Prudential Drive, Jacksonville, FL 32207, USA

Perhaps the biggest news in the immunization world over the past 2 years was the 2009 (H1N1) novel influenza A virus outbreak. The virus was initially identified to be the cause of influenza-like illness in two children in the United States during March and April 2009 and the cause of respiratory illness outbreaks in Mexico [1,2]. The virus spread rapidly and within weeks cases were identified across the United States and in several countries around the world. On June 11, 2009 the Director General of the World Health Organization (WHO) Dr Margaret Chan declared a global pandemic. As of August 10, 2010, this has been updated to postpandemic status. This review focuses on discussing the 2009 pandemic briefly along with the global response in terms of vaccine development, recommendations for vaccination for the 2010–2011 influenza season, followed by other recent updates in adolescent and pediatric vaccines.

INFLUENZA VACCINES

2009 (H1N1) novel influenza A

As part of the family Orthomyxoviridae, influenza viruses are single-stranded RNA viruses with 3 types: A, B, and C. Influenza A viruses circulate in more than 18 mammalian species (including pigs and humans, although the main reservoir is aquatic wildfowl, including migratory birds) and are responsible for all known major epidemics and pandemics [3]. The influenza A virus genome contains 8 separate gene segments that have the ability to "reassort" or "mix" with other influenza A virus gene segments and thus "shift" antigenic characteristics [3–5]. These viruses are classified according to the subtypes of surface proteins, hemagglutinin (HA) and neuraminidase (NA) that they possess. HA is a surface glycoprotein essential for viral binding and entry into host cells. HA contains the primary epitopes for protective neutralizing antibodies, whereas NA has a somewhat lesser role in protective immunity and is primarily required for viral release [6]. Thus antibody against HA confers protection against infection and illness whereas antibody against NA

*Corresponding author. Department of Pediatrics, 653-1 West 8th Street, LRC 3rd Floor, Jacksonville, FL 32209. *E-mail address*: mobeen.rathore@jax.ufl.edu

0065-3101/11/$ – see front matter
doi:10.1016/j.yapd.2011.03.006

can reduce the severity of illness. Annual changes in the HA epitopes lend themselves to a "drift" in protective immunity to circulating strains, hence the need for yearly review of the antigenic content of circulating influenza viruses. Pandemics occur when influenza viruses with HA for which there is little or no protective immunity emerge in the human population and transmit virus efficiently from person to person.

Since the global influenza A(H1N1) virus pandemic of 1918 (Spanish flu), influenza virus gene reassortment has been well documented and observed to occur frequently between human virus subtypes, between human and avian, and among avian influenza viruses [7,8]. Such reassortments led to the global pandemics of 1957 (H2N2) (Asian flu) and 1968 (H3N2) (Hong Kong flu) [8,9]. To have an idea of the magnitude of these epidemics, more Americans died as a result of the 1918 (Spanish flu) pandemic than were killed during World Wars I and II, the Korean, Vietnam, Gulf, Afghanistan, and Iraq wars combined [10].

Nearly all human influenza A infections worldwide since 1918 have been caused by descendants of the 1918 pandemic virus [7]. While influenza A(H1N1) viruses continue to circulate among humans, seasonal epidemics of influenza A virus from 1968 to 2009 were dominated by A(H3N2) virus variants generated by antigenic drift. However, in early April 2009 a new influenza A(H1N1) virus (originally referred to as swine-origin influenza A virus) emerged among humans in California and in Mexico, quickly spreading worldwide through human-to-human transmission, and generating the first influenza pandemic of the twenty-first century. Molecular studies of the new influenza A(H1N1) pandemic virus genome showed that it was antigenically unrelated to human seasonal influenza viruses but genetically derived from several viruses which had been circulating in pigs for a long time [8]. Initial transmission to humans is believed to have taken place at least several months before recognition of the first outbreak, and phylogenetic data suggest that the reassortment of swine lineages may have occurred years before emergence in humans. The 2009 H1N1 is a quadruple-reassortant virus containing gene segments from North American as well as Asian and European swine influenza viruses, some gene segments from North American avian influenza viruses, and one gene segment from a human influenza virus (Fig 1) [3–8]. During the current epidemic, however, there was no evidence that swine were playing any role in the epidemiology or in the worldwide spread of the virus in human populations [9].

Novel influenza A(H1N1), henceforth referred to as 2009 H1N1, for the most part presented as a mild, self-limiting upper respiratory tract illness with (or at times without) fever, cough, sore throat, body aches, fatigue, chills, rhinorrhea, conjunctivitis, headache, and shortness of breath [9,11]. Up to 50% of patients had gastrointestinal symptoms at presentation including diarrhea and vomiting. The spectrum of clinical presentation varied from asymptomatic cases to primary viral pneumonia resulting in respiratory failure, acute respiratory distress, multiorgan failure, and death [12]. While fewer than 1% of

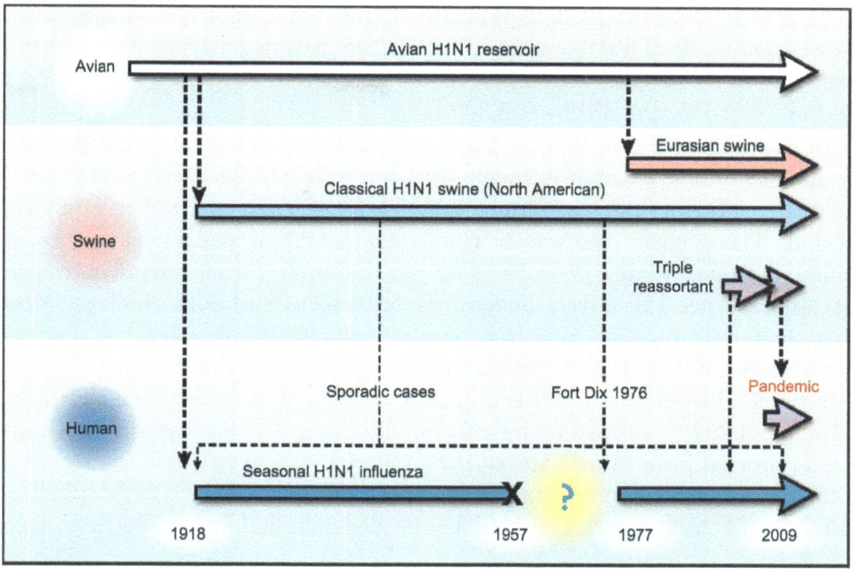

Fig. 1. Emergence of influenza A (H1N1) viruses from birds and swine into humans. The diagram shows the important events and processes in the emergence of influenza A (H1N1) viruses during the past 91 years. Avian, swine, and human populations are represented in the top, middle, and bottom of the diagram, respectively. Epidemic or zoonotic viruses are shown as wide horizontal arrows (*white* for avian viruses, *light blue* or *pink* for swine viruses, and *dark blue* for human viruses). Cross-species transmissions are shown as vertical dashed lines, with thick lines for transfers that gave rise to sustained transmission in the new host and thin lines for those that were transient and resulted in a self-limited number of cases. Principal dates are shown along the bottom of the diagram. The disappearance of H1N1 in 1957 most likely represents competition by the emerging pandemic H2N2 strain in the face of population immunity to H1N1. The reemergence in 1977 is unexplained and probably represents reintroduction to humans from a laboratory source. (*From* Zimmer SM, Burke DS. Historical perspective—emergence of influenza A (H1N1) viruses. N Engl J Med 2009;361(3):279–85; with permission.)

estimated cases of 2009 H1N1 in the United States resulted in hospitalization, a quarter of those hospitalized required admission to the intensive care unit (ICU), and more than half required mechanical ventilation. The presence of underlying conditions was common among hospitalized patients; up to 60% of children, and 83% of adults admitted with 2009 H1N1 infection had at least one underlying chronic medical condition (CMC) (asthma, diabetes, cardiovascular disease, neurologic and developmental disorders, the latter 2 being more common in children). Eleven percent of hospitalized adults with 2009 H1N1 were pregnant [13].

The United States experienced its first wave of 2009 H1N1 pandemic activity in the spring of 2009, followed by a second wave of 2009 H1N1 activity in the fall. Activity peaked during the second week in October and then declined quickly to below baseline levels in January. The early increase in flu activity in October is in contrast to nonpandemic influenza seasons. From April 2009 to April 2010, a total of 61 million cases were reported, estimated range 43 to 89 million, with an estimated 195,000 to 403,000 hospitalizations and estimated deaths 8870 to 18,300 [14].

In the United States reports from around the country for pediatric cases seemed to follow a common theme. In California 345 children younger than 18 years with laboratory-confirmed 2009 H1N1 were reported over a 3-month period. The median age was 6 years; hospitalization rates were highest in infants younger than 6 months (13.9 per 100,000) versus overall rates (3.5 per 100,000 per 110 days). Two-thirds (230; 67%) had comorbidities. More than half (163 of 278; 59%) had pneumonia, 94 (27%) required intensive care, and 9 (3%) died; in 3 fatal cases (33%), children had secondary bacterial infections. More than two-thirds (221 of 319; 69%) received antiviral treatment, 44% (88 of 202) within 48 hours of symptom onset [15]. Similar numbers have been reported from other parts of the country [16].

In the authors' own hospital in Northeast Florida, of the 119 hospitalized children, 25 (21%) were admitted to the pediatric ICU and 94 (79%) were admitted to the general medical ward [17]. Mean age was 6.4 years with 52 (44%) patients younger than 5 years. More than 70% of patients had at least one CMC, with the 3 most common being pulmonary, immunosuppression, and neurodevelopmental. The incidence of microbiologically proven coinfections and mortality rate were 6.7% and 0.8%, respectively. Comparison showed statistically that patients in the pediatric ICU had a significantly higher rate of CMCs, complications, and longer length of stay than patients admitted to the general medical ward. Minority populations also seemed to be affected disproportionately. This result may be partly related to the fact that they seemed to suffer more from underlying conditions, putting them at higher risk [18].

Review of reports published from countries in both the northern and southern hemispheres corroborated reports from across the United States that 2009 H1N1 occurred more frequently in young and middle-aged adolescents followed by older children and adolescents [19,20]. This course differs from that of seasonal influenza, which tends to affect people at the two extremes of life, namely the very young and the elderly. It is hypothesized that elderly individuals may have substantial levels of protective antibody against 2009 H1N1 due to past encounters with influenza virus with antigenic epitopes similar to the pandemic strain. Surveys of serum collected before 2009 showed that 4% of United States residents born after 1980 had preexisting neutralizing antibody titers of $\geq$40 against 2009 H1N1 whereas 34% of those born before 1950 and 57% of those born before 1940 had neutralizing antibody titers of $\geq$80 [21]. Fatal outcomes were seen at any age, however, and were more frequent in those with an underlying CMC.

Groups at risk for particularly severe infection included pregnant women as well as those with obesity. In the United States more than one-third of pregnant women with confirmed 2009 H1N1 infection had to be hospitalized because of acute respiratory distress syndrome. Pregnancy is known to increase the risk for severe influenza infection because of the physiologic changes of decreased pulmonary tidal volume and increased cardiac output. Suppressed T-helper cell-mediated immune responses also impair maternal responses to infection with several viruses. Seasonal influenza related hospitalization in healthy pregnant women occurs at a rate of 1 to 2 per 1000, a risk that is 18-fold greater than that for healthy nonpregnant women [22]. Obese individuals may also have been at increased risk related to changes in physiology as a result of altered body composition. It should also be noted that while the vast majority of cases reported in the literature were those of hospitalized patients, many cases of 2009 H1N1 influenza probably remained unrecognized in the community with a mild unrecognized respiratory illness; therefore, the true extent of the pandemic may actually be underreported.

The propensity to primarily affect children and young adults as well as its rapid spread made the 2009 H1N1 virus unique from other reassortant viruses. One theory is that the H1N1 virus binds α2,3-sialic acid receptors found on the surface of cells located deep in the lungs that seasonal influenza virus cannot bind, suggesting why people with the pandemic influenza seemed to experience more severe pulmonary symptoms [23].

The development of a vaccine against 2009 H1N1 was a top priority for public health officials globally. The threat of a possible increase in pathogenicity through further reassortment with avian or human virus strains as well as the total lack of cross-immune reactivity observed between the 2009 H1N1 and seasonal influenza virus strains (which made the 2009 seasonal vaccine ineffective against the 2009 H1N1 virus) were just two of the reasons why this became a global emergency.

Production of a pandemic influenza vaccine, however, raised several challenges, and public health officials were faced with several daunting issues as they began to make preparations for a vaccine against 2009 H1N1. These problems included ensuring that sufficient seasonal influenza vaccine would still be available before the start of seasonal influenza. This in turn required estimating with accuracy the production capacity of different producers for both seasonal and pandemic influenza vaccines. In addition, early on it was not clear whether one or two doses of pandemic vaccine would be required to induce full protection. Further, because influenza vaccines are made using eggs, it was imperative that there be a sufficient supply of healthy poultry and ultimately healthy eggs.

Influenza vaccines are licensed based on immunogenicity and not efficacy. Seasonal influenza vaccines contain 3 strains: A(H1N1), A(H3N2), and influenza B. Antibodies specific to HA are believed to be the best correlate of protection against influenza virus protection, and are the primary end point used to determine vaccine immunogenicity. The accepted correlate of protection is a hemagglutination inhibition (HI) titer of 1:40 or more (this test measures the ability of serum to compete with the binding of influenza virus to red blood cells) [24]. Influenza vaccines are made using the same reassortment process that leads to pandemic strains [25]. A virus seed strain adapted for growth in eggs using reassortment techniques is made and then serially passaged in eggs. This process gives way to the development of a high growth variant. This process clearly is extremely time consuming, depends on the egg supply, and is fraught with other technical challenges [26]. Cell culture–based vaccines may eventually be the way to overcome these issues.

Preliminary reports from a study done in Australia indicated that a single 15-μg dose of an inactivated split influenza A 2009 H1N1 vaccine induced a HI assay titer of 1:40 or more in 95% of 18- to 64-year-old healthy, nonpregnant subjects [27]. The robust immune response observed in the 18- to 49-year-old volunteer cohort was surprising. The findings suggested that there may be some cross-protection from previous exposure to antigenically drifted strains of H1N1 subtype. In addition, 2009 H1N1 shares 3 gene sequences with circulating seasonal H1N1, suggesting that there was more similarity between the 2009 H1N1 virus and the prevailing seasonal virus strains than had been recognized. Similarly, another randomized, observer-blind, age-stratified, parallel group study in 370 healthy infants aged 6 months to children under 9 years old in Australia, using 2 doses of either 15 μg HA or 30 μg HA monovalent, unadjuvanted 2009 H1N1 vaccine showed that a single 15-μg dose was immunogenic in children in this age group. No significant adverse events were reported [28].

In a United States phase 2 trial on 410 children and 724 adults who received a single dose (15 μg HA) of inactivated 2009 H1N1 vaccine, protective serologic titers of greater than 1:40 were detected at 21 days after vaccination in 45% to 50% of 6- to 35-month-old infants, 69% to 75% of 3- to 9-year-old children, 95% to 100% of 18- to 64-year-old adults, and 93% to 95% of adults older than 64 years. No vaccine-related severe adverse events were reported, but about 50% of every age and vaccine group reported injection-site and systemic reactions with no noticeable differences in the vaccine as compared with the placebo group [29]. Similarly, a multicenter, double-blind, randomized trial on 12,691 individuals 3 years of age and older in China receiving a single dose (7.5 μg HA) of a split virion 2009 H1N1 vaccine showed that protective serologic titers were detected on day 21 in 76.7% of 3- to 12-year-old children, 96.8% of 12- to 18-year-old adolescents, 89.5% of 18- to 60-year-old adults, and 80.3% of adults older than 60 years. In children, the administration of a second dose of the 7.5-μg formulation increased the seroprotection rate to 97.7%. Adverse reactions were mild to moderate [30].

Most recently another phase 2, multicenter, randomized, placebo-controlled, observer-blind, clinical trial using 2009 H1N1 vaccine in 1313 young adults (18–64 years) and older (≥65 years) conducted in 11 sites across the United States demonstrated that a single 7.5-μg dose of a monovalent, unadjuvanted 2009 H1N1 vaccine induced protective HI antibody levels in adults of all ages, including elderly adults [31]. Also, at baseline, 28.8% of young adults (18–64 years), 43.9% of younger elderly adults (65–74 years), and 62.9% of very elderly adults (≥75 years) had HI titers to 2009 H1N1 vaccine. Both older age (≥75 years) and receipt of the seasonal influenza vaccine in the previous season contributed independently to the antibody titer at baseline. Other studies in adults and children also suggest that receipt of seasonal influenza vaccine did have some cross-protection against 2009 H1N1 [32–35]. The Centers for Disease Control and Prevention (CDC) recommends immunization against both seasonal and 2009 H1N1 infection [36].

Given the safety and immunogenicity of the 2009 H1N1 vaccine in multiple trials around the world as well as the documented increased risk of complications from influenza and influenza-related illness, vaccination during pregnancy as well as in individuals with CMCs was considered high priority during the pandemic [37,38]. Vaccination of pregnant women was also seen as an effective strategy to prevent infection in infants too young to be vaccinated [39,40]. Health care workers were another group targeted for priority vaccination during the first round of immunizations. In fact, mandatory 2009 H1N1 vaccination was ordered in New York State for health care workers who had direct contact with patients or who had the potential to expose patients to the seasonal and 2009 H1N1 influenza. Ultimately this order was rescinded because of a shortage of both seasonal and 2009 H1N1 vaccine and opposition from some professional organizations. This mandatory vaccination policy raised several ethical questions and since then has come under much scrutiny [41]. Recently the American Academy of Pediatrics (AAP), the Society for Healthcare Epidemiology of America (SHEA), and the Infectious Diseases Society of America (IDSA) endorsed mandatory vaccination of health care workers to reduce the risk of infection among patients and employees [42,43]. The only exceptions would be people with medical contraindications for receipt of the vaccine. It was noted that the benefits of immunization would include prevention of disease from health care workers to patients, decrease health care workers' risk of infection, create herd immunity, prevent excessive absenteeism during outbreaks, and set an example among the general public regarding the importance of immunization. Other priority groups included individuals with an underlying cardiovascular or respiratory medical condition including asthma, autoimmune disorders, and diabetes, as well as young children.

Studies of intranasal, live-attenuated, monovalent 2009 H1N1 influenza vaccine in children and adults have also demonstrated similar safety and immunogenicity when compared with similar seasonal influenza vaccine [44].

That it is possible to induce protective antibody levels against A(H1N1) infection in adults within 2 weeks of administration of a single dose of vaccine has now been confirmed with every pandemic H1N1 vaccine tested, whether split-inactivated vaccines, or whole virion vaccines. The same one-dose schedule applies to intranasal live-attenuated influenza virus (LAIV) vaccines. The Advisory Committee on Immunization Practices (ACIP) and AAP have recommended that young children should receive a 2-dose schedule, as is the case for seasonal influenza vaccines, but immunogenicity data from the aforementioned clinical trials indicate that a single dose induces appropriate levels of immune responses.

The safety of the 2009 H1N1 vaccines continues to be thoroughly monitored. Current data show that the vaccines are well tolerated and behave just as the corresponding seasonal influenza vaccines in terms of safety and lack of severe adverse events. It is of importance that the 2009 H1N1 vaccines are manufactured in exactly the same way as the seasonal influenza vaccines and therefore are not really "new" vaccines. A small number of Guillain-Barré syndrome (GBS) cases have been reported to be temporally associated after H1N1 vaccine administration in large-scale vaccination campaigns, but they all reverted quickly [45,46]. Clinical trials are still in progress in certain at-risk subpopulations.

Vaccination against 2009 H1N1 influenza was first implemented in China, followed by a large number of countries [47]. In the United States, the Food and Drug Administration (FDA) licensed the first 2009 H1N1 vaccines on September 15, 2009 [48]. None of these vaccines contained any adjuvants. The WHO was responsible for coordinating the effort to ensure adequate supply and access to 2009 H1N1 vaccine in underresourced countries.

A total of 26 vaccine manufacturers from America, Europe, Russia, Australia, and Asia have now developed or are presently developing pandemic A(H1N1) vaccines, whether inactivated whole-virus vaccines, split inactivated vaccines, subunit vaccines, live-attenuated vaccines, or other formulations. The silver lining to this pandemic was the emergence of several new vaccine manufacturers in China, India, Thailand, and South America [49].

Despite the widespread publicity as well as education campaigns by the CDC and state and local public health officials, public attitudes toward 2009 H1N1 immunization at best remained lukewarm both in the United States and globally. Despite all the available safety data from multiple studies the public, including individuals at high risk, remained skeptical about vaccine safety [50–54]. This situation continues to highlight the need for ongoing education and public health campaigns. Immunization remains the key to the control of future disease outbreaks. Concerns over the development of resistance to antiviral medications currently used for the treatment of influenza are beyond the scope of this discussion, yet remain another important reason why prevention is so critical. One recent study suggested that any practice visits during October through January as well as evening/weekend influenza vaccine clinics seemed to improve influenza vaccine uptake in young children. This study looked at simultaneous practice and child characteristics as well as practice strategies that are associated with influenza vaccination in geographically different states [55].

Other issues that have implications for future public health policy regarding influenza immunization include school-based immunization as well as immunization within households. There are mixed data regarding transmission within households. It does not appear that 2009 H1N1 transmission was any different from seasonal influenza [56–58]. Similarly, transmission within schools also depended on several factors including rapid identification of cases, implementation of prophylaxis, and school closure in certain instances [59]. It is imperative that we consider the implications of secondary cases due to household and school contacts when formulating public health policy during future pandemics and when formulating future strategies for immunization and containment [60,61].

Seasonal influenza

In the United States, 2009 H1N1 remained the dominant circulating virus during 2009. Few seasonal influenza viral infections were reported, the most being due to influenza A/H3N2 or influenza B. Seasonal influenza A/H1N1 almost seemed to disappear. Similar trends were seen worldwide [62].

Immunization recommendations for the current influenza season include immunization of all high-risk groups previously identified for seasonal influenza immunization (Box 1) [63,64]. An algorithm for immunization in children who may or may not have received the 2009–2010 seasonal as well as 2009 H1N1 vaccine is also outlined in the policy statement by the AAP. Recommendations that are new this year include expansion of routine immunization to include adults 19 to 49 years regardless of any underlying medical condition. Vaccines available for the 2010–2011 influenza season are listed in Table 1.

While influenza vaccines generally are not licensed for use in infants younger than 6 months, an age when they are as vulnerable to complications related to influenza as the elderly, a double-blind, randomized, placebo-controlled trial conducted in 1375 healthy United States infants 6 to 12 weeks of age, receiving 2 doses of trivalent inactivated influenza vaccine 1 month apart in combination with other age-appropriate vaccines, demonstrated that at least 90% of vaccine recipients had antibody titers of 1:40 or more for at least one vaccine strain and 49.6% for 2 strains, versus 16.4% and 0.9% in placebo recipients. The investigators concluded that the vaccine was safe and immunogenic for use in infants aged 6 to 12 weeks [65].

So far in 2010, between June 13 and September 25, the United States has experienced low levels of influenza activity, and the southern hemisphere has

Box 1: AAP influenza vaccine recommendations for the 2010–2011 season

All children 6 months of age and older

Household contacts and out-of-home providers for children with high-risk conditions[a] and healthy children younger than 5 years

Health care personnel

Pregnant women

[a]These conditions include chronic systemic disorders including but not limited to asthma, diabetes mellitus, immunosuppressive disorders, those on long-term aspirin therapy, residents of long-term care facilities, certain ethnic groups (ie, American Indian, Alaskan natives), morbid obesity (body mass index 40 kg/m^2).

Table 1
Currently available influenza vaccines, 2010–2011 season

Vaccine and Manufacturer	Age Labeling and Thimerosol Content (μg mercury per 0.5 mL dose)
Afluria (inactivated) CSL Biotherapeutics Ltd	≥6 mo Not for use in children 6 mo–8 y (due to increased risk of fever and seizures) May be given in children 5–8 y if no other influenza vaccine available 25 μg mercury for multidose vial, 0 μg for prefilled syringes
Fluarix (inactivated) GSK Biologicals	≥3 y No mercury
Flulaval[a] (inactivated) ID Biomedical Corp. of Quebec	≥18 y 25 μg mercury
Flumist (live attenuated) MedImmune LLC	2–49 y No mercury
Agriflu[a] (inactivated) Novartis Vaccines and Diagnostics Inc	≥18 y 0 μg mercury (prefilled syringe)
Fluvirin (inactivated) Novartis Vaccines and Diagnostics Inc	≥4 y 25 μg mercury for multidose vial and <1 μg for prefilled syringe
Fluzone (inactivated) Sanofi Pasteur, Inc	6 mo and older New high dose licensed for ≥65 y 25 μg for 5 mL multidose vial, 0 μg for prefilled syringe

[a]Adult labeling.

experienced seasonal patterns of influenza activity and a mix of 2009 H1N1, influenza A/H3N2, and influenza B viruses cocirculated in tropical regions [66].

Adolescent immunizations

Estimated vaccination coverage among adolescents 13 to 17 years of age continued to improve during 2009 although it remains well below the Healthy People 2010 objectives [67]. Immunization coverage did vary among states, with 4 states achieving greater than 60% coverage for the 3 routine adolescent vaccines (meningococcal conjugate MenACWY, tetanus-diphtheria-acellular pertussis Tdap, and human papilloma virus HPV). During the 2009–2010 school years, on entry into middle school 27 states required Tdap, 7 required MenACWY, and 2 required HPV with opt-out provisions.

Tetanus, diphtheria, and acellular pertussis containing vaccine: Tdap

Even though immunization rates continue to increase, it is important that providers not become complacent but continue to educate their patients about the risks of vaccine-preventable diseases. The 2010 outbreak of pertussis in California, as well as the increased numbers of cases being reported in Michigan, Pennsylvania, New York, and South Carolina, continue to serve as reminders that vaccine-preventable diseases have been far from eradicated [68]. Adolescents and young adults who have not received the booster doses of Tdap continue to serve as carriers within schools, households, and the community [69,70]. A school-based immunization strategy has been used to control an outbreak in a school previously, and seems to be a logical approach when large numbers of individuals need immunization in an outbreak situation [71].

From January 1 through December 2011, 9,477 confirmed, probable and suspect cases of pertussis have been reported to the California Department of Health for a state rate of 24.2 cases/100,000 [72]; this is the highest number of cases reported since 1945. At the time of writing of this article 10 deaths have been reported, 9 of them in Hispanic infants. Nine fatalities were in infants younger than 2 months at the time of disease onset and who had not received any pertussis containing vaccine. Highest rates of diseases were seen in infants younger than 6 months, predominantly of Hispanic ethnicity. This outbreak highlights the importance of immunization for not only young children but also young adults. Household contacts including mothers of newborns have been documented as the primary source of disease for young infants [73]. The case for maternal immunization is important. Not only does it protect young infants from acquiring disease, but transplacental acquisition of maternal antibody is also the mainstay of protection for young infants until they are old enough to be immunized themselves [74]. Current recommendations in the United States call for immunization of mothers not previously immunized to be given Tdap vaccination as soon as possible in the postpartum period and before discharge from the hospital [75].

Following the California outbreak, the ACIP voted to recommend the "off-label" use of Tdap in two patient groups to try to capture those who might be at risk of passing disease to young infants. The first group is children 7 to 9 years who may not have completed the primary childhood series, and the second group is adults aged 65 and older who have contact with young infants. A dose of Tdap may also be given to people in this age group who have not previously received the vaccine [76]. California also issued expanded pertussis immunization recommendations to include immunization of the two groups as recommended by the ACIP in addition to immunization of pregnant women during or after pregnancy, as well as immunization of individuals who had contact with pregnant women or infants.

Meningococcal vaccines

The first tetravalent conjugate meningococcal vaccine (Menactra, MCV4; Sanofi Pasteur, Swiftwater, PA, USA) was approved for use in adolescents 11 through 55 years of age in 2005 [77]. Since then a second conjugate meningococcal vaccine (Menveo, MenACWY-CRM; Novartis Vaccines and Diagnostics, Sovicille, Italy) was licensed by the FDA on February 10, 2010 [78]. The two vaccines contain serogroups A/C/Y/W 135. The vaccines differ in the carrier to which the meningococcal polysaccharide capsule is conjugated:

MenACWY-diphtheria CRM 197 and MCV4-diphtheria toxoids. MCV4 is approved for use for ages 2 through 55 years whereas MenACWY-CRM is approved for ages 11 through 55 years. Neither vaccine provides protection against serogroup B disease.

A recently published study looked to determine the immunogenicity and safety of MenACWY-CRM compared with MCV4 in 2- to 10-year-olds. A total of 2907 children were divided in to two groups (2–5 years and 6–10 years) and were randomized to receive a single dose of MenACWY-CRM or MCV4. Seroresponse to MenACWY-CRM showed statistical superiority for groups W and Y and was noninferior for group C in both groups. For group A, noninferiority criteria were not met. When the two age groups were combined, MenACWY-CRM was noninferior to MCV4 for all 4 serogroups and statistically superior for groups C/W/Y. There was no difference in safety parameters for both vaccines across both age groups [79]. Licensure for MenACWY-CRM for the 2- to 10-year-old age group is pending FDA licensure. Of the two licensed vaccines Menveo (MenACWY-CRM) is the only one that is Halal certified, and should be given to all Muslims needing meningococcal vaccine especially before embarking on the annual Haj pilgrimage to Makkah.

Prelicensure studies did not show an increase in cases of GBS with either vaccine. Initial postmarketing studies suggested a temporal association and a potential increased risk for GBS with the use of MCV4; however, ongoing studies have not been able to confirm a causal relationship, therefore either meningococcal vaccine may be used when meningococcal immunization is indicated. A history of GBS is a precaution to administration of MCV4 [80].

During the October 2010 meeting, the ACIP recommended changes for meningococcal vaccination as well. For children in high-risk groups it was already recommended that they receive MCV4 at age 2 years; now they would receive a booster 3 to 5 years following the initial immunization. The committee also voted to recommend a booster dose for adolescents at age 16 if they received the first dose at the 11- to 12-year visit. For those who received the immunization at ages 13 to 15, the booster dose would be 5 years after the initial immunization [81]. The basis for these recommendations is increasing evidence that levels of protective antibody decline with time since vaccination; invasive disease develops rapidly, therefore immune memory alone cannot be relied on for protection, and one cannot rely on herd immunity for protection of adolescents [82].

The quadrivalent meningococcal polysaccharide vaccine (MPSV4) remains available for use in children older than 2 years and older individuals at high risk for meningococcal disease. Periodic case reports have also linked MPSV4 to the development of Henoch-Schönlein purpura (HSP). A recent review of the Vaccine Safety Datalink cohort did not show any association of HSP with the vaccine in the 16- to 20-year age cohort [83]. No cases were seen in the 42 days following MPSV4 after 42,027 doses.

While there are several candidate meningococcal serogroup B vaccines in development, none has been licensed for routine clinical use as yet. Given that this is a significant cause of meningitis and septicemia in many industrialized countries, this remains a challenge. Issues faced in the development of a suitable vaccine are mainly that the polysaccharide capsule of serogroup B, being a homopolymer of α2-8 linked sialic acid, contains epitopes that are cross-reactive with the polysialylated form of the neural cell adhesion molecule. Because this is expressed by several host tissues, it is a poor immunogen even when conjugated to a carrier protein, and any anticapsular antibodies elicited have the potential to cross-react with host antigens and contribute to autoimmune disease. Efforts have therefore focused on using noncapsular antigens; however, the difficulty has been to find surface-exposed noncapsular antigens that are safe, antigenically conserved, and can elicit serum bactericidal antibodies. Various technologies using outer membrane vesicles (OMV) from the meningococcus as well as recombinant proteins alone or in combination with OMV are being used for different candidate vaccines in development [84]. An investigational recombinant vaccine that contains 3 central neisserial proteins with and without OMV from the New Zealand epidemic strain is currently in phase 2 and phase 3 clinical trials in young infants [85,86].

Human papilloma virus vaccines

The second HPV vaccine (HPV2) (Cervarix; GlaxoSmithKline Biologicals, Rixensart, Belgium) was licensed by the FDA on October 16, 2009 [87]. This bivalent vaccine contains types 16 and 18, and is indicated for the prevention of cervical cancer, cervical intraepithelial neoplasia (CIN) grade 2 or worse, adenocarcinoma in situ, and CIN grade 1 caused by HPV types 16 and 18 in females aged 10 through 25 years. Prior to this a quadrivalent HPV vaccine (HPV4 contains types 6/11/16/18) (Gardasil; Merck & Co. Inc, West Point, PA, USA) was licensed in June 2006. Like HPV4, HPV2 is composed of noninfectious, recombinant, virus-like particles (VLP) [88]. The VLP are composed of the viral L1 protein, which is the major capsid protein of the virus and has been shown to elicit strong systemic immune responses, eliciting antibodies that are highly effective in preventing native viral particles from entering epithelial cells and causing infection. Both vaccines can be given as early as 9 years of age. Catch-up vaccination is recommended for females 13 through 26 years old who have not been previously vaccinated, and the series can be completed if the female turns 26 before the series is complete [89].

Given the fact that HPV infections are most often sexually transmitted, that there are approximately 500,000 cases per year of genital warts in the United States in sexually active men and women, 90% being caused by types 6 and 11, that there are 600,000 cases of cancer caused by HPV annually in the United States, the majority being cervical, vaginal, and vulvar cancers in women (70% of cervical cancers are caused by types 16 and 18), and that HPV-associated cancers in men are caused primarily by type 16, it made sense to consider HPV vaccination for men as well. On October 16, 2010 the FDA licensed HPV4 for use in men aged 9 through 26 years old for prevention of HPV 6/11/16/18-related outcomes (genital warts and cancer). Following licensure, the ACIP issued a *permissive* recommendation that the quadrivalent vaccine may be given to males 9 through 26 years of age to reduce their likelihood of acquiring genital cancers [90]. In a permissive recommendation the ACIP states that administering the vaccine may be beneficial but that it is not an affirmative recommendation. The vaccine is available through the Vaccines for Children (VFC) Program, and VFC providers are required to administer the vaccine if requested by a VFC-eligible patient. Mathematical modeling suggests that adding male HPV vaccination to a female-only HPV vaccination program is not the most cost-effective immunization strategy for reducing HPV-related disease when immunization coverage for females is high (>80%). It may be more beneficial when female immunization rates are less than 80% [91].

Several barriers to HPV immunization leading to suboptimal immunization rates have been identified, Some of these are common to all adolescent vaccines; that is, the fact that adolescents do not visit the doctor as frequently as young children has decreased parental as well as public awareness about adolescent vaccines as opposed to routine childhood vaccines, as well as less acceptance of minor vaccine-related side effects such as injection-site soreness. There have also been specific parental concerns about HPV vaccine. Some parents have been reluctant to have their children vaccinated, fearing it will create a false sense of security about engaging in sexual activity. There has also been some stigma associated with HPV vaccine for similar reasons. Both provider and parental as well as patient education will go a long way toward dispelling some of these fears, therefore ongoing education remains crucial [92–94]. Acceptance and knowledge about HPV vaccine among male patients is also varied [95].

Routine HPV immunization for 12-year-old girls was introduced in the United Kingdom in 2008 and has had uptake rates between 80% and 90% [96]. In the United States the vaccine was recommended for use by the ACIP in 2006, shortly after licensure; however, in 2009 estimated vaccine coverage in 13- to 17-year-old girls for one dose of the vaccine was 44% and only 27% for 3 doses [67]. These rates are an improvement over the 2008 numbers, but still far below what is being reported in the United Kingdom. A recently published survey of physicians nationwide showed that while nearly all physicians surveyed started using the quadrivalent vaccine shortly after licensure, physician recommendation for older adolescents (19–26 years) was greater than for younger adolescents (11–12 years). Parents of younger adolescents also seemed more reluctant to vaccinate their girls [97]. Reasons for refusal have been mentioned in the previous section. Financial concerns were also perceived as a barrier to vaccination.

Apart from routinely administered vaccines recommended at the 11- to 12-year visit, physicians should also ensure that adolescents are current with other vaccines including hepatitis A and varicella, because recommendations for immunization for these vaccines have changed over the last several years, and include inclusion in the routine immunization schedule as well as addition of a second booster dose for varicella vaccine.

PEDIATRIC VACCINES

Pneumococcal conjugate vaccines

Introduction of 7-valent pneumococcal conjugate vaccine (PCV7) to the primary childhood immunization schedule in 2000 resulted in a significant reduction in invasive pneumococcal diseases in children as well as adults. A decrease in pneumococcal infections in unvaccinated children and adults due to indirect effects (herd immunity) was also seen, in addition a decline in diseases due to antibiotic resistant serotypes [98–103]. However, increase in invasive disease due to replacement serotypes was seen, particularly serotype 19A [104]. On February 24, 2010 the FDA licensed the 13-valent pneumococcal conjugate vaccine for use in place of the 7-valent vaccine [105]. This 13-valent vaccine (Prevnar 13; Wyeth Pharmaceuticals Inc, Philadelphia, PA, USA) contains serotypes 1/3/4/5/6A/6B/7F/9V/14/18C/19A/19F/23F. It is licensed for the prevention of invasive serotypes mentioned as well as for the prevention of otitis media caused by serotypes 4/6B/9V/14/18C/19F/23F in children 6 weeks through 5 years of age. Following licensure, the ACIP issued recommendations for use of PCV13 to include routine immunization of all children aged 2 to 59 months, vaccination of children 60 to 71 months with underlying medical conditions placing them at increased risk for invasive pneumococcal disease, and for those children who have previously received one or more doses of PCV7. For children 14 to 59 months who have received 4 or more doses of PCV7, a single supplemental dose is recommended. In addition, a single dose of PCV13 is also recommended for children younger than 71 months with underlying medical conditions, including children who have previously received 23-valent pneumococcal polysaccharide vaccine (PPSV23). PCV13 should be given after an interval of 8 weeks following PCV7 or PPSV23 [106]. Prelicensure studies demonstrated that the safety and immunogenicity of PCV13 were comparable with those of PCV7. The AAP has issued guidelines for the use of PCV13 and recommends replacement of PCV7 with PCV13 [107]. While it is beyond the scope of this review, the ACIP has also issued updated recommendations for the use of PPSV23 in adults [108]. Postlicensure surveillance data in the coming years will hopefully demonstrate changes in the epidemiology of pneumococcal isolates in children as well as adults. The effect on hospitalization due to invasive disease as well as usage of antibiotics in pediatric practices is also expected as we continue to see the anticipated decline in pneumococcal disease.

Rotavirus vaccines

On April 3, 2008, the second rotavirus vaccine was licensed in the United States (Rotarix; GlaxoSmith Kline, Rixensart, Belgium) [109]. Several studies have demonstrated the effectiveness and safety of both rotavirus vaccines since licensure [110–114]. In March 2010, the FDA recommended suspension of Rotarix after it was learnt that the vaccine contained DNA from porcine circovirus 1. Later it was discovered that Rotateq also has small quantities of porcine circovirus 2. However, these viruses cannot be grown in human cell lines and do not infect or cause disease in humans. Later in May 2010 the FDA recommended that use of Rotarix resume and Rotateq continue, because the risk of using these vaccines did not outweigh their benefits [115]. There is no question that these two vaccines have been extensively studied for safety and efficacy, and the AAP considers both vaccines to be equivalent. The FDA did, however, add the use of both rotavirus vaccines as a contraindication to the package insert following reports to the Vaccine Adverse Event Reporting System regarding the development of vaccine-associated diarrhea and prolonged virus shedding in 5 infants with severe combined immunodeficiency. Live-attenuated vaccines are contraindicated in the setting of severe immunodeficiency states involving cellular immunity [116]. Postmarketing surveillance data from Mexico showed a possible increased risk of intussusception of about 1.8-fold in the 30-day period following the first dose of Rotarix, with a clustering of cases in the first week after vaccination. Similar studies from Australia reported an increase in intussusception cases in the first week after vaccination with both rotavirus vaccines [117]. These findings are based on a small number of cases and have all been reported outside the United States. Based on these data, 1 case of intussusception per approximately 100,000 doses of rotavirus vaccine would occur in infants vaccinated according to age-appropriate recommendations. Following these reports, the ACIP recommends that while a small risk of intussusception is possible, given the benefit of rotavirus vaccines immunization with both rotavirus vaccines for prevention of severe rotavirus disease in United States infants and children should continue as recommended. The FDA advised a labeling change for Rotarix to inform health care providers about the potential risk of intussusception. Postmarketing surveillance studies for both rotavirus vaccines are ongoing.

OTHER CHILDHOOD COMBINATION VACCINES ON THE HORIZON

Combined *haemophilus influenzae* type B-*neisseria meningitidis* serogroups C and Y-tetanus toxoid conjugate vaccine

Given the large number of vaccines that are now part of the routine immunization schedule, combination vaccines have become increasingly popular. A new conjugate, combined *Haemophilus influenzae* type B (Hib)-*Neisseria meningitidis* Serogroups C and Y (MenCY)-Tetanus Toxoid (TT) vaccine (HibMenCY-TT), is on the horizon, currently awaiting FDA review. So far this vaccine has shown noninferiority compared with monovalent MenC and Hib conjugate vaccines, with a comparable safety profile. Bactericidal antibodies against MenC/Y were induced after 2 doses of HibMenCY-TT [118,119].

In the United States, Tdap-inactivated polio vaccine (IPV)/Hib and Tdap-IPV combination vaccines have been available since 2008. Combination vaccines containing Hib were recommended for use by the CDC in 2008 following the Hib vaccine shortage in 2008 and the death of 5 children due to invasive Hib disease in Minnesota [120]. Combination vaccines available in other countries but not licensed in the United States include Tdap-HBV-IPV/Hib. This vaccine is currently being evaluated in 2-, 4-, and 6-month-old infants in Canada for safety and immunogenicity [121].

Changes in recommendations for vaccines used in special circumstances

Given the increasing number of international adoptions over the last several years in the United States, readers are reminded that immunization schedules vary widely depending on the country of origin of the adoptee. In addition, vaccine-induced immunity may vary depending on several factors, therefore all internationally adopted children should be evaluated carefully once in the United States. As an example, a recently published study looking at hepatitis A virus (HAV) immunity at an international adoption clinic showed that prevalence of immunity to HAV was lowest in children born in the Asia/Pacific Rim (17%) and highest in children born in Africa (72%) [122]. Young children may also remain asymptomatic with acute infection and have prolonged shedding, placing their new families and close contacts at risk for infection. All international adoptees should therefore have a thorough evaluation of their immunization status within a few weeks on arrival in the United States [123].

Readers are also reminded that despite immunization recommendations, several parents either refuse or alter the routine schedule, preferring to give vaccines in a "staggered" fashion for. Concerns about vaccine safety, religious beliefs, and the parents' belief that their child may not be at risk are just some reasons a child may not have received all age-appropriate vaccines. Physicians should inquire about specific immunization history in any child presenting for evaluation of fever following travel or if visiting from another country. The authors recently dealt with a case of severe varicella infection in a child traveling to the United States from the United Kingdom who had not been immunized. This child was initially admitted to the general pediatric floor with fever. Accurate knowledge of a child's immunization status in such cases will aid in timely diagnosis, avoid unnecessary testing, and also be invaluable for infection control purposes if such children require hospitalization.

INTERNATIONAL VACCINE NEWS

Eradication of poliomyelitis still remains elusive, as cases of polio continue to occur in endemic countries (Pakistan, India, Afghanistan, and Nigeria) as well as in countries that have reestablished transmission (Angola, Chad, Republic of Congo) and in 13 other countries mainly in Africa, central Asia, and the former Soviet Republics with importation of the virus. Despite continuous setbacks, global poliomyelitis eradication efforts continue. It is estimated that the economic benefits of polio eradication will be approximately US$40 to 50 billion [124]. The global alliance for vaccines and immunization (GAVI), a private-public partnership supported by country and donor agreements, WHO, UNICEF, the World Bank, the global pharmaceutical industry, the Bill and Melinda gates Foundation, as well as private philanthropists, continues to provide vital support to developing countries in their efforts to support and sustain critically needed immunization programs in their respective countries.

For example, in GAVI-supported countries, immunization coverage rates for diphtheria-tetanus-pertussis, hepatitis B, and Hib disease have gone from 60%/20%/0% in 2000 to 80%/ just under 60%/30%, respectively. Funding support for pneumococcal and rotavirus vaccines has also been provided, and efforts are ongoing to extend support to more countries to implement immunization programs for these diseases. Plans are also in place to provide future support for immunization programs for HPV vaccines, HAV, Japanese encephalitis, meningitis A, rubella, and typhoid [125].

As of November 2009, 130 of 193 WHO member states have introduced rubella-containing vaccine into their national immunization schedules. It is interesting that while two-thirds of WHO member states have incorporated rubella vaccine into their programs, these member states only represent less than half of the global birth cohort [126].

SUMMARY

Childhood immunization rates are one of the leading indicators of a nation's health. As more vaccines are added to the growing list of requirements for children, adolescents, and adults, it is imperative that clinicians keep abreast of continuous changes and updates in immunization recommendations based on ongoing evidence-based research and science. It is also crucial that we keep ourselves abreast of issues that may affect immunization delivery such as vaccine acquisition costs, reimbursement, disruptions in vaccine supply, and safety concerns both real and perceived by the public. Health care providers must continually strive to improve the health of their communities, and the one sure way to accomplish this is by improving immunization rates in our communities and educating ourselves, our patients, and their families.

References

[1] CDC. Swine influenza A (H1N1) infection in two children—Southern California, March-April 2009. MMWR Morb Mortal Wkly Rep 2009;58(15):400–2.
[2] CDC. Outbreak of swine-origin influenza A (H1N1) virus infection—Mexico, March-April 2009. MMWR Morb Mortal Wkly Rep 2009;58(17):467–70.
[3] Gatherer D. The 2009 H1N1 influenza outbreak in its historical context. J Clin Virol 2009;45(3):174–8.
[4] Zimmer SM, Burke DS. Historical perspective-emergence of influenza A (H1N1) viruses. N Engl J Med 2009;361(3):279–85.
[5] Novel swine-origin influenza A (H1N1) virus investigation team. Emergence of a novel swine-origin influenza A (H1N1) virus in humans. N Engl J Med 2010;360(25):2605–15.
[6] Farley MM. 2009 H1N1 influenza: a twenty-first century pandemic with roots in the early twentieth century. Am J Med Sci 2010;340(3):202–8.
[7] Taubenberger JK, Reid AH, Lourens RM, et al. Characterization of the 1918 influenza virus polymerase genes. Nature 2005;437(7060):889–93.
[8] Garten RJ, Davis CT, Russell CA, et al. Antigenic and genetic characteristics of swine-origin 2009 A(H1N1) influenza viruses circulating in humans. Science 2009;325(5937):197–201.
[9] Acute Respiratory Infections. The A/2009 H1N1 influenza virus pandemic (update September 2009) Available at: http://www.who.int/vaccine_research/diseases/ari/en/index5.html. Accessed November 8, 2010.

[10] Johnson NP, Mueller J. Updating the accounts: global mortality of the 1918–1920 ''Spanish'' influenza pandemic. Bull Hist Med 2002;76(1):105–15.
[11] Cao B, Li XW, Mao Y, et al. Clinical features of the initial cases of 2009 pandemic influenza A (H1N1) virus infection in China. N Engl J Med 2009;361(26):2507–17.
[12] Jain R, Goldman RD. Novel influenza A (H1N1): clinical presentation, diagnosis and management. Pediatr Emerg Care 2009;25(11):791–6.
[13] Hain S, Kamimoto L, Bramley AM, et al. Hospitalized patients with 2009 H1N1 influenza in the United States, April-June 2009. N Engl J Med 2009;361(20):1935–44.
[14] Updated CDC estimates of 2009 H1N1 influenza cases, hospitalizations and deaths in the United States. April 2009-April 10, 2010. Available at. http://www.cdc.gov/h1n1flu/estimates_2009_h1n1.htm. Accessed November 22, 2010.
[15] Louie JK, Gavali S, Acosta M, et al. (California Pandemic (H1N1) working group). Children hospitalized with 2009 novel influenza A(H1N1) in California. Arch Pediatr Adolesc Med 2010;164(11):1023–31.
[16] Kumar S, Havens PL, Chusid MJ. Clinical and epidemiologic characteristics of children hospitalized with 2009 pandemic H1N1 influenza A infection. Pediatr Infect Dis J 2010;29(7):591–4.
[17] Custodio H, Carmen M, Bailey C, et al. Hospitalized children infected with the novel H1N1 (nH1N1) influenza: comparison of the ICU to non-ICU patients. Poster presentation, Infectious Diseases Society of America Annual Meeting. Vancouver British Columbia (Canada); October 21–24, 2010.
[18] Chitnis AS, Truelove SA, Druckenmiller JK. Epidemiologic and clinical features among patients hospitalized in Wisconsin with 2009 H1N1 influenza A virus infections, April to August 2009. WMJ 2010;109(4):201–8.
[19] Falagus ME, Koletsi PK, Baskouta E, et al. Pandemic A (H1N1) 2009 influenza; a review of the southern hemisphere experience. Epidemiol Infect 2011;139(1):27–40.
[20] Falagas ME, Chovelas NV, Kapaskelis AM, et al. Epidemiological aspects of 2009 H1N1 influenza: the accumulating experience from the northern hemisphere. Eur J Clin Microbiol Infect Dis 2010;29(11):1327–47.
[21] Hancock K, Veguilla V, Lu X, et al. Cross reactive antibody responses to the 2009 pandemic H1N1 influenza virus. N Engl J Med 2009;361(20):1945–52.
[22] Mak TK, Mangtani P, Leese J, et al. Influenza vaccination in pregnancy: current evidence and selected national policies. Lancet Infect Dis 2008;8(1):44–52.
[23] Childs RA, Palma AS, Wharton S, et al. Receptor-binding specificity of pandemic influenza A (H1N1) 2009 virus determined by carbohydrate microarray. Nat Biotechnol 2009;27(9):797–9.
[24] Plotkin SA. Correlates of protection induced by vaccination. Clin Vaccine Immunol 2010;17(7):1055–65.
[25] Treanor J. Influenza vaccine-outmaneuvering antigenic shift and drift. N Engl J Med 2004;350(3):218–20.
[26] Neuzil KM, Bright RA. Influenza vaccine manufacture: keeping up with the change. J Infect Dis 2009;200(6):835–7.
[27] Greenburg ME, Lai MH, Hartel GF, et al. Response to a monovalent 2009 influenza A (H1N1) vaccine. N Engl J Med 2009;361(25):2405–13.
[28] Nolan T, McVernon J, Skeljo M, et al. Immunogenicity of a monovalent 2009 influenza A(H1N1) in infants and children: a randomized trial. JAMA 2010;303(1): 37–46.
[29] Plennevaux E, Sheldon E, Blatter M, et al. Immune response after a single vaccination against 2009 influenza A H1N1 in the USA: a preliminary report of two randomized controlled phase 2 trials. Lancet 2010;375(9708):41–8.
[30] Liang XF, Wang HQ, Wang JZ, et al. Safety and immunogenicity of 2009 pandemic influenza A H1N1 vaccines in China: a multi-center, double-blind, randomized, placebo-controlled trial. Lancet 2010;375(9708):56–66.

[31] Talaat KR, Greenburg ME, Lai MH. A single dose of unadjuvanted novel 2009H1N1 vaccine is immunogenic and well tolerated in young and elderly adults. J Infect Dis 2010;202(9):1327–37.
[32] Garcia-Garcia L, Valdespino-Gómez JL, Lazcano-Ponce E, et al. Partial protection of seasonal trivalent inactivated vaccine against novel pandemic influenza A/H1N1 2009: case control study in Mexico City. BMJ 2009;339:b3928.
[33] Cowling BJ, Ng S, Ma ES, et al. Protective efficacy of seasonal influenza vaccination against seasonal and pandemic influenza virus infection during 2009 in Hong Kong. Clin Infect Dis 2010;51(12):1370–9.
[34] Subbramanian RA, Basha S, Shata MT, et al. Pandemic and seasonal H1N1 influenza haemagglutinin-specific T cell responses elicited by seasonal influenza vaccination. Vaccine 2010;28(52):8258–67.
[35] Marcelin G, Bland HM, Negovetich NJ, et al. Inactivated seasonal influenza vaccines increase serum antibodies to the neuraminidase of pandemic influenza A (H1N1)2009 virus in an age-dependant manner. J Infect Dis 2010;202(11):1634–8.
[36] Centers for Disease Control and Prevention. Effectiveness of 2008–2009 trivalent influenza against 2009 pandemic influenza A (H1N1)—United States, May-June 2009. MMWR Morb Mortal Wkly Rep 2009;58(44):1241–5.
[37] Lim SH, Lee JH, Kim BC. Adverse reaction of influenza A (H1N1) 2009 virus vaccination in pregnant women and its effect on newborns. Vaccine 2010;28(47):7455–6.
[38] Centers for Disease Control and Prevention. Surveillance for pediatric deaths associated with 2009 pandemic influenza A (H1N1) virus infection-United States, April-August 2009. MMWR Morb Mortal Wkly Rep 2009;58(34):941–7.
[39] Schlaudecker EP, Steinhoff MC. Helping mothers prevent influenza illness in their infants. Pediatrics 2010;126(5):1008–11.
[40] Eick AA, Uyeki TM, Klimov A, et al. Maternal influenza vaccination and effect on influenza virus infection in young infants. Arch Pediatr Adolesc Med 2011;165(2): 104–1110.1001/archpediatrics.2010.192.
[41] Stewart AM. Mandatory vaccination of health care workers. N Engl J Med 2009;361(21): 2015–7.
[42] AAP COID. Policy statement—recommendation for mandatory influenza immunization of all health care personnel. Pediatrics 2010;126(4):809–15.
[43] Talbot TR, Babcock H, Caplan AL, et al. Revised SHEA position paper: influenza vaccination of healthcare personnel. Infect Control Hosp Epidemiol 2010;31(10): 987–95.
[44] Mallory RM, Malkin E, Ambrose CS, et al. Safety and immunogenicity following administration of a live attenuated monovalent 2009 H1N1 influenza vaccine to children and adults in two randomized controlled trials. PLoS One 2010;5(10):e13755.
[45] Vellozi C, Broder KR, Haber P, et al. Adverse events following influenza A (H1N1) 2009 monovalent vaccines reported to the Vaccine Adverse Event Reporting System, United States, October 1, 2009-January 31, 2010. Vaccine 2010;28(45):7248–55.
[46] Centers for Disease Control and Prevention. Preliminary results: surveillance for Guillain-Barre syndrome after receipt of influenza A (H1N1) 2009 monovalent vaccine-United States 2009-2010. MMWR Morb Mortal Wkly Rep 2010;59(21):657–61.
[47] Stone R. Swine flu outbreak. China first to vaccinate against novel H1N1 virus. Science 2009;325(5947):1482–3.
[48] FDA 2009 H1N1 vaccine questions and answers. Available at: http://www.fda.gov/BiologicsBloodVaccines/Vaccines/QuestionsaboutVaccines/ucm182335.htm. Accessed November 25, 2010.
[49] Girard MP, Tam JS, Assossou OM, et al. The 2009 A (H1N1) influenza virus pandemic: a review. Vaccine 2010;28(31):4895–905.
[50] Hilton S, Smith E. Public views of the UK media and government reaction to the 2009 swine flu pandemic. BMC Public Health 2010;10(1):697.

[51] Bone A, Guthman JP, Nicolau J, et al. Population and risk group uptake of H1N1 influenza vaccine in mainland France 2009–2010: results of a national vaccination campaign. Vaccine 2010;28(51):8157–61.
[52] White SW, Peterson RW, Quinlivan JA. Pandemic (H1N1) 2009 influenza vaccine uptake in pregnant women entering the 2010 influenza season in Western Australia. Med J Aust 2010;193(7):405–7.
[53] Savas E, Tanriverdi D. Knowledge, attitudes and anxiety toward influenza A/H1N1 vaccination of healthcare workers in Turkey. BMC Infect Dis 2010;10:281.
[54] Maurer J, Uscher-Pines L, Harris KM. Perceived seriousness of seasonal and A(H1N1) influenzas, attitude toward vaccination and vaccine uptake among US adults: does the source of information matter? Prev Med 2010;51(2):185–7.
[55] Poehling KA, Fairbrother G, Zhu Y, et al. Practice and child characteristics associated with influenza vaccine uptake in young children. Pediatrics 2010;126(4):665–73.
[56] Papenburg J, Baz M, Hamelin ME, et al. Household transmission of the 2009 pandemic A/H1N1 influenza virus: elevated laboratory-confirmed secondary attack rates and evidence of asymptomatic infections. Clin Infect Dis 2010;51(9):1033–41.
[57] Cauchemez S, Donnelly CA, Reed C, et al. Household transmission of 2009 pandemic influenza A (H1N1) virus in the United States. N Engl J Med 2009;361(27):2619–27.
[58] Cowling BJ, Chan KH, Fang VJ, et al. Comparative epidemiology of pandemic and seasonal influenza A in households. N Engl J Med 2010;362(23):2175–84.
[59] Calatayud L, Kurkela S, Neave PE, et al. Pandemic (H1N1) 2009 virus outbreak in a school in London, April-May 2009: an observational study. Epidemiol Infect 2010;138(2): 183–91.
[60] France AM, Jackson M, Schrag S, et al. Household transmission of 2009 influenza A (H1N1) virus after a school based outbreak In New York City, April-May 2009. J Infect Dis 2010;201(7):984–92.
[61] Cauchemez S, Ferguson NM, Wachtel C, et al. Closure of schools during an influenza pandemic. Lancet Infect Dis 2009;9(8):473–81.
[62] Centers for Disease Control and Prevention. Update: influenza activity—United States 2009-10 season. MMWR Morb Mortal Wkly Rep 2010;59(29):901–8.
[63] Fiore AE, Uyeki TM, Broder K, et al. Prevention and control of influenza with vaccines: recommendations of the Advisory Committee on Immunization Practices (ACIP), 2010. MMWR Recomm Rep 2010;59(RR-8):1–62.
[64] AAP COID. Policy statement—recommendations for prevention and control of influenza in children, 2010-2011. Pediatrics 2010;126(4):816–26.
[65] Englund JA, Walter E, Black S. Safety and immunogenicity of trivalent and inactivated influenza vaccine in infants: a randomized, double-blind, placebo-controlled study. Pediatr Infect Dis J 2010;29(2):105–10.
[66] Centers for Disease Control and Prevention. Influenza activity—United States and worldwide, June 13-September 25, 2010. MMWR Morb Mortal Wkly Rep 2010;59(39): 1270–3.
[67] Centers for Disease Control and Prevention. National, state and local area vaccination coverage among adolescents aged 13–17 years—United States, 2009. MMWR Morb Mortal Wkly Rep 2010;59(32):1018–23.
[68] Roehr B. Whooping cough outbreak hits several US states. BMJ 2010;341:c4627.
[69] Baptista PN, Magalhães VS, Rodrigues LC. The role of adults in household outbreaks of pertussis. Int J Infect Dis 2010;14(2):e111–4.
[70] Berger F, Njamkepo E, Minaberry S, et al. Investigation on a pertussis outbreak in a military school: risk factors and approach to vaccine efficacy. Vaccine 2010;28(32): 5147–52.
[71] Centers for Disease Control and Prevention. Use of mass Tdap vaccination to control an outbreak of pertussis in a high school—Cook County, Illinois, September 2006-January 2007. MMWR Morb Mortal Wkly Rep 2008;57(29):796–9.

[72] Pertussis Report. California Department of Health. Available at: http://www.cdph.ca.gov/programs/immunize/Documents/PertussisReport2011-03-09.pdf. Accessed April 13, 2011.
[73] Bisgard KM, Pascual FB, Ehresmann KR, et al. Infant pertussis: who was the source? Pediatr Infect Dis J 2004;23(11):985–9.
[74] Mooi FR, de Greef SC. The case for maternal vaccination against pertussis. Lancet Infect Dis 2007;7(9):614–24.
[75] Murphy TV, Slade BA, Border KR, et al. Prevention of pertussis, tetanus and diphtheria among pregnant and post partum women and their infants: recommendations of the Advisory Committee on Immunization Practices. MMWR Recomm Rep 2008;57(RR-4):1–51.
[76] Centers for Disease Control and Prevention. ACIP Presentation slides: October 2010 meeting. Available at: http://www.cdc.gov/vaccines/recs/acip/slides-oct10.htm#pertussis. Accessed November 25, 2010.
[77] FDA Approval Letter-Menactra. Available at: http://www.fda.gov/BiologicsBloodVaccines/Vaccines/ApprovedProducts/ucm131181.htm. Accessed November 25, 2010.
[78] FDA Approval Letter-Menveo. Available at: http://www.fda.gov/BiologicsBlood Vaccines/Vaccines/ApprovedProducts/ucm201343.htm. Accessed November 25, 2010.
[79] Halperin SA, Gupta A, Jeanfreau R, et al. Comparison of the safety and immunogenicity of an investigational and a licensed quadrivalent meningococcal conjugate vaccine in children 2–10 years of age. Vaccine 2010;28(50):7865–72.
[80] Centers for Disease Control and prevention. Revised recommendations of the Advisory Committee on Immunization Practices to vaccinate all persons aged 11–18 years with meningococcal conjugate vaccine. MMWR Morb Mortal Wkly Rep 2007;56:794–5.
[81] Centers for Disease Control and Prevention. ACIP Presentation Slides October 2010. Available at: http://www.cdc.gov/vaccines/recs/acip/downloads/mtg-slides-oct10/02-5-mening-mcv4.pdf. Accessed November 25, 2010.
[82] Centers for Disease Control and Prevention. Revised Recommendations from the Advisory Committee on Immunization Practices (ACIP) for revaccination of persons at prolonged increased risk for meningococcal disease. MMWR Morb Mortal Wkly Rep 2010;58(37):1042–3.
[83] Goodman MJ, Nordin JD, Belongia EA. Henoch-Schonlein purpura and polysaccharide meningococcal vaccine. Pediatrics 2010;126(2):e325–9.
[84] Granoff DM. Review of meningococcal group B vaccines. Clin Infect Dis 2010;50(S2):S54–65.
[85] Findlow J, Borrow R, Snape MD, et al. Multicenter, open-label, randomized phase II controlled trial of an investigational recombinant Meningococcal serogroup B vaccine with and without outer membrane vesicles, administered in infancy. Clin Infect Dis 2010;51(10):1127–37.
[86] Snape MD, Dawson T, Oster P, et al. Immunogenicity of two investigational serogroup B meningococcal vaccines in the first year of life: a randomized comparative trial. Pediatr Infect Dis J 2010;29(11):e71–9.
[87] FDA Approval Letter-Cervarix. Available at: http://www.fda.gov/BiologicsBloodVaccines/Vaccines/ApprovedProducts/ucm186959.htm. Accessed November 27, 2010.
[88] Cutts FT, Franceschi S, Goldie S, et al. Human papillomavirus and HPV vaccines: a review. Bull World Health Organ 2007;85(9):719–26.
[89] Centers for Diseases Control and Prevention. FDA licensure of bivalent human papillomavirus (HPV2, Cervarix) for use in females and updated HPV vaccination recommendations from the Advisory Committee on Immunization Practices. MMWR Morb Mortal Wkly Rep 2010;59(20):626–9.
[90] Centers for Disease Control and Prevention. FDA licensure of quadrivalent human papillomavirus vaccine (HPV4, Gardasil) for use in males and guidance from the Advisory Committee on Immunization Practices. MMWR Morb Mortal Wkly Rep 2010;59(20):630–2.

[91] Brisson M, Van de Velde N, Boily MC. Economic evaluation of human papillomavirus vaccination in developed countries. Public Health Genomics 2009;12:343–51.
[92] Brewer NT, Fazekas KI. Predictors of HPV vaccine acceptability: a theory-informed systematic review. Prev Med 2007;45(2–3):107–14.
[93] Allen JD, Othus MK, Shelton RC. Parental decision making about HPV vaccine. Cancer Epidemiol Biomarkers Prev 2010;19(9):2187–98.
[94] Zimet GD, Weiss TW, Rosenthal SL, et al. Reasons for non vaccination against HPV and future vaccination intentions in 19-26-year-old women. BMC Womens Health 2010;10:27.
[95] Liddon N, Hood J, Wynn BA, et al. Acceptability of human papillomavirus vaccine for males: a review of the literature. J Adolesc Health 2010;46(2):113–23.
[96] Finn A, Clarke E, Mytton J. Adolescent immunization: the next big thing? Arch Dis Child 2010;10.1136/adc.2010.192070. Accessed online November 28, 2010.
[97] Daley MF, Crane LA, Markowitz LE, et al. Human papillomavirus vaccination practices: a survey of US physicians 18 months after licensure. Pediatrics 2010;126(3):425–33.
[98] Whitney CG, Farley MM, Hadler J, et al. Decline in invasive pneumococcal disease after the introduction of protein-polysaccharide conjugate vaccine. N Engl J Med 2003; 348(18):1737–46.
[99] Flannery B, Schrag S, Bennett NM, et al. Impact of childhood vaccination on racial disparities in invasive *Streptococcus pneumoniae* infections. JAMA 2004;291(18): 2197–203.
[100] Lezau CA, Lynfield R, Danila R, et al. Changing epidemiology of invasive pneumococcal disease among older adult in the era of pediatric pneumococcal conjugate vaccine. JAMA 2005;294(16):2043–51.
[101] Kyaw MH, Lynfield MH, Schaffner W, et al. Effect of introduction of the pneumococcal vaccine on drug-resistant *Streptococcus pneumoniae*. N Engl J Med 2006;354(14): 1455–63.
[102] Poehling KA, Talbot TR, Griffin MR, et al. Invasive pneumococcal disease among infants before and after introduction of pneumococcal conjugate vaccine. JAMA 2006; 295(14):1668–74.
[103] Pilishvili T, Zell ER, Farley MM, et al. Sustained reductions in invasive pneumococcal disease in the era of conjugate vaccine. J Infect Dis 2010;201(1):32–41.
[104] Hicks LA, Harrison LH, Flannery B, et al. Incidence of pneumococcal disease due to non-pneumococcal conjugate vaccine (PCV7) serotypes in the United States during the era of widespread PCV7 vaccination, 1998–2004. J Infect Dis 2007;196(9):1346–54.
[105] FDA Approval Letter- Prevnar 13. Available at: http://www.fda.gov/BiologicsBloodVaccines/Vaccines/ApprovedProducts/ucm201741.htm. Accessed November 28, 2010.
[106] Centers for Disease Control and Prevention. Licensure of a 13-valent pneumococcal conjugate vaccine (PCV13) and recommendations for use among children—Advisory Committee on Immunization Practices (ACIP), 2010. MMWR Morb Mortal Wkly Rep 2010;59(9):258–61.
[107] American Academy of Pediatrics Committee on Infectious Diseases. Recommendations for the prevention of invasive *Streptococcus pneumoniae* infections in infants and children: use of 13-valent pneumococcal conjugate vaccine (PCV13) and pneumococcal polysaccharide vaccine (PPSV23). Pediatrics 2010;126(1):186–90.
[108] Centers for Disease Control and Prevention. Updated recommendations for prevention of invasive pneumococcal disease among adults using the 23-valent pneumococcal polysaccharide vaccine (PPSV23). MMWR Morb Mortal Wkly Rep 2010;59(34):1102–6.
[109] FDA US Food and Drug Administration. Rotavirus Approval. 2008 Biologicals License Applications Approval. Available at: http://www.fda.gov/BiologicsBloodVaccines/DevelopmentApprovalProcess/BiologicalApprovalsbyYear/ucm173571.htm. Accessed November 29, 2010.

[110] Wang FT, Mast TC, Glass RJ, et al. Effectiveness of the pentavalent rotavirus vaccine in preventing gastroenteritis in the United States. Pediatrics 2010;125(2):e208–13.

[111] Boom JA, Tate JE, Sahni LC, et al. Effectiveness of pentavalent rotavirus vaccine in a large urban population in the United States. Pediatrics 2010;125(2):e199–207.

[112] Zaman K, Dang DA, Victor JC, et al. Efficacy of pentavalent rotavirus vaccine against severe rotavirus gastroenteritis in infants in developing countries in Asia: a randomized double-blind placebo controlled trial. Lancet 2010;376(9741):615–23.

[113] Pawinski R, Debrus S, Delem A, et al. Rotarix in developing countries: paving the way for inclusion in national childhood immunization programs in Africa. J Infect Dis 2010;202: S80–6.

[114] Desai SN, Vásquez M. Update on rotavirus trends and the importance of surveillance. Pediatr Infect Dis J 2010;29(12):1130–2.

[115] Kuehn BM. FDA: benefits of rotavirus vaccination outweigh potential contamination risk. JAMA 2010;304(1):30–1.

[116] Centers for Disease Control and Prevention. Addition of severe combined immunodeficiency as a contraindication for administration of rotavirus vaccine. MMWR Morb Mortal Wkly Rep 2010;59(22):687–8.

[117] Centers for Disease Control and Prevention. Vaccine preventable diseases: statement regarding Rotarix and Rotateq rotavirus vaccines and intussusception. Available at: http://www.cdc.gov/vaccines/vpd-vac/rotavirus/intussusception-studies-acip.htm. Accessed December 8, 2010.

[118] Nolan T, Richmond P, Marshall H, et al. Immunogenicity and safety of an investigational combined *Haemophilus influenzae* type B—*Neisseria meningitis* serogroups C and Y-tetanus toxoid conjugate vaccine. Pediatr Infect Dis J 2010;. Available at: http://www.ncbi.nlm.nih.gov.lp.hscl.ufl.edu/pubmed/20948453. Accessed November 27, 2010.

[119] Habermehl P, Leroux-Roels G, Sanger R, et al. Combined *Haemophilus* type b and *Neisseria meningitides* serogroup C (HibMenC) or serogroup C and Y-tetanus toxoid conjugate (and HibMenCY) vaccines are well tolerated and immunogenic when administered according to the 2,3,4 months schedule with a fourth dose at 12–18 months of age. Hum Vaccin 2010;6(8):640–51.

[120] Centers for Disease Control and Prevention. Invasive *Haemophilus influenza* type B disease in five children—Minnesota, 2008. MMWR Morb Mortal Wkly Rep 2009; 58(3):58–60.

[121] Immunogenicity and safety of GSK Biologicals' Infanrix Haxa in infants. Available at: http://clinicaltrials.gov/ct2/show/NCT00753649. Accessed November 28, 2010.

[122] Abdulla RY, Rice MA, Donauer S, et al. Hepatitis A in internationally adopted children: screening for acute and previous infections. Pediatrics 2010;126(5):e1039–44.

[123] American Academy of Pediatrics. Medical evaluation of internationally adopted children for infectious diseases. In: Pickering LK, Baker CJ, Kimberlin DW, et al, editors. Red Book 2009: Report of the Committee on Infectious Diseases. Elk Grove Village (IL): American Academy of Pediatrics; 2009. p. 177–84.

[124] Global Polio Eradication Initiative. Infected countries. Available at: http://www.polioeradication.org/Infectedcountries.aspx. Accessed November 28, 2010.

[125] The GAVI Alliance. Available at: http://www.gavialliance.org/resources/GAVI_Alliance_Nov_2010.pdf. Accessed November 28, 2010.

[126] Centers for Disease Control and Prevention. Progress towards control of rubella and prevention of congenital rubella syndrome—worldwide, 2009. MMWR Morb Mortal Wkly Rep 2010;59(40):1307–10.

Advances in Pediatrics 58 (2011) 65–85

ADVANCES IN PEDIATRICS

The Human Parechoviruses: An Overview

José R. Romero, MD[a,*], Rangaraj Selvarangan, BVSc, PhD[b]

[a]Pediatric Infectious Diseases Section, Arkansas Children's Hospital, University of Arkansas for Medical Sciences, 1 Children's Way, Slot 512-11, Little Rock, AR 72202-3591, USA
[b]Children's Mercy Hospital, University of Missouri-School of Medicine, 2401 Gillham Road, Kansas City, MO 64108, USA

In the summer of 1956, the first two members of the *Parechovirus* genus were isolated from Ohio children with diarrhea [1]. Human parechoviruses (HPeVs) types 1 and 2, as they would eventually become known, were originally designated as the 22nd and 23rd members (Harris and Williamson strains, respectively) of the "enteric cytopathic human orphan (ECHO) group" or echoviruses (E22 and E23, respectively) [2]. Over the next 50 years, the advent of molecular and genomic virology would provide tools for their in-depth characterization and the identification of other members of the *Parechovirus* genus [3]. This article reviews past and current medical literature concerning the virology, epidemiology, clinical significance, and diagnosis of the HPeV.

HISTORICAL BACKGROUND

The human *Parechoviruses* (HPeVs) constitute a genus within the *Picornaviridae* family of RNA viruses [3]. The family currently comprises 12 genera. Of these, the *Enteroviruses*, *Hepatoviruses*, and *Parechoviruses* are commonly pathogenic for humans. The traditional approach to the taxonomic classification of the *Enteroviruses* was based on schemes using pathogenicity in humans and animals, patterns of replication in cell culture, and neutralization testing [2,4,5]. The ultimate measure of antigenic relatedness of new viral isolates was based on the generation of antisera against a new serotype and reciprocal cross-neutralization testing using a complete panel of prototype enterovirus strains and antisera [5]. Although useful, this approach resulted in the inclusion of non-enteroviral isolates and misclassification of enterovirus strains within the four original species (Poliovirus, Coxsackievirus type A, Coxsackievirus type B, Echovirus) that constituted the genus *Enterovirus*.

This misclassification occurred with E22 and E23. Although originally classified as echoviruses, HPeV 1 and 2 exhibited growth characteristics that

*Corresponding author. *E-mail address:* RomeroJose@uams.edu

0065-3101/11/$ – see front matter
doi:10.1016/j.yapd.2011.03.008

differed from those of other members of the species [1,6]. The development of experimental and computational methodologies to study the molecular biology and genomic analysis provided further evidence that E22 and E23 were atypical among members of the echovirus species, and other members of the genus in general [7–13]. The inability to hybridize subgenomic probes, pan-reactive with members from all species of the *Enterovirus* genus, to the genomes of E22 and E23 raised the possibility that their genomes differed significantly from those of other enteroviruses [7,8,13]. Ultimately, the elucidation of their genome sequences and their phylogenetic relationship to other enteroviruses confirmed that they where genetically distinct and merited classification into a novel genus: *Parechovirus* [3,10–12]. This genus currently consists of 16 types and, most likely, will continue to increase in number [14].

VIROLOGY

As with other *Picornaviridae*, the HPeVs are small (28 nm in diameter), nonenveloped RNA viruses [3,10,15,16]. The HPeV genome is a single-stranded, positive (messenger) sense RNA molecule approximately 7.35 kb in length (Fig. 1) [10–12,14,17–19]. The organization of the HPeV genome is consistent with that of other *Picornaviridae* [20]. A covalently linked protein, VPg (also designated 3B), is attached to the extreme 5' end of the genome immediately preceding a long nontranslated region (NTR), constituting approximately 10% of the viral genome's length. The 5'NTR precedes a single open reading frame (ORF) that is subdivided into three regions (P1–3) and codes for a polyprotein of approximately 2180 amino acids, depending on the type and strain [14,20]. The ORF is followed by a short 3'NTR and a terminal polyadenylated tail.

The 5'NTR of the *Picornaviridae* plays critical roles in viral replication and translation of the viral genome [20]. Multiple lines of evidence support the existence of higher-order structures, formed by short- and long-distance RNA–RNA interactions, within the picornaviral 5'NTR [20]. Experimental and computation data also support this for the HPeV [12,18,21]. A stem-loop structure (SLS) and pseudoknot at the extreme upstream end of the HPeV 5'NTR, shown to be essential for replication of the viral genome, have been computationally shown to exist in multiple HPeV types [18,22].

A series of SLSs, downstream of the replication-essential SLS, that constitute an internal ribosome entry site (IRES) exist in the HPeV [18,22]. The IRES is essential for efficient translation of the picornavirus genome [20]. The HPeV IRES seems to be more closely related to those of the *Cardiovirus* and *Aphthovirus*

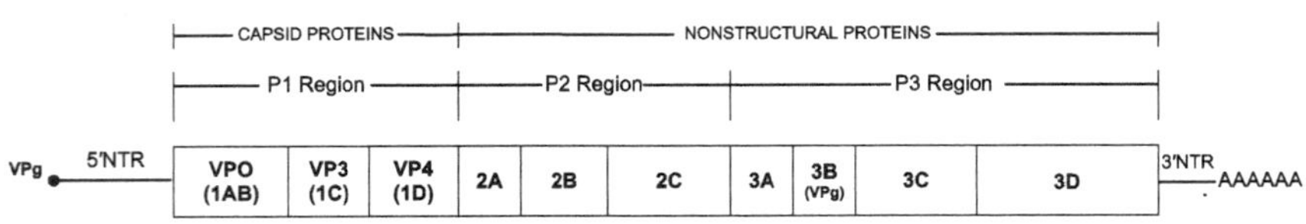

Fig. 1. Organization of the human parechovirus genome.

genera than to the *Enteroviruses*. Within the HPeV 5'NTR are conserved regions of nucleotide identity that are shared among members of the genus. These regions can be used to develop nucleic acid amplification tests (NAATs) for HPeV detection in clinical specimens.

The 3'NTR of the enteroviruses contains higher-order structures important in viral replication. Genomic analysis of HPeV types 1 through 5 revealed the existence of a predicted SLS in the 3'NTR [18], raising the possibility that it also plays a role in HPeV replication.

Translation of the ORF results in the generation of a large polyprotein that undergoes immediate posttranslational modification to yield the structural (capsid) and nonstructural proteins essential to HPeV replication and viral assembly (see Fig. 1) [20]. The structure and functions of all of the HPeV proteins have not been extensively studied. Although many have functions similar to enteroviral cognate proteins, differences are emerging. Unlike most of the *Picornaviridae*, in HPeV the P1 region codes for three rather than four capsid proteins (see Fig. 1). The capsid protein coding sequences are organized contiguously and without intervening stop codons as VP0 (1AB), VP3 (1C), VP1 (1D) in the 5' to 3' orientation [10–12,16–19]. The HPeV VP0 protein is not maturationally cleaved to form the VP2 and VP4 capsid proteins, as is typical of other enteroviruses, resulting in a capsid that is composed of three, rather than four, proteins in the mature virion [10–12,16–19]. The VP0 protein has been found to contain an SLS that may function as a *cis*-acting replication element (CRE) [18]. The CRE is critical for RNA replication in poliovirus where it is located within the 2C protein coding sequence. The C-terminal region of VP1 of several of the HPeV types contains an arginine–glycine-aspartic acid (RGD) motif that has been shown to be functional in binding to host cell integrins, which serve as receptors for some members of the genus [10,12,16,18,23,24]. The cell receptors used by HPeV lacking the RGD motif are currently unknown. The VP1 protein is also important for molecular typing of the HPeV [25,26]. The VP3 of HPeV characteristically varies from that of the enteroviruses because of the *N*-terminal extension of 28 to 34 amino acid residues [27].

The P2 and P3 regions code for seven nonstructural proteins (5'-2A, 2B, 2C, 3A, 3B, 3C, and 3D-3') and their intermediates required for the viral lifecycle (see Fig. 1) [20]. The HPeV 2A protein seems to differ functionally from that of the enteroviruses in that it lacks proteolytic activity. Evidence indicates that it is incapable of mediating the cleavage between the 1D and 2A proteins [28,29]. In addition, the HPeV fail to shut off host cell protein synthesis [8,9,23], a function mediated in enteroviruses by 2A cleavage of eIF4G [20], which confers a replication advantage to the virus. The HPeV 2A protein also binds to RNA and may play a role in RNA replication [30]. The 2C protein of the HPeV also seems to differ from its cognate enterovirus protein. Like the enterovirus 2C, it localizes to endoplasmic reticulum membrane–associated replication complexes, supporting its role in viral replication. However, it is also associated with cellular structures not directly involved in replication [31,32]. The 2C protein also has AMP kinase activity, but the significance of this property is currently unknown.

EPIDEMIOLOGY

HPeVs have been reported worldwide [18,27,33–45]. When discussing the epidemiology of the HPeV, one must understand that until 2004 only 2 HPeV types were known to exist. Since then, 14 new types have been recognized [14]. Additionally, most of what is known about the epidemiology of the HPeV is based on cell culture detection of these agents, a methodology that has poor sensitivity for the detecting HPeV. Therefore, understanding of the epidemiology of the HPeV continues to evolve as new types are identified and molecular methodologies (eg, NAATs) are used for their detection.

The contribution of each of the 16 known HPeV types to the total burden of HPeV-related disease is yet unclear. Similarly, the worldwide distribution of each of the types is still being defined. Evaluation of longitudinal data spanning 39 years indicates that in the United States, HePV1 accounts for 1.8% (880/49,637) of all typed enterovirus isolates reported to the Centers for Disease Control and Prevention (CDC) [37,46]. During that period, HPeV 1 numbered among the top 15 isolates for 74% of all years. In contrast, HPeV 2 accounted for only 0.1% of all enteroviruses isolated. The contribution of HPeV 1 to the burden of enterovirus disease in the neonate seems to be similarly low: 0.8% (19/2356 typeable isolates) over a 21-year period [47]. However, because of multiple factors, these data may not represent the true burden of HPeV disease [37,46].

A report from Niigata, Japan documented that over a 15-year period, 41 HPeV isolates where identified using cell culture from stool, throat swabs, and cerebrospinal fluid (CSF) specimens [19]. In comparison, during that same period, 1437 enterovirus isolates were identified. Thus, approximately 2.8% of all enteroviruses isolated were HPeV. Typing showed that HPeV 1, 3, 4, and 6 constituted approximately 34%, 39%, 2%, and 24% of the total isolates, respectively. A second report from Japan found that 110 (2.2%) of 4976 stool specimens collected over a 9-year period from children with suspected viral infections were positive for HPeV [16]. HPeV 1 and 3 accounted for 57% (n = 63) and 40% (n = 44) of isolates, respectively. The remaining three isolates were HPeV 4 (n = 2) and HPeV 6 (n = 1).

A Swedish study also documented a low incidence of HPeV 2–related disease, with only five cases identified among 1000 enteroviruses over a 33-year period [34]. A Canadian report found that among 28 HPeV isolates identified over a 20-year period, types 1, 2, and 3 accounted for 71.4% (n = 20), 10.7% (n = 3), and 17.9% (n = 5), respectively [27].

The current data appear to indicate that overall the HPeV account for approximately 2% of all enteroviruses isolated by clinical laboratories using traditional methods. HPeV 1 is the most frequently identified member of the genus, followed by HPeV 3. Currently, other members seem to make minor contributions to the total burden of HPeV-related disease. However, as NAATs are used more frequently for their detection, this may change.

Evidence indicates that HPeV infections are acquired early in life and that geographic variations may contribute to the predominant serotypes initially encountered. A report summarizing data from the World Health Organization (WHO) Virus Unit from 1967 to 1974 documented that 61% of reported HPeV 1 infections occurred in infants younger than 1 year [48]. In the United States, most cases of HPeV 1 and 2 reported to the CDC have occurred in infants younger than 1 year (73% and 67.6%, respectively) [37]. Children younger than 5 years accounted for 95.6% and 88.2% of all HPeV 1 and 2 isolates, respectively [37].

Although available seroprevalence data are sparse and focus on a limited number of HPeV types, they too support that early infection with HPeV and geographic variation factor into what type is encountered [16,36,49–51]. Studies conducted in Finland documented that 72% to 89% of infants 2 years of age possessed antibodies to HPeV 1 [36,50]. A small study of Israeli infants showed that 89% of subjects had antibodies to HePV 1 through 3 at the same age [51]. The same study also showed that 70% of Canadian children younger than 5 years possessed antibodies to the same HPeV types [51].

Two studies conducted in Japan suggest that seroprevalence rates to HPeV 1 and HPeV 3 in children vary at different ages when adjusted for a similar definition of significant titers (>1:8) to the virus in question [16,49]. Among children aged 4 to 6 years from Hiroshima (n = 195) and Aichi (n = 207) Prefectures, the seroprevalence of antibodies to HPeV 1 and HPeV 3 was approximately equal (80% and 85%, respectively). However, the age at which seropositivity occurred to the specific serotypes varied between studies. In infants 7 to 12 months of age from Hiroshima Prefecture, 66% had antibodies to HPeV 1. In contrast, only 15% of infants of the same age from Aichi Prefecture showed presence of antibodies to HPeV 3. Among children aged 2 to 3 years from Hiroshima Prefecture, 80% had antibodies to HPeV 1. In comparison, only 45% of similarly aged children from Aichi Prefecture had antibodies to HPeV 3.

A Canadian study of 28 children, retrospectively identified as having HPeV infection, documented variations in the mean age at which infants had infections with various HPeV types [27]. The mean age at which HPeV 3 infection occurred was 0.7 months compared with 14.6 and 6.3 months for HPeV 1 and 2, respectively. In dramatic counterpoint to the previous study, a limited serologic survey of the prevalence of HPeV 3 among adults in the Milwaukee, Wisconsin area failed to detect any seropositive individuals [52].

A prospective, longitudinal study of HPeV infection, determined through stool culture, in 102 Norwegian infants followed up for 36 months documented that the cumulative incidence of infection was 86% by 24 months of age and 94% at 36 months [38]. The incidence rate of infection increased with increasing age: 11.6 versus 20 to 23 infections per 100 person months for infants aged 4 months and infants older than 15 months of age, respectively.

The specific HPeV serotypes were not determined. Of the infants in one cohort, 55% had more than one HPeV infection during the period of observation, indicating that sequential HPeV infections are common [38].

Taken together, these studies indicate that for individual HPeV types, differences may exist regarding how soon after birth infants become infected. These differences may be a reflection of factors such as modes of transmission for a given HPeV type, prevalence of HPeV types in the community, and variations in patterns of exposure to HPeV types.

Although HPeV infections may occur throughout the year, they exhibit a strong seasonal epidemiology. Around the world, the peak incidence of infections occurs during the summer and fall months [27,35,38,44,50,53–61]. Several reports have documented a biennial pattern of HPeV 3 infection [40,56,57,62]. Other reports, however, have specifically failed to support this finding [19,38,42,59]. Cocirculation of multiple HPeV types within a community or geographic region is common [38,41,42,44,55,59,60,62,63]. HPeVs have been associated with community [58] and nosocomial outbreaks in pediatric and neonatal units [34,35,45,64,65].

CLINICAL SYNDROMES

Transmission of the HPeV seems to occur via the fecal–oral and respiratory routes. Fecal–oral transmission is favored by high viral titers in stool. In one report, the median HPeV titer was 502,380 copies/mL (range, 3,170–503,377,290 copies/mL) [55]. Reports of neonates with HPeV infections occurring in the first 2 days of life may support the possibility of in utero transmission [45,56].

After infection, the virus is shed from the gastrointestinal and upper respiratory tracts [38,54,66]. The duration of shedding from these sites is still poorly characterized but may range from less than 2 weeks to 5 months [38,66] in stool and 1 to 3 weeks in the upper respiratory tract [54,66]. The median duration of HPeV shedding in stool has been shown to be 51 days [38]. Approximately 10% of infected children shed virus in stool for more than 3 months.

The detection of HPeV from the stool of healthy, asymptomatic infants, and high seroprevalence rates among infants and children in the general population support that many, if not most, infections are subclinical [16,38,45,55]. A comparison of symptoms from longitudinally followed infants showed that no symptom (cough, sneezing, fever [>38°C], diarrhea) was significantly associated with HPeV detection in stool when compared with children not shedding virus [38]. Additionally, given the high prevalence of HPeV infections, severe infections are probably rare.

CENTRAL NERVOUS SYSTEM INFECTIONS

The HPeVs have been linked to various central nervous system (CNS) syndromes, including acute flaccid paralysis [16,19,33], encephalitis [57,61,67–69], and meningitis [33,59,61,69].

Meningitis

Detection of HPeV from permissive (upper respiratory and gastrointestinal tracts) [19,42,53,58,62] and nonpermissive (CSF, blood) sites [40,57,58] supports that the HPeVs and, in particular HPeV 3, contribute to the burden of viral meningitis worldwide. A retrospective study of CSF specimens previously found to be negative for enteroviruses from 761 Dutch children 5 years of age, collected from 2004 to 2006, showed that 4.6% had HPeV genome present (typing was not attempted) [57]. Of these, 97% were younger than 24 months, with infants younger than 28 days constituting 46% of all positive children. The prevalence of HPeV-positive specimens fluctuated annually: 8.2%, 0.4% and 5.7% for 2004, 2005 and 2006, respectively.

A Scottish study examined CSF samples from 1480 individuals collected from 2006 to 2008 [40]. In 14 (0.9%) individuals, HPeV was detected by reverse transcription-polymerase chain reaction (RT-PCR); all were type 3. The prevalence of positive specimens varied by year: 0.7% in 2006, 0% in 2007, and 7.2% in 2008. All 14 patients were younger than 3 months. The frequency of detection for subjects in this age cohort was 2.9%.

A retrospective analysis of 780 CSF nucleic acid extracts from United States children, previously shown to be negative for enteroviruses, documented that 7.4% (n = 58) harbored HPeV genome [61]. Of these subjects, 81% were 2 months of age or younger and 26% were 1 month of age or younger. Genotyping showed HPeV 3 in 52 and HPeV 1 in 1. The prevalence of positive specimens varied significantly by year of the study: 1.8% in 2006, 16.9% in 2007, and 0% in 2008.

A review of archival CSF specimens from 397 Spanish infants younger than 12 months, obtained to exclude CNS infection, found that 2.3% (n = 9) were positive for the HPeV genome [59]. All but one of the infants were younger than 2 months and 4 infants (44%) were younger than 30 days. In 8 subjects, genotyping showed that the HPeV was type 3. Lastly, during an HPeV 3 epidemic in Hiroshima, Japan, 4% of CSF specimens evaluated were positive [58].

These reports indicate that HPeV, and particularly HPeV 3, may be detectable in 2.3% to 7.4% of all infants undergoing CSF evaluation for possible infection. Most cases occurred in infants younger than 3 months. As point of comparison, several of the studies documented that enterovirus was detected in 5.3% to 25.7% of CSF samples evaluated [40,59,61]. Considerable annual variation was observed (0%–16.9%) in the prevalence of HPeV-positive CSF samples. Despite the presence of other HPeV types circulating in the community, HPeV 3 was the overwhelmingly dominant cause of HPeV-related meningitis [40].

Review of clinical and laboratory data from 96 infants (including 2 with proven or possible encephalitis) from the three largest reports of patients with unequivocal HPeV 3 CSF infection indicate that fever is present in more than 95% of infants [57,59,61]. Irritability was also reported in more than 95% of cases. In all reports, males accounted for most cases (55%–71%). An exanthem was reported in 17% to 60% of infants, and was characterized as maculopapular in nature in one report [61]. Gastrointestinal signs (emesis, diarrhea, distention) were reported in approximately one-quarter to half of cases. Respiratory symptoms ("rhinorrhea, cough, tachypnea, apnea, wheezing, and/or abnormalities on radiograph of the thorax") were present in 36% in one series [57]. Conspicuously absent in all reports were findings indicating increased intracranial pressure (bulging fontanelle) or meningeal irritation (nuchal stiffness, Kernig or Brudzinski signs).

The CSF cytochemical evaluation showed that most patients had no or minimal abnormalities [57,59,61]. Only 12% of 67 infants had a white blood cell count above the norm for age [59,61], and in only 2 was the pleocytosis greater than 25 cells/mm^3. Hypoglycorrhachia was reported in only 2 infants and the CSF protein was increased above age-adjusted normal values in only 7.5% [59,61]. Similar CSF findings to those described in the previous large series have been reported in case reports of HPeV meningitis [70].

Ninety-eight percent of infants were hospitalized. Of the two infants not admitted, one was observed in the emergency room for 24 hours and the other discharged home [57,59,61]. Antibiotics were administered to 82% to 100% of infants. In a cohort of infants from the United States, 17% also received acyclovir [61]. Although 54% of infants in one report were felt to have a sepsis-like clinical presentation, only one required admission to an intensive care unit [57]. The mean duration of hospitalization varied from 3.6 to 7.4 days [57,59,61]. No deaths were reported in any of the studies [57,59,61]. Long-term outcome data were not provided.

Acute flaccid paralysis

The HPeVs have been etiologically linked to cases of acute flaccid paralysis [16,19,33,71]. The original identification of HPeV 3 was from a 1-year-old female with fever, diarrhea, and transient paralysis [16]. Other HPeV types associated with acute flaccid paralysis include 1 and 6 [19,33].

The sole recorded outbreak of HPeV-related acute flaccid paralysis occurred in Jamaica and was the result of HPeV 1 [33]. Two adults (26 and 27 years) and 4 children (21 months and 4, 7, and 13 years) were involved. Three children were fully immunized against polio and the fourth had received two doses of oral polio vaccine. All had acute onset of flaccid paralysis with inability to walk and one child also had involvement of the muscles of respiration and required mechanical ventilation. Two of three older children reported paraesthesias of extremities. Cranial nerve involvement occurred in one child. All children had areflexia and two had signs of meningeal irritation. CSF pleocytosis was present in only one child, but protein was increased in all. Although all children recovered, two required admission to the intensive care unit and three had lower extremity weakness as sequelae.

A case involving a 10-month-old male, reported as encephalomyelitis with residual paralysis, may have been acute flaccid paralysis [71]. The clinical presentation consisted of fever, emesis, generalized hypotonia, and decreased tendon reflexes. No pleocytosis was observed on examination of the CSF.

Type 1 HPeV genome was detected in the CSF. Recovery was complicated by residual upper extremity paralysis.

Encephalitis

Reports of HPeV-related encephalitis have exclusively involved neonates and young infants [56,57,61,68,69]. HPeV types 1 and 3 have been isolated from confirmed cases, with HPeV 3 dominating [68,69].

Evaluation of cases for which sufficient information is provided indicates that most cases have occurred in full-term neonates, with onset of symptoms occurring in the first 2 weeks of life [56,68,69]. Among cases in prematurely born infants, the onset of illness was later: at 50 to 90 days of life [68]. Seizures constituted the predominant clinical finding (82%). In one-third, recurrent seizures persisted for more than 24 hours. Fever and irritability were each present in 73% of infants. Rash was present in approximately two-thirds and apnea in 55%. Approximately one-third had hypotension that required inotropic support. Additional findings included diarrhea, hypertonia, and photophobia. CSF evaluation was abnormal in only one patient and showed moderate pleocytosis [68].

All infants showed abnormalities on neuroimaging using MRI or cranial ultrasound [68,69]. MRI detected white matter changes consisting of high signal intensity and punctate lesions in 90%. These consisted of high signal intensity and punctate lesions. MRI detected white matter changes in two infants without seizures [68,69]. Severe periventricular echogenicity was detected with cranial ultrasound in all infants.

No deaths occurred [68,69]. Although long-term neurologic outcome data were not available for all patients, only 64% were neurologically normal at the time of the clinical report. Neurologic sequelae included epilepsy, cerebral palsy, visual impairment, learning disability, and mild distal hypotonia [68]. Repetitive seizures and a discontinuous background detected on amplitude-integrated electroencephalogram were found to correlate with poor neurodevelopmental outcome [68].

NEONATAL DISEASE

As with enteroviral infections in neonates, most HPeV infections in this age group are likely asymptomatic or result in benign, self-limited febrile illness [72,73]. However, similar to their viral cousins, HPeVs have the potential to cause severe life-threatening disease in the newborn [52,56].

Undifferentiated febrile illness

The HPeV have frequently been isolated from the stools of neonates and infants with undifferentiated febrile illness [42,70,74]. A small but well-documented case series has been published describing the clinical, laboratory, and radiologic findings in three neonates, aged 7 to 21 days, with HPeV 3 infection presenting as a febrile illness without a discernable cause [70]. Fever ($\geq$39° C) and irritability were presenting complaints in all infants. Rhinorrhea in association with cough and poor feeding were reported in one infant each.

All had exposure histories significant for contact with family members with upper respiratory tract infections before the onset of illness. At admission, one infant each was tachypneic and tachycardic. An erythematous rash, present at admission or developing the next day, occurred in all infants. CSF and chest radiographs were normal in all. After admission, all infants developed worsened respiratory status consisting of tachypnea and oxygen desaturation singly or in combination; prompting admission to the intensive care unit. All infants became afebrile by the fourth day after admission. HPeV 3 was detected from nasopharyngeal aspirates of all infants. Given the similarity of the clinical and CSF findings of these infants to those described previously with meningitis, one or all may have had CNS infection. However, CSF was not evaluated for the presence of HPeV using NAAT in any patient.

The clinical findings described in this case series are similar to those described in neonates with enterovirus infections [75]. However, additional studies with larger numbers of patients are necessary to fully characterize this syndrome.

Hemorrhage-hepatitis syndrome

A report of severe HPeV infections in neonates included two infants with hepatitis and associated thrombocytopenia [56]. Although specific details are not provided, the latter two infants may have had hemorrhage-hepatitis syndrome [47], a condition often associated with echovirus 11 infections in neonates [75]. A well-documented case of HPeV 3–related hemorrhage-hepatitis syndrome has been reported [69]. Onset of illness occurred at 24 days of age with fever and irritability. Admission aspartate and alanine aminotransferases (alanine aminotransferase [ALT] and aspartate aminotransferase [AST], respectively) levels and platelet count were initially normal. On the fourth day of hospitalization the ALT and AST levels increased to 5421 U/L and 1207 U/L, respectively. The infant developed prolonged prothrombin and partial thromboplastin times and thrombocytopenia. Although none of the infants died, one required a liver transplant at 3 years of age as a result of severe liver necrosis [56].

Necrotizing enterocolitis

Neonatal HPeV 1 infection has been associated with necrotizing enterocolitis [35,45]. In an outbreak of gastroenteritis involving 19 infants being cared for in a neonatal intensive care unit, 7 with bloody diarrhea had abdominal radiograph findings of early necrotizing enterocolitis. One was found to have pneumatosis intestinalis.

In addition to the constellation of signs and symptoms associated with the specific clinical syndromes discussed previously, manifestations reported in single or combined association with HPeV infection in neonates include fever, apnea, tachypnea, respiratory distress, rhinorrhea, conjunctivitis, and rash [45,70].

GASTROINTESTINAL DISEASE

Diarrhea is a component of the symptom complex of almost every syndrome associated with HPeV infection. Multiple studies, varying in stringency, controls, and clinical venues, have examined the role of HPeV in the origin of acute gastroenteritis in children [41,42,44,55,60,63] and adults [55].

Using RT-PCR, a study conducted in Germany examined the presence of HPeV in the stool of patients of all ages with acute enteritis [55]. Only specimens negative for rota-, adeno-, astro-, noro-, and enteroviruses were included. No HPeVs were detected in a cohort of 118 patients comprised of hospitalized young children and older children and adults evaluated in the context of enteritis outbreaks. A second cohort consisted of 499 nonhospitalized subjects with community-acquired enteritis and 39 controls without enteritis [55]. Eight subjects in the former group and one control subject were found to have HPeV. All positive subjects were children, and all but one was younger than 2 years. The prevalence of HPeV among the enteritis and control groups was not statistically significant: 1.6% (8/499) versus 2.6% (1/39), respectively. Prevalence was 11.6% (7/60) when only children younger than 2 years of age were included. The authors concluded that the HPeVs were not responsible for epidemic enteritis but rather were causes of endemic disease [55].

An RT-PCR evaluation for rota-, adeno-, saporo-, noro- and astroviruses in 82 fecal specimens collected from Thai children with acute gastroenteritis found HPeV genome in 12 (14.6%) [44]. Patients in whom HPeV was identified ranged in age from 6 to 24 months. Typing was possible in 9 and revealed types 1 (n = 5), 2 (n = 1), 3 (N = 2), and 4 (n = 1). Clinical findings and venue of collection were not provided.

A study conducted in Sri Lankan children hospitalized with acute gastroenteritis examined 362 fecal specimens for the presence of HPeV genome using RT-PCR [60]. All specimens positive for HPeV were also tested for the presence of rota-, adeno-, saporo-, noro-, and astroviruses. HPeV was detected in 8.3% (n = 30). Among the 27 specimens that were typed, HPeV types 1 (n = 11), 3 (n = 1), 4 (n = 5), 5 (n = 3), 10 (n = 5), and 11 (n = 2) were identified. Coinfection with other viral enteric pathogens was found in 67%. The 10 patients solely infected with HPeV ranged in age from 2 to 26 months. Fever and emesis were present in 30% and 40% of patients, respectively. Respiratory symptoms (wheezing, cough, and coryza) were present in 30% [60].

A study of Japanese children aged 2 months to 15 years with acute gastroenteritis examined stool specimens collected at pediatric clinics for the presence of HPeV genome using RT-PCR [63]. Of 477 stool specimens, 247 were found to be negative for rota-, adeno-, saporo-, noro-, and astroviruses and were tested for HPeV genome using RT-PCR. HPeV was detected in 8.1% (n = 20) of samples. Typing was possible in 17 specimens, and identified HePV 1 (n = 15) and HPeV 3 (n = 2). Patients with HPeV ranged in age from 5 to 51 months. Fever and emesis were present in 30% and 15%, respectively. Respiratory symptoms consisting of cough and coryza were noted in 10% and 5% of patients, respectively.

A study designed to identify novel HPeVs evaluated stool samples from 335 Brazilian children aged 6 years or younger evaluated as outpatients or hospitalized for acute diarrhea lasting 13 days or less with associated dehydration [41]. RT-PCR detected HPeV in 16.1% (n = 54) of samples. Typing was possible in only 11 samples and identified types 1, 5, 6, and 8. HPeV 1 was the most frequently identified (n = 7). Information regarding coinfection with other diarrheal agents and clinical data were not provided.

Based on available information, HPeVs seem to be associated with endemic cases of diarrheal illness restricted to infants and young children. This finding is not surprising given the high prevalence of seropositivity (>80%–85%) to various HPeV types found in older children and adults, as discussed previously. In addition to diarrhea, fever, vomiting, or respiratory symptoms may be present in up to one-third of cases. The studies summarized earlier seem to indicate that no significant differences exist in the prevalence of HPeV infection in children between industrialized (8.2%–11.6%) [55,63] and developing (8.3%–14.6%) nations [44,60]. The finding of significant coinfection (66.7%) with other enteric viral pathogens [60] raises questions as to whether dual infections result in more severe disease.

RESPIRATORY DISEASE

Multiple reports have described respiratory symptoms alone or in combination with other syndrome complexes in patients in whom HPeV has been detected through culture, serology, or NAATs [45,48,55,57,60,63,64,70]. Data from the WHO Virus Unit indicated that approximately one-quarter of cases of HPeV 1 presented with respiratory disease [48]. A 15-year review of HPeV-related cases from a university center in Japan showed that 14.6% of 41 cases were respiratory tract infections [19]. HPeV types identified included 1 (n = 2), 3 (n = 3), and 6 (n = 1). A series of outbreaks of HPeV 1–related respiratory tract disease were reported from a neonatal unit in the United States. Although the report included 64 premature infants, only 28% had virologic or serologic criteria sufficient to support acute HPeV infection [64].

Although these studies seem to support a role for HPeV as the etiologic agents of respiratory tract disease, a large Scottish study raises questions concerning the causal role of at least some types [54]. This study evaluated 3844 respiratory specimens, collected from 2200 individuals, for the presence of traditional respiratory viral pathogens (respiratory syncytial virus, influenza viruses A and B, parainfluenza viruses 1 through 3, adenovirus and bocavirus), and HPeV using NAAT. HPeVs were detected in only 34 specimens (0.9% sample prevalence) collected from 27 individuals (1.2% person prevalence).Of those in whom any respiratory virus was identified (n = 930), HPeV accounted for 2.9% of cases. All HPeV infections occurred in children aged 6 months to 5 years of age, 89% were younger than 3 years of age. Typing was possible in 33 specimens; only HPeV types 1 (n = 25) and 6 (n = 8) were identified. Coinfection with one or more of the traditional respiratory viral pathogens was noted in 76% of children in whom HPeV was detected. The authors concluded that the findings failed to provide evidence supporting the proposed role of HPeV as a cause of respiratory disease in children [54]. The observed incidence of HPeV infections in children younger than 5 years was within the expected frequency of the general population. Lastly, the clinical profile, in terms of nonspecific and upper and lower respiratory tract symptoms, of those in whom HPeV was detected coincided more closely to the profiles of individuals with negative samples.

SUDDEN UNEXPLAINED INFANT DEATH

Reports of pediatric fatalities associated with HPeV infection are rare [16,17,52,76]. The HPeVs have been recovered from autopsy specimens obtained from pediatric decedents diagnosed with sudden unexplained infant death [52]. A review of autopsy reports from 1263 infants and children found that viruses were identified in 34% (n = 426). HPeVs were identified in 24 (5.6%). Typing identified 20 as HPeV 1; 3 as HPeV 3; and 1 as HPeV 6. The isolate of HPeV 6 was obtained from an infant who died of blunt force trauma and one HPeV 3 isolate came from an infant who died of asphyxiation secondary to loss of tracheal airway. In these instances, HPeV was not deemed causal in the deaths. The remaining HPeV 3 isolates were obtained from two female infants aged 4 weeks and 4 months, respectively. Both had viral-like upper respiratory tract symptoms at the time of death or 1 week preceding it. HPeV 3 was isolated from lung and in swabs of the nasopharynx and colon. The authors concluded that HPeV 3 may have contributed to their deaths.

MISCELLANEOUS CLINICAL ASSOCIATIONS

Two reports document the isolation of HPeV types 6 and 5 from the CSF and stool from children with Reye syndrome [18,19,77]. HPeVs have been isolated from infants and children with a wide array of illnesses and syndromes (Table 1). A causal link may exist between the HPeV and those conditions. However, in most of the reports, the HPeVs were detected from

Table 1
Miscellaneous syndromes reported with HPeV infection

Condition	HPeV Type	Source	References
Hydrocephalus	Unknown	Urine	[18,77]
TORCH syndrome	4	Rectum, throat	[18,77]
"Cardiac"	4	Throat	[18,77]
Hand-foot-mouth disease	1, 3	Throat, stool	[19,42]
Myositis	3	Throat	[19]
Lymphadenitis	4	Stool	[19]
Myocarditis	1	Myocardium	[76]
Hemolytic uremic syndrome	1	Stool	[78]
Herpangina	6	Stool	[42]
Otitis	1	Middle ear fluid	[79]

sites where prolonged shedding is known to occur and not from the involved organ system or tissue. Additionally, reports fail to detail whether other infectious agents, known to be associated with the syndrome, were conclusively excluded. Further adding to the complexity of ascribing a causal relationship between HPeV and an illness is the codetection of a second agent, known to be linked to the disease in question [42,54,63].

Diagnosis

Several approaches (NAAT, cell culture, or serology) have been used to diagnose HPeV infections. Routine use of these tests in the clinical laboratory is generally limited by the lack of commercially available reagents.

NUCLEIC ACID AMPLIFICATION

Currently, RT-PCR is the preferred methodology for detecting HPeV because of its sensitivity and ability to detect all known HPeV types in a clinically meaningful time frame. Although the HPeVs are related to the enteroviruses, RT-PCR assays used for detecting the latter do not detect HPeVs because of sequence heterogeneity within the 5'NTR of members of the two genera.

Detection of the HPeV using RT-PCR has relied on amplification of portions of the HPeV 5'NTR flanked by stretches of conserved nucleic acid sequence. The initially described assays detected the amplified region using agarose gel electrophoresis or liquid hybridization [36,54,80–82]. The advent of real-time amplification systems has led to the development of several highly sensitive HPeV real-time RT-PCR (rRT-PCR) assays capable of simultaneous amplification and detection of amplification products [54,83–85]. One- and two-step rRT-PCR assays have been described for HPeV detection [54,83,85]. In a two-step RT-PCR, the conversion of the HPeV RNA genome target area into a complimentary DNA (cDNA) copy (ie, reverse transcription) is performed initially. An aliquot of the cDNA reaction is then transferred to a second reaction vessel for amplification of the target region (ie, PCR). The one-step RT-PCR combines the cDNA synthesis and PCR in a single reaction vessel.

rRT-PCR assays have been shown to be significantly more sensitive than cell culture for detecting the HPeV. One-step HPeV rRT-PCRs and a two-step rRT-PCR have been developed that show approximately 100- to 1000-fold greater sensitivity than culture for detection of HPeV [83,85]. Using stool specimens, one report documented that cell culture failed to identify HPeV in 64% of specimens found to be positive using rRT-PCR [86]. A two-step rRT-PCR assay using clinical specimens (CSF, blood, stool, and throat swabs) showed superior detection of the HPeV rRT-PCR over cell culture [87]. All patients with positive CSF specimens (n = 3) also had positive results from blood. Fourteen patients who had positive HPeV results from blood or CSF also had positive results from feces or throat. The rRT-PCR detected 19 additional positive specimens (16/159 feces and 3/57 throat swabs) that were missed by culture.

Optimum diagnostic RT-PCR assays targeting the 5'NTR for detection of HPeV are not type-specific. They are designed for increased sensitivity and to broadly detect all known HPeV types from clinical specimens. Type-specific HPeV identification relies on phylogenetic evaluation of the VP1 coding region, and is considered to be the criterion standard for HPeV typing [26,86]. HPeV strains of the same genotype share 77% or more nucleotide sequence identity or 87% or more amino acid identity of VP1 [26]. A recent report described an assay for amplification of the complete VP1 sequences from HPeV 1 through 7 and 9 through 14 for use in genotyping [26]. The VP1 assays are less sensitive than the rRT-PCR assays targeting the 5'NTR region, and hence some of low-titer clinical specimens may be potentially missed by the VP1 assays [26,86]. Although genotyping is not necessary for clinical purposes, it may be a useful adjunct to diagnosis for epidemiologic purposes and to gain a better understanding of genotype–disease association.

Currently only a limited number of clinical and reference laboratories in the United States offer RT-PCR testing for HPeV [88]. In the absence of RT-PCR assays approved by the U.S. Food and Drug Administration for HPeV detection, clinical laboratories that elect to develop in-house RT-PCR assays for detection or genotyping should carefully validate assays intended for clinic use. Validation of RT-PCR detection systems is complex and should include careful selection of the primers and probes for amplification, analysis of the polymerase enzymes, amplification conditions, platforms, and specimen types to be tested.

CELL CULTURE

The HPeV can produce enterovirus-like cytopathic effect on appropriate cell lines [86]. However, not all HPeV types replicate equally on the same primary cells or cell lines. A recent study documented that HT29 (primary colorectal adenocarcinoma) cells recovered 75% of all cultivable HPeV types 1, 4, and 6 from stool specimens [86]. HPeV 1 and 4 could also be cultured using tm (tertiary cynomolgus monkey kidney), Vero (African green monkey kidney), A549 (human lung adenocarcinoma), and RD (rhabdomyosarcoma) cells. In contrast, HPeV 3 grew only on Vero and A549 cells. An earlier study noted tm cells could also detect HPeV 3 isolates from stool specimens [89]. Thus, optimal recovery of HPeV requires the use of multiple cell lines.

The use of cell culture for clinical detection of HPeV is limited by several factors. As indicated, the detection of HPeV using traditional cell culture methodologies lacks sensitivity because not all cell lines support their growth equally [36,86]. Furthermore, many of the primary cells or cell lines required for optimum detection of the HPeV are not part of routine cell culture systems used in clinical laboratories. Even using the widest combination of cells known to support the growth of HPeV, many types grow poorly, if at all, in cell culture (eg, HPeV types 11 to 14). The ability to propagate the HPeV in cell culture is also dependant on viral load in the specimen being tested, so that specimens containing lower viral titers may fail to yield HPeV [86]. Cell culture detection of HPeV may take several days, hence limiting its clinical usefulness in the acute management of the patient. Lastly, the lack of commercial immunostaining reagents for confirmation and type-specific identification of isolated HPeV strains necessitates the use of neutralization assays with a panel of standardized serotype-specific antiserum pools; a process that is laborious, time-consuming, and limited by the availability of reagents. All of these limitations have constrained the use of appropriate cell culture HPeV detection to research, reference, and a few commercial laboratories.

Specimen selection and interpretation of results

Specimen types selected for testing should be based on disease condition and organ system involved. Stool, throat swabs, and CSF are good choices for detecting gastrointestinal, respiratory, and CNS infections, respectively. Similar to RT-PCR detection of enteroviruses using blood, limited data suggest that additional testing of blood may improve the diagnostic yield for detecting CNS infection.

Several important concepts should be borne in mind when interpreting RT-PCR or cell culture results. Because HPeV are excreted from the throat and gastrointestinal tract for prolonged periods [38,66], their detection in these sites should not be taken as prima facie proof of a causal role in illnesses being evaluated. Their presence may represent shedding from an infection that occurred weeks earlier and have no relationship to the medical problem being evaluated. The same is not the case for HPeV detected in CSF and blood, which their detection is considered diagnostic. Additionally, detection of an HPeV in the stool or throat specimen of a neonate may be considered supportive evidence for the cause of an HPeV-related syndrome.

Serology

Serologic assays can be used to detect HPeV-specific antibody responses in infected individuals. However, the time required to perform them, lack of standardization, and commercial reagents make them impractical for clinically relevant use. Therefore, they are generally restricted to use as epidemiologic research tools. Enzyme immunoassays (EIAs) using synthetic peptides derived from the capsid proteins VP0 and VP3 have been developed [51,90]. An EIA using a recombinant VP3 protein showed 96% sensitivity and 100% specificity in detecting HPeV antibodies in previously characterized sera from HPeV 1–positive adults. Antibodies to VP0 and VP1 have been useful for immunostaining of HPeV-infected cells in cell culture. The immunogenic epitope on VP3 is suited for use as an antigen in EIAs to determine seroimmunity. As with other viral infections, demonstration of either HPeV-specific IgM or a fourfold rise in HPeV IgG antibodies in paired acute and convalescent sera collected 3 to 4 weeks apart is considered indicative of acute infection. Currently available serologic assays cannot differentiate antibodies elicited by infection with different HPeV serotypes and, therefore, are unable to determine HPeV type-specific infection.

PREVENTION AND CONTROL

No vaccine is currently available for the prevention of HPeV disease. The HPeVs are spread primarily by the lack of adequate hand hygiene. Hand washing prevents their spread because their major mode of transmission is via the fecal–oral route. During nursery outbreaks, cohorting infected neonates may be effective in limiting the outbreak. For patients hospitalized with HPeV-related syndromes, infection control measures similar to those for the enteroviruses, consisting of standard precautions, are sufficient [91].

SUMMARY

The HPeVs have emerged as increasingly recognized causes of several important clinical syndromes in neonates and young infants. Understanding of their epidemiology and the ability to diagnose infections caused by these agents have been greatly improved through the development of NAATs. Although much has been learned, additional well-designed studies are necessary to better define the epidemiology and clinical syndromes associated with the HPeV and their contribution to the burden of childhood disease.

References

[1] Wigand R, Sabin AB. Properties of ECHO types 22, 23 and 24 viruses. Arch Gesamte Virusforsch 1961;11:224–47.
[2] Enteric cytopathogenic human orphan (ECHO) viruses. Science 1955;122:1187–8.
[3] Knowles NJ, Hovi T, King AMQ, et al. Overview of taxonomy. In: Ehrenfeld E, Domingo E, Roos RP, editors. The picornaviruses. Washington, DC: American Society for Microbiology Press; 2010. p. 19–32.
[4] Committee on the enteroviruses. The enteroviruses. Am J Public Health Nations Health 1957;47:1556–66.
[5] Committee on enteroviruses. Classification of human enteroviruses. Virology 1962;16: 501–4.
[6] Shaver DN, Barron AL, Karzon DT. Distinctive cytopathology of ECHO viruses type 22 and 23. Proc Soc Exp Biol Med 1961;106:648–52.
[7] Rotbart HA, Levin MJ, Villareal L. Use of subgenomic poliovirus DNA hybridization probes to detect the major subgroup of enteroviruses. J Clin Microbiol 1984;20:1105–8.
[8] Coller BA, Chapman NM, Beck MA, et al. Echovirus 22 is an atypical enterovirus. J Virol 1990;64:2692–701.
[9] Coller BG, Tracy SM, Etchison D. Cap-binding complex protein p220 is not cleaved during echovirus 22 replication in HeLa cells. J Virol 1991;65:3903–5.
[10] Hyypia T, Horsnell C, Maaronen M, et al. A distinct picornavirus group identified by sequence analysis. Proc Natl Acad Sci U S A 1992;89:8847–51.
[11] Oberste MS, Maher K, Pallansch MA. Complete sequence of echovirus 23 and its relationship to echovirus 22 and other human enteroviruses. Virus Res 1998;56:217–23.
[12] Ghazi F, Hughes PJ, Hyypia T, et al. Molecular analysis of human parechovirus type 2 (formerly echovirus 23). J Gen Virol 1998;79:2641–50.
[13] Auvinen P, Stanway G, Hyypia T. Genetic diversity of enterovirus subgroups. Arch Virol 1989;104:175–86.
[14] Picornaviridae study group. Human parechoviruses. Available at: http://www.picornastudygroup.com/types/parechovirus/hpev.htm. Accessed April 13, 2011.
[15] Jamison RM. Morphology of echovirus 22. J Virol 1969;4:904–6.
[16] Ito M, Yamashita T, Tsuzuki H, et al. Isolation and identification of a novel human parechovirus. J Gen Virol 2004;85:391–8.

[17] Abed Y, Boivin G. Molecular characterization of a Canadian human parechovirus (HPeV)-3 isolate and its relationship to other HPeVs. J Med Virol 2005;77:566–70.
[18] Al-Sunaidi M, Williams CH, Hughes PJ, et al. Analysis of a new human parechovirus allows the definition of parechovirus types and the identification of RNA structural domains. J Virol 2007;81:1013–21.
[19] Watanabe K, Oie M, Higuchi M, et al. Isolation and characterization of novel human parechovirus from clinical samples. Emerg Infect Dis 2007;13:889–95.
[20] Racaniello VR. Picornaviridae: the viruses and their replication. In: Knipe DM, Howley PM, editors. Field's virology. Philadelphia: Lippincott, Williams & Wilkins; 2007. p. 795–838.
[21] Seal LA, Jamison RM. Evidence for secondary structure within the virion RNA of echovirus 22. J Virol 1984;50:641–4.
[22] Nateri AS, Hughes PJ, Stanway G. In vivo and in vitro identification of structural and sequence elements of the human parechovirus 5′ untranslated region required for internal initiation. J Virol 2000;74:6269–77.
[23] Stanway G, Kalkkinen N, Roivainen M, et al. Molecular and biological characteristics of echovirus 22, a representative of a new picornavirus group. J Virol 1994;68:8232–8.
[24] Seitsonen J, Susi P, Heikkilä O, et al. Interaction of alphaVbeta3 and alphaVbeta6 integrins with human parechovirus 1. J Virol 2010;84:8509–19.
[25] Oberste MS, Nix WA, Maher K, et al. Improved molecular identification of enteroviruses by RT-PCR and amplicon sequencing. J Clin Virol 2003;26:375–7.
[26] Nix WA, Maher K, Pallansch MA, et al. Parechovirus typing in clinical specimens by nested or semi-nested PCR coupled with sequencing. J Clin Virol 2010;48:202–7.
[27] Abed Y, Boivin G. Human parechovirus infections in Canada. Emerg Infect Dis 2006;12: 969–75.
[28] Schultheiss T, Emerson SU, Purcell RH, et al. Polyprotein processing in echovirus 22: a first assessment. Biochem Biophys Res Commun 1995;217:1120–7.
[29] Martinez-Salas E, Ryan MD. Translation and protein processing. In: Ehrenfeld E, Domingo E, Roos RP, editors. The picornaviruses. Washington, DC: American Society for Microbiology Press; 2010. p. 141–61.
[30] Samuilova O, Krogerus C, Pöyry T, et al. Specific interaction between human parechovirus nonstructural 2A protein and viral RNA. Biol Chem 2004;279:37822–31.
[31] Krogerus C, Egger D, Samuilova O, et al. Replication complex of human parechovirus 1. J Virol 2003;77:8512–23.
[32] Krogerus C, Samuilova O, Pöyry T, et al. Intracellular localization and effects of individually expressed human parechovirus 1 non-structural proteins. J Gen Virol 2007;88: 831–41.
[33] Figueroa JP, Ashley D, King D, et al. An outbreak of acute flaccid paralysis in Jamaica associated with echovirus type 22. J Med Virol 1989;29:315–9.
[34] Ehrnst A, Eriksson M. Echovirus 23 Observed as a nosocomial infection in infants. Scand J Infect Dis 1996;28:205–6.
[35] Birenbaum E, Handsher R, Kuint J, et al. Echovirus type 22 outbreak associated with gastrointestinal disease in a neonatal intensive care unit. Am J Perinatol 1997;14:469–73.
[36] Joki-Korpela P, Hyypiä T. Diagnosis and epidemiology of echovirus 22 infections. Clin Infect Dis 1998;27:129–36.
[37] Khetsuriani N, Lamonte-Fowlkes A, Oberste S, et al. Enterovirus surveillance—United States, 1970–2005. MMWR Surveill Summ 2006;55:1–20.
[38] Tapia G, Cinek O, Witsø E, et al. Longitudinal observation of parechovirus in stool samples from Norwegian infants. J Med Virol 2008;80:1835–42.
[39] Shan TL, Guo W, Cui L, et al. The first detection of human parechovirus infections in China. J Clin Virol 2009;45:371–2.
[40] Harvala H, Robertson I, Chieochansin T, et al. Specific association of human parechovirus type 3 with sepsis and fever in young infants, as identified by direct typing of cerebrospinal fluid samples. J Infect Dis 2009;199:1753–60.

[41] Drexler JF, Grywna K, Stöcker A, et al. Novel human parechovirus from Brazil. Emerg Infect Dis 2009;15:310–3.
[42] Ito M, Yamashita T, Tsuzuki H, et al. Detection of human parechoviruses from clinical stool samples in Aichi, Japan. J Clin Microbiol 2010;48:2683–8.
[43] Boros A, Uj M, Pankovics P, et al. Detection and characterization of human parechoviruses in archived cell cultures, in Hungary. J Clin Virol 2010;47:379–81.
[44] Pham NTK, Trinh QD, Khamrin P, et al. Diversity of human parechoviruses isolated from stool samples collected from Thai children with acute gastroenteritis. J Clin Microbiol 2010;48: 115–9.
[45] Ljubin-Sternak S, Juretić E, Šantak M, et al. Clinical and molecular characterization of a parechovirus type 1 outbreak in neonates in Croatia. J Med Virol 2011;83:137–41.
[46] Centers for Disease Control and Prevention. Nonpolio enterovirus and human parechovirus surveillance—United States, 2006–2008. MMWR Morb Mortal Wkly Rep 2010;59: 1577–80.
[47] Khetsuriani N, Lamonte A, Oberste MS, et al. Neonatal enterovirus infections reported to the national enterovirus surveillance system in the United States, 1983–2003. Pediatr Infect Dis J 2006;25:889–93.
[48] Grist NR, Bell EJ, Assaad F. Enteroviruses in human disease. Prog Med Virol 1978;24: 114–57.
[49] Takao S, Shimazu Y, Fukuda S, et al. Seroepidemiological study of human parechovirus 1. Jpn J Infect Dis 2001;54:85–7.
[50] Tauriainen S, Martiskainen M, Oikarinen S, et al. Human parechovirus 1 infections in young children–no association with type 1 diabetes. J Med Virol 2007;79:457–62.
[51] Abed Y, Wolf D, Dagan R, et al. Development of a serological assay based on a synthetic peptide selected from the VP0 capsid protein for detection of human parechoviruses. J Clin Microbiol 2007;45:2037–9.
[52] Sedmak G, Nix WA, Jentzen J, et al. Infant deaths associated with human parechovirus infection in Wisconsin. Clin Infect Dis 2010;50:357–61.
[53] Benschop KS, Schinkel J, Minnaar RP, et al. Human parechovirus infections in Dutch children and the association between serotype and disease severity. Clin Infect Dis 2006;42: 204–10.
[54] Harvala H, Robertson I, McWilliam Leitch EC, et al. Epidemiology and clinical associations of human parechovirus respiratory infections. J Clin Microbiol 2008;46:3446–53.
[55] Baumgarte S, Kleber de Souza Luna L, Grywna K, et al. Prevalence, types, and RNA concentrations of human parechoviruses, including a sixth parechovirus type, in stool samples from patients with acute enteritis. J Clin Microbiol 2008;46:242–8.
[56] Verboon-Maciolek MA, Krediet TG, Gerards LJ, et al. Severe neonatal parechovirus infection and similarity with enterovirus infection. Pediatr Infect Dis J 2008;27:241–5.
[57] Wolthers KC, Benschop KS, Schinkel J, et al. Human parechoviruses as an important viral cause of sepsis like illness and meningitis in young children. Clin Infect Dis 2008;47:358–63.
[58] Yamamoto M, Abe K, Kuniyori K, et al. Epidemic of human parechovirus type 3 in Hiroshima City, Japan in 2008. Jpn J Infect Dis 2009;62:244–5.
[59] Piñeiro L, Vicente D, Montes M, et al. Human parechovirus in infants with systemic infection. J Med Virol 2010;82:1790–6.
[60] Pham NT, Takanashi S, Tran DN, et al. Human parechovirus infection in children hospitalized with acute gastroenteritis in Sri Lanka. J Clin Microbiol 2011;49:364–6.
[61] Selvarangan R, Nzabi M, Selvaraju SB, et al. Human parechovirus 3 causing sepsis-like illness in children from Midwestern United States. Pediatr Infect Dis 2011;30(3):238–42.
[62] van der Sanden S, de Bruin E, Vennema H, et al. Prevalence of human parechovirus in The Netherlands in 2000 to 2007. J Clin Virol 2008;46:2884–9.
[63] Pham NT, Chan-It W, Khamrin P, et al. Detection of human parechovirus in stool samples collected from children with acute gastroenteritis in Japan during 2007–2008. J Med Virol 2011;83:331–6.

[64] Berkovich S, Pangan J. Recoveries of virus form premature outbreaks of respiratory disease: the relation of ECHO virus type 22 to disease of the upper and lower respiratory tract in the premature infant. Bull N Y Acad Med 1968;44:377–87.
[65] Barbi Guidotti M, Cappellini D, Pedretti CC, et al. Spread of echovirus 23 in a neonatal pathology unit. Ann Sclavo 1982;24:76–84.
[66] Pajkrt D, Benschop KS, Westerhuis B, et al. Clinical characteristics of human parechoviruses 4–6 infections in young children. Pediatr Infect Dis J 2009;28:1008–10.
[67] Koskiniemi M, Paetau R, Linnavuori K. Severe encephalitis associated with disseminated echovirus 22 infection. Scand J Infect Dis 1989;21:463–6.
[68] Verboon-Maciolek MA, Groenendaal F, Hahn CD, et al. Human parechovirus causes encephalitis with white matter injury in neonates. Ann Neurol 2008;64:266–73.
[69] Levorson RE, Jantausch BA, Wiedermann BL, et al. Human parechovirus-3 infection: emerging pathogen in neonatal sepsis. Pediatr Infect Dis J 2009;28:545–7.
[70] Boivin G, Abed Y, Boucher FD. Human parechovirus 3 and neonatal infections. Emerg Infect Dis 2005;11:103–7.
[71] Legay V, Chomel JJ, Fernandez E, et al. Encephalomyelitis due to human parechovirus type 1. J Clin Virol 2002;25:193–5.
[72] Jenista JA, Powell KR, Menegus MA. Epidemiology of neonatal enterovirus infection. J Pediatr 1984;104:685–90.
[73] Modlin J. Update on enterovirus infections in infants and children. Adv Pediatr Infect Dis 1996;12:155–80.
[74] Benschop KS, Schinkel J, Luken ME, et al. Fourth human parechovirus serotype. Emerg Infect Dis 2006;12:1572–5.
[75] Abzug M. Presentation, diagnosis, and management of enterovirus infections in neonates. Paediatr Drugs 2004;6:1–10.
[76] Maller HM, Powars DF, Horowitz RE, et al. Fatal myocarditis associated with ECHO virus, type 22, infection, in a child with apparent immunological deficiency. J Pediatr 1967;71:204–10.
[77] Schnurr D, Dondero M, Holland D, et al. Characterization of echovirus 22 variants. Arch Virol 1996;141:1749–56.
[78] O'Regan S, Robitaille P, Mongeau JG, et al. The hemolytic uremic syndrome associated with ECHO 22 infection. Clin Pediatr (Phila) 1980;19:125–7.
[79] Tauriainen S, Oikarinen S, Taimen K, et al. Temporal relationship between human parechovirus 1 infection and otitis media in young children. J Infect Dis 2008;198:35–40.
[80] Oberste MS, Maher K, Pallansch MA. Specific detection of echoviruses 22 and 23 in cell culture supernatants by RT-PCR. J Med Virol 1999;58:178–81.
[81] Legay V, Chomel, Lina B. Specific RT-PCR procedure for the detection of human parechovirus type 1 genome in clinical samples. J Virol Methods 2002;102:157–60.
[82] Jokela P, Joki-Korpela P, Maaronen M, et al. Detection of human picornaviruses by multiplex reverse transcription-PCR and liquid hybridization. J Clin Microbiol 2005;43:1239–45.
[83] Corless CE, Guiver M, Borrow R, et al. Development and evaluation of a 'real-time' RT-PCR for the detection of enterovirus and parechovirus RNA in CSF and throat swab samples. J Med Virol 2002;67:555–62.
[84] Benschop K, Molenkamp R, van der Ham A, et al. Rapid detection of human parechoviruses in clinical samples by real-time PCR. J Clin Virol 2008;41:69–74.
[85] Nix WA, Maher K, Johansson ES, et al. Detection of all known parechoviruses by real-time PCR. J Clin Microbiol 2008;46:2519–24.
[86] Benschop K, Minnaar R, Koen G, et al. Detection of human enterovirus and human parechovirus (HPeV) genotypes from clinical stool samples: polymerase chain reaction and direct molecular typing, culture characteristics, and serotyping. Diagn Microbiol Infect Dis 2010;68:166–73.

[87] Noordhoek GT, Weel JF, Poelstra E, et al. Clinical validation of a new real-time PCR assay for detection of enteroviruses and parechoviruses, and implications for diagnostic procedures. J Clin Virol 2008;41:75–80.
[88] Landry ML. The molecular diagnosis of parechovirus infection: has the time come? Clin Infect Dis 2010;50:362–3.
[89] de Vries M, Pyrc K, Berkhout R, et al. Human parechovirus type 1, 3, 4, 5, and 6 detection in picornavirus cultures. J Clin Microbiol 2008;46:759–62.
[90] Alho A, Marttila J, Ilonen J, et al. Diagnostic potential of parechovirus capsid proteins. J Clin Microbiol 2003;41:2294–9.
[91] Siegel JD, Rhinehart E, Jackson M, et al. Guideline for isolation precautions: preventing transmission of infectious agents in healthcare settings 2007. Available at: www.cdc.gov/hicpac/pub.html. Accessed April 13, 2010.

Advances in Pediatrics 58 (2011) 87–111
ADVANCES IN PEDIATRICS

Care of the Foster Child: A Primer for the Pediatrician

Claudia Wang, MD[a,*], Susan B. Edelstein, LCSW[b], Lori Waldinger, MA[c], Caroline M. Lee, MA, CCC-SLP[c], Eraka Bath, MD[d]

[a]UCLA Department of Pediatrics, UCLA Suspected Child Abuse and Neglect (SCAN) Team, UCLA TIES for Families, Mattel Children's Hospital at UCLA, David Geffen School of Medicine at UCLA, 10833 Le Conte Avenue, Los Angeles, CA 90095, USA
[b]UCLA Department of Pediatrics, UCLA TIES for Families, 1000 Veteran Avenue, Box 957142, Los Angeles, CA 90095-7142, USA
[c]UCLA TIES for Families, 1000 Veteran Avenue, Box 957142, Los Angeles, CA 90095-7142, USA
[d]Child Forensic Services, UCLA Department of Psychiatry, UCLA Neuropsychiatric Institute, David Geffen School of Medicine at UCLA, 300 Medical Plaza, Room 1243, Los Angeles, CA 90095, USA

Foster care was designed to provide temporary, nurturing environments to children while their caregivers (usually birth parents) receive services to help them facilitate eventual reunification. The number of children in foster care in the United States has been steadily increasing in the past 2 decades with more than 500,000 children in care on any given day [1–3]. However, according to the US Department of Health and Human Services, Adoption and Foster Care Analysis and Reporting System (AFCARS), there has been a gradual decline in numbers since fiscal year (FY) 2007. In AFCARS Report #17, an estimated 424,000 children were in foster care in the United States on September 30, 2009. Since 2007, the number of foster children exiting the system has been greater than those entering. Overall, the number of children in foster care has declined to its lowest level since 2002, and the number of adoptions has increased to its highest level [1,4]. The recent trend has been to (1) attempt to keep children with their birth families while providing family preservation services, (2) push for more timely reunification of families, and (3) commence concurrent planning early with the aim of expediting termination of parental rights and permanency preparation in cases where reunification is not possible [5,6]. Despite this progress, there still are a large number of children in foster care who require quality health care assessments, treatment, and close monitoring.

*Corresponding author. *E-mail address*: claudiawang@mednet.ucla.edu

0065-3101/11/$ – see front matter
doi:10.1016/j.yapd.2011.03.009

Training, Intervention, Education and Services (TIES) for Families is a University of California, Los Angeles (UCLA) program consisting of a multidisciplinary team of social workers, psychologists, psychiatrists, education and speech/language consultants, and a pediatrician who use a team approach to assist the integration of children within their new foster family, school, and community. The lead author has served as the pediatric consultant on this team since its inception in 1995. Families interested in becoming foster/adoptive parents are provided psychoeducation and other services before, during, and following a child's placement into their home. This article was written by specialists on our team and provides primers for the primary care physician (PCP) focusing on the areas of health care, speech and language, education, mental health, and psychosocial functioning of the foster child.

MEDICAL FOCUS ON THE FOSTER CHILD

Environmental risk factors for the foster child

Children can be adversely affected by their environment while in utero. Maternal malnutrition and poor prenatal care (both often associated with poverty), substance abuse, intimate partner violence, and serious parental developmental disabilities and/or mental illness can all have a significant impact on the fetus, leading to an increased risk of morbidity (eg, low birth weight, preterm delivery) and mortality [2,7]. Children come to the attention of the child welfare system either shortly after birth because of prenatal substance exposure (PSE) or severe maternal developmental disability and/or mental illness, or they may present later because of abuse or neglect, often in association with these same factors [8].

The National Survey on Drug Use and Health estimates that more than 1 in 10 minors reside in homes with a substance-dependent or substance-abusing parent [9]. It is estimated that more than 400,000 infants are born in the United States each year prenatally exposed to alcohol or illicit substances [10]. Most maternal drug abuse can be categorized as polysubstance abuse. Drugs, alcohol, and tobacco use during pregnancy, especially in the first trimester, can have deleterious effects on the fetus. Research regarding the effects of drugs on the fetus is challenging because of difficulties in identifying users by self-reports; the combined effects of polysubstance use itself; unreliable estimations in the timing and dosage of drug and alcohol exposure; and variations in an individual's metabolism of substances. The impact of other prenatal high-risk factors (eg, poor prenatal care, poor nutrition) as well as the influence of genetics and postnatal environmental factors also contribute to making it impossible to predict the outcome for any particular child.

The drug with the most deleterious effects on a fetus is alcohol. The most recent estimates of the prevalence of fetal alcohol syndrome (FAS) in the United States are 2 to 7 per 1000 live births [11]. Alcohol consumed in significant quantities during the first trimester can lead to FAS. FAS is the leading cause of preventable mental retardation in the Western hemisphere [12].

This diagnosis can be elusive at times. The characteristic facial features of small eyes measured from inner to outer canthus, smooth philtrum, and thin upper lip may not be apparent in infancy. Other findings include prenatal and postnatal growth retardation, central nervous system involvement, and prenatal alcohol exposure. The spectrum of disorders can be categorized using the fetal alcohol spectrum disorders classification system [13]. Use of this classification system has shown the prevalence of FAS in the foster care population to be 10 to 15 per 1000 [14]. Even though FAS is a permanent birth defect, establishing the diagnosis early in a foster child can assist in preparing caregivers in meeting the child's needs, leading to more stability and fewer placements. A referral to a team with expertise in identification of FAS may be indicated when the diagnosis is entertained.

The early extremely negative predictions as to the future for children with PSE have not been supported by research. At birth, children with PSE may be at risk for smaller head circumferences, lower birth weights, and may be small for gestational age [15–17]. During infancy they may have sleep difficulties as well as problems with state regulation (ie, inability to remain quiet, calm, and alert). Gross and fine motor delays as well as coordination difficulties noted early have been shown to improve with interventional services with potential resolution by 18 months of age [18]. Children with PSE may be at risk for difficulties in behavior, attention, language, and learning [19]. Although longitudinal studies examining long-term outcomes for children are ongoing, initial findings show that, early on, children who have been exposed to cocaine, methamphetamines, or opiates typically have an intelligence quotient (IQ) within the normal range [15,19,20]. Potential differences do exist, but have been found to be minimal. Even though studies show some relationship between PSE and outcomes, it does not mean that every child with PSE will be affected. Additional research is needed to evaluate the impact of environmental factors as well as services on outcome. The significance of postnatal environmental influences was noted in one study in which the IQ scores of children exposed to cocaine placed in more stimulating environments were found to be similar to scores of nonexposed children [20]. The importance of protective factors and early interventional services cannot be overemphasized. In summary, there is a range of outcomes for children with PSE. A host of factors, including genetics and postnatal environment, can influence these outcomes. It is prudent that the PCPs become familiar with the special needs of this vulnerable population and submit timely referrals for early assessment and interventional services to improve the foster child's future.

Postplacement comprehensive medical care

Children placed in out-of-home care require a thorough medical assessment preceding or shortly following their first placement and any changes thereafter. The timing of this initial examination varies from state to state [21]. Many foster parents select their local community physicians for initial and ongoing health care [22]. The PCP plays a central role in caring for foster children and therefore it is imperative for them to be familiar with current guidelines for health care evaluation recommended by the Child Welfare League of America (CWLA) and American Academy of Pediatrics (AAP) [23,24] as well as those of their own state and locality. This examination is significant to ensure that (1) existing acute or chronic medical problems are identified and treated, (2) injuries and/or infections caused by physical or sexual abuse are documented and treated, (3) needed medications or medical equipment are supplied, and (4) referrals are made for urgent developmental or mental health issues.

The inability to interview birth parents, absence of records, and/or the lack of prior medical care can hinder the new PCP's assessment. Foster children can present with growth indices concerning for short stature, failure to thrive, or even obesity [25]. Assessment of these disorders relies heavily on an accurate medical history for the child as well as a complete family history. Many children in foster care are inadequately immunized [2,26], with only two-thirds of them receiving necessary immunizations while in foster care [2,27]. Poor access to health records aggravates this problem. The use of a medical passport has proved helpful in maintaining an ongoing record of the foster child's medical care [5,28]. Advocates may also use school immunization records as a source of information. If no records are located, many of these children may need to be reimmunized. Contacting the child's caseworker to seek out additional records and information from the birth parents can be beneficial.

There is an increased incidence of acute and chronic health problems for foster children [25,29]. Commonly diagnosed conditions within the foster care population include respiratory (including asthma); ear, nose and throat (including otitis media); skin; and dental issues [21,30]. Many foster children have not received routine hearing and vision screens. Deficits in these areas can affect speech and language development as well as behavioral and school functioning. A referral for a hearing screen or evaluation is also recommended as soon as any speech, language, or hearing problem is suspected [31]. Studies have shown that unidentified vision impairments plague the foster care population at rates of more than 30% [30,32]. The adolescent population seems to be at risk for these common maladies as well as tuberculosis exposure, substance abuse, sexually transmitted infections, and pregnancy [32]. The PCP should be knowledgeable about and comfortable with the needs of adolescents, including issues surrounding confidentiality and consents. At times, referral to an adolescent medicine specialist may be appropriate.

Children in foster care are at high risk for human immunodeficiency virus (HIV). Estimates reveal that up to 78% of foster children could be at risk for HIV, with only 9% tested [26]. Routes of acquisition include perinatal transmission from HIV-positive mothers, infection via sexual abuse, and, as for adolescents, secondary to their own sexual activity and drug use. Perinatal HIV infection may remain asymptomatic for years or present with mild symptoms. Studies have noted some asymptomatic carriers presenting at or beyond 4 years of age [33–35] with 1 case report of an asymptomatic 13-year-old child with perinatal HIV acquisition [36]. It is recommended by the AAP that foster care agencies attempt to obtain information regarding maternal HIV status and for all foster children to undergo an HIV risk assessment [37]. If maternal status is unknown or the child is at high risk, then testing should be pursued. Early diagnosis, placement on antiviral regimens, and close follow-up can delay symptoms. In addition to HIV, these children are at risk for transmission of hepatitis B and C, which should also be investigated.

Most children in foster care are referred because of allegations of abuse or neglect. A meticulous physical examination during the initial assessment may reveal evidence of abuse and/or neglect that not only assists investigating agencies in substantiating allegations but also safeguards the new foster home placement from false accusations. Discovery and documentation of the presence or absence of injuries at every health care visit is imperative to ensure that foster children are safe and not subjected to additional abuse by foster parents, birth parents during visitations, or by siblings (birth or foster) [38,39]. A history of sexual and physical abuse, as well as other stressors such as witnessing intimate partner violence, places children and adolescents at risk for developing sexualized behaviors as well as an increased risk of victimization and/or perpetration of sexual acts on others, especially younger children [40,41]. Inappropriate sexual behaviors should be referred for mental health evaluation and services for the child and caregivers. For a review of normal versus abnormal childhood sexualized behaviors, please refer to Kellogg [42]. Children exposed to abusive and dysfunctional home environments may also have an increased risk for long-term medical and psychosocial issues in adulthood, as noted in the Adverse Childhood Experiences (ACE) study [43].

Enuresis and encopresis, both common problems in the foster care population [29,44,45], can lead to significant distress for both caregiver and child and disruptions in placement. Children struggle with anxiety, grief, distress, as well as shame, fear of being exposed, and issues of poor self-esteem that, if unresolved, may continue into adulthood. The magnitude of family distress can lead to a lack of empathy, harsh punishments, and can be a trigger for maltreatment, sometimes fatal [38,46,47]. The incidence of enuresis for children 5 years and older in out-of-home care can be as high as 17.9% [44]. Enuresis and encopresis lacking any organic cause have been associated with psychosocial stressors (ie, abuse and neglect) [44,48], developmental delays [47], and attention-deficit/hyperactivity disorder (ADHD) [49–52], findings frequently observed within the foster care population. For the PCP, urgent evaluation, treatment, and close follow-up of foster children with these issues are critical.

Early childhood experiences can profoundly affect the development of the brain during infancy and youth [53]. Delays in one domain (ie, language) can affect other domains (ie, cognitive and social) and areas of functioning (ie, education and mental health). In FY 2009, AFCARS estimated that more than 40% of children entering foster care in the United States were less than

5 years of age [1]. It is estimated that up to 60% of children in foster care have developmental delays [30,54]. Early assessment, identification, and interventional services can help those with delays. Screening for developmental delays is the responsibility of the PCP; however, PCPs are more likely to identify and refer issues related to physical health disorders versus developmental and mental health impairments [55]. Utilization of a validated screening instrument such as the Ages and Stages Questionnaire (0–5 years) can double the detection rate of developmental problems before school entry [56]. This questionnaire can easily be completed by caregivers before their appointment and can complement the physician's office assessment and be factored in the decision of whether a more formal evaluation by a developmental specialist is necessary.

Mental health screening and referral for treatment when indicated is strongly recommended because of the prevalence of mental health issues in this population [24,25,29]. Information regarding this important area is covered later in this article.

In addition to the AAP preventative health care schedule, visits are recommended monthly up to 6 months of age, semiannually after 2 years of age, and into adolescence, as well as during periods of transitions [5,23,24].

As a final note, regarding confidentiality and consent issues surrounding foster children, the federal Health Insurance Portability and Accountability Act (HIPAA) of 1996 was enacted to protect health insurance, as well as to protect the privacy of patient health care data. In general, HIPAA regulations override state laws unless the state law is more stringent than HIPAA. For the PCP, questions as to who can provide medical consent for a foster care child, in which conditions, and to whom to release information may be confusing. HIPAA addresses issues regarding release of information of minors who are the suspected victims of child abuse and neglect [57]. All PCPs should be familiar with HIPAA regulations as well as their own state laws and the policies of their local agencies governing confidentiality. For a review, please refer to Refs. [24,57,58]. Most states prefer that birth parents retain medical consent [59]. However, in controversial situations, it is prudent for the PCP to clarify who holds the right for medical consent by consulting with legal counsel and the child's caseworker.

COMMUNICATION SKILLS AND THE FOSTER CHILD

Developmental delays, including speech and language delays, are common among children who enter foster care. The rate of speech and/or language impairment in this population is 12.25% [60], twice the rate of speech-language impairments in the general pediatric population, which is 6.34% [61]. These numbers exclude children who present with a communication disorder secondary to primary developmental disabilities, such as mental retardation, autism, and sensory impairments, such as hearing loss. A review of the literature by CWLA in 2006 noted that the estimated prevalence of language delays amongst foster children is even higher; from 35% to 73% [62]. Despite the CWLA and AAP guidelines, 43.2% of children in foster care are not receiving developmental assessments at intake [22]. Given the high rate of communication disorders in children in foster care and the negative impact that these disorders have on their social and learning outcomes, PCPs need to be aware of how communication disorders are identified so that timely assessments and interventional services are provided.

Speech disorders

Speech disorders in a child include the areas of articulation (eg, speech sound substitution errors), fluency (eg, stuttering), and voice (eg, hypernasal voice). They may be developmental (eg, mental retardation) or acquired (eg, stroke) [63]. The prevalence of articulation delays in the general population is estimated to be 3.8% for children aged 6 years [63]. There are currently no prevalence estimates of articulation delays for foster children. Risk factors for articulation delays and disorders may include significantly less than normal intelligence, male gender, socioeconomic disadvantage, lower birth order/sibling status, delayed language development, delayed motor skills, poor auditory discrimination, hearing loss, and oral-facial structural anomalies [64]. We are most concerned about children who present with multiple speech sound errors and poor speech clarity. Children with poor articulation skills and intelligibility should be referred for speech, as well as language, testing to rule out receptive and expressive language delays, because poor speech intelligibility may mask delays in language development. Approximately 11% to 15% of children with articulation delays have a comorbid diagnosis of a language delay [63].

Language disorders

Language disorders are divided into receptive language disorders, expressive language disorders, and pragmatic language disorders. Difficulty understanding spoken language is a receptive language disorder. Difficulty using a spoken language system is an expressive language disorder. A pragmatic language disorder reflects difficulties coordinating verbal (eg, auditory comprehension and expressive skills) and nonverbal (eg, use of gestures, eye contact, facial expression) language skills for social interaction.

Screening for language delays

The rate of language-only impairments (specific language impairment) in the foster care population is reportedly a little more than 15% [65], whereas specific language impairment in the general pediatric population is 7.40% [66]. Studies have documented that both parents and medical professionals often rely on expressive language delays to identify language impairments. Concerns for delay typically arise if there are no verbalizations by age 1 years, or if speech or language is different from that of other children the same age [67]. Cohen and colleagues [68] studied unsuspected language impairment in children from psychiatric outpatient populations and found that, of 288 children referred solely for a psychiatric disorder, 99 (34.4%) had a language impairment that was not identified until a routine systematic assessment had been completed. Although this study did not directly address children in foster care, it is relevant to this population because a significant number of children entering foster care have emotional and behavioral health problems, with estimates ranging from 35% to 50% [22]. Therefore, when screening the foster child for possible language disorders, it is important to remember that (1) a high percentage of children with mental health disorders also have language disorders, (2) mixed receptive-expressive language and receptive-language–only delays are more common than expressive-language–only delays, and (3) their language impairments are often missed because they are more difficult to discern by adults or are overshadowed by more salient externalizing behavior problems (such as symptoms of delinquency and aggression) [68].

Although children continue to develop their vocabulary skills and more complex sentence forms in the school years, most children have acquired the basic forms and functions of language by 5 or 6 years of age, an accomplishment that has led some researchers to believe that language development is essentially complete by school entry [64,69].

The following findings in young children are never normal:

- Lack of gesture use, such as, pointing, waving, and showing behaviors, at 12 months
- Inconsistent response to name (12 months and older)
- Poor vocal and social imitative play (18 months)
- Less than 50 words, and no 2-word combinations at 2 years old
- Does not show objects (12 months), make comments to share what is seen (24 months), or share thoughts and personal experiences frequently and spontaneously (3 years and older)
- Does not respond to yes/no questions (2 years), accurately (3 years and older)
- Does not answer who, what, where, when questions directly and/or accurately (4 years and older).

Inconsistent language stimulation and exposure

Children in foster care may be at risk for inconsistent language stimulation and may be exposed to multiple languages, both of which may affect normal language acquisition and/or development. Children who enter foster care tend to come from minority groups and impoverished backgrounds [70]. They have been separated from their families and are frequently placed with caregivers of different cultural backgrounds. The language used in their foster home might be different from that of their biologic home. Given the changes and stresses of removal, separation, new rules, and possibly a new language, it is common for the foster child to present with developmental regression [71]. Therefore, when screening for language delays in young children who have been newly placed in foster care, the screening guidelines mentioned earlier apply. A wait-and-see approach should only be taken if the child is not talking and does not show any other problems in the areas of auditory comprehension, social interaction, behavior, attention, or development. Such a child needs to be rescreened and referred for a comprehensive evaluation of speech and language if delays persist.

For bilingual language exposure, children who are exposed to multiple languages are not normally delayed in their acquisition of language. When a child is in an environment in which more than 1 language is used, the child is expected to develop multiple linguistic systems and become proficient in the language, or languages, that they use most. Children who are exposed to 2 languages at the same time before the age of 3 years are expected to acquire both languages at the same rate [72]. There are some variations to consider: language structure variations are normal (ie, the child transfers the language structure of one language for use in another language) and vocabulary is counted as if it were 1 language (ie, a Spanish-English 2-year-old speaker is expected to have a total of 50 English and Spanish words). For the child who was speaking 1 language and then introduced to a second language later in life, the first language is expected to develop dominance and reach language milestones per age expectation. Ideally, the use of the child's first language is maintained and reinforced while the second language is being introduced and developed. If the first language is not reinforced, there could be a loss of language that can be detrimental and frustrating for a child [73]. The child who exhibits delays in the acquisition of the dominant language or both languages likely has a language delay. It is recommended that this child be referred for a speech-language evaluation, and helped to develop a firm language base in the dominant language before a second language is introduced [72].

Abuse and neglect

The most common reason for a child's placement in foster care is neglect (44%), followed by abuse (13%) [70,71]. Culp and colleagues [74] studied the effects of different forms of maltreatment on speech and language development and found that child neglect was the form of maltreatment most detrimental to the development of both receptive and expressive language skills. Their findings showed that neglected children were delayed by 6 to 9 months and abused children were delayed by 0 to 2 months compared with normative expectations. The linguistic skills of children who had experienced both abuse and neglect were at a level between the abused group and the neglected group on measures of language ability.

The consensus amongst researchers is that there is an association between neglect and language delays that may be attributed to a general lack of stimulation within the child's environment. It is believed that abused children show comparatively minimal language delays because language development is particularly vulnerable to disruption in parent-child interaction, and that the verbal negotiation that may occur in abusive parent-child relationships protects linguistic growth in a way that a neglecting environment does not [74]. Therefore, when screening and referring maltreated children to rule out language delays, it is important to remember that child neglect is significantly more detrimental to language development than is child abuse.

Prenatal alcohol and drug exposure

It is estimated that nearly 80% of children in foster care are prenatally exposed to alcohol and/or other drugs [75]. PSE may be associated with subtle (or not so subtle) neurobehavioral impairments (ie, attention), which may in turn disrupt an infant's ability to extract, process, or use linguistic information. Second, drug and/or alcohol abuse by parent(s) may cause impairments that may disrupt a parent's ability to initiate and sustain the affective, social, and linguistic interaction with the infant that is critical to normal development. Third, in the child welfare system families in which parents use drugs are likely to be poor, homeless, and unstable, conditions that potentially result in an impoverished social-linguistic environment, which has a negative impacts on language growth and development [76–78].

The effects of prenatal alcohol exposure on language development are well documented. Studies have shown that children exposed to large amounts of alcohol in utero display communication deficits on measures of word comprehension, naming ability, grammar, pragmatics, and verbal learning, whether or not they present with characteristics of FAS [79–81]. Recent longitudinal prospective research on prenatal cocaine exposure and its effect on language supports the possibility that prenatal cocaine exposure is associated with subtle but stable negative effects on speech and language development during early childhood [82–84]. Children with prenatal cocaine exposure were more likely than controls to have mild receptive language delays and poorer expressive language abilities [83]. With increasing severity of prenatal cocaine exposure was an incremental decrement in expressive language function [84]. Further decrements in language function were found if the fetus was additionally exposed to alcohol [82], marijuana [83], or tobacco [83]. Language scores in children who were prenatally exposed to cocaine as well as controls also declined with time, suggesting that factors that were common to both groups, including low socioeconomic status, education, and poverty also have negative impacts on language development [83]. The quality and quantity of stimulation and support available to a child in the home environment and maternal vocabulary scores are positively related to child language outcomes in children who were cocaine exposed prenatally [83]. Therefore, although children placed in foster care tended to be more heavily exposed to cocaine prenatally than exposed children who remained in relative or maternal care, their language skills were found to be better at age 4 years than their counterparts who remained in the care of birth families, possibly because of a more stimulating environment for language development as shown by the higher Home Observation of the Environment (HOME) scores and verbal IQ scores of the adoptive-foster mothers [83]. Therefore, it is recommended that children who have confirmed exposure be thoroughly screened, and those with suspected delays be referred for further testing to confirm the presence of language delays as soon as possible, so that they be able to receive treatment and services accordingly.

EDUCATIONAL ADVOCACY

Research indicates that foster children are less likely to perform at or better than grade level compared with their peers in the general population. Up to 55% of foster youth fail to obtain a high school diploma or acquire a General Education Diploma (GED), which affects their chances for success when transitioning out of foster care and seeking employment [85]. Negative educational impacts can be traced to a foster child's early lack of fulfillment of basic needs (food, clothing, shelter, stimulation, and consistent parenting), multiple placement and school changes, higher rate of absenteeism, lack of a consistent advocate, numerous profound losses with resulting emotional problems, and the stigma and loneliness children often perceive related to their status as a foster child [86]. The PCP is in a prime position to identify potential factors that could negatively affect a child's educational performance and to provide assistance to the caregiver on ways to promote better educational outcomes [87].

Children with established educational delays and those at risk for such delays because of the existence of a disability or developmental vulnerability have better educational outcomes if their needs are addressed as early as possible through early intervention services. Misdiagnoses and lack of genetic and educational background information are commonplace, but it is essential that PCPs acquire family, developmental, and educational histories that are as thorough as possible to make appropriate recommendations. PCPs should screen all foster children at the earliest possible age for potential developmental and learning disabilities. PCPs can identify and make appropriate referrals for conditions such as a learning disability, ADHD, or speech and language impediments that may have gone undetected and that could potentially affect the child's future educational progress. If those conditions adversely interfere with the child's educational progress, they could qualify a child for special education services [88]. In accordance with federal law, each state has developed a definition of those conditions and identifies which agency in the state is classified as the lead agency for infants and toddlers between the ages of birth and 3 years. In addition, many states have included as eligible for early intervention services children who are identified as at risk for certain conditions, such as those children who show developmental delays in the general areas of speech and language, large and fine motor skills, social and emotional behavior, and cognitive and/or adaptive skills, or who have vision or hearing losses [89].

Public schools have a federal requirement to seek out and serve students between the ages of birth and 21 years with suspected disabilities. Congress has enacted laws that mandate the educational rights of children with disabilities to ensure that they receive a free appropriate public education. The Federal Individuals with Disabilities Education Improvement Act (IDEIA) requires school districts and all educational agencies to protect the rights of disabled children. IDEIA defines eligibility for children who are within 1 or more of the following disability categories and who require special education and related services to make educational progress.

The following categories are disabilities that may qualify a child for special services if the disability negatively affects the child's education [89]:

1. Autism
2. Other health impaired (OHI): the child exhibits limited strength, vitality, and alertness because of acute or chronic health problems including, but not limited to, ADHD, asthma, cancer, cardiac condition, diabetes, epilepsy, hemophilia, lead poisoning, leukemia, nephritis, rheumatic fever, sickle cell anemia, and Tourette syndrome. The list of acute or chronic health conditions is not exhaustive, but provides examples of problems that could make children eligible if their medical conditions adversely affect their educational performance
3. Intellectual disability (formerly mental retardation): defined as significantly less than average general functioning with deficits in adaptive behavior
4. Emotional disturbance (ED)
5. Deafness
6. Hearing impairment
7. Visual impairment
8. Deaf-blindness
9. Specific learning disability (SLD)
10. Multiple disabilities: the child exhibits 2 or more severe disabilities, 1 of which is intellectual disability
11. Orthopedic impairment: displays severe impairments that are the result of congenital anomaly, developmental, or other causes (such as cerebral palsy) that negatively affect the child's education
12. Speech or language impairment: exhibits a communication disorder, such as stuttering, impaired articulation, or a receptive and/or expressive language disorder
13. Traumatic brain injury: the child has an external injury to his/her brain resulting in total or partial functional disability. The term does not apply to brain injuries that are congenital or degenerative, or to brain injuries induced by birth trauma, because these students may qualify for special education services in the Other Health Impairment category
14. Development disability: a delay in 1 or more of the following areas: physical development, cognitive development, communication, social or emotional development, or adaptive [behavioral] development.

PCPs are in a position to support and collaborate with caregivers and school staff regarding a student's medical condition. Chronic health conditions or disabilities can interfere with school attendance, participation, and achievement. Many students with stable conditions such as ADHD or mild intermittent asthma may require basic school nursing services, such as health care monitoring or medication administration. Advanced medical technology in conjunction with legislation (IDEIA mandates), has allowed a greater number of students with medical needs to attend school. Services once believed to be clearly outside the responsibility of schools are now legally mandated by state and federal statutes for all children who require these services. Schools should be able to assist with managing more complex medical regimens and/or treatments (eg, tracheostomy suctioning) to meet the child's health-related needs.

Medical equipment and devices allow more students to attend their neighborhood schools who previously were home or institutional-bound. PCPs can assist the school by providing comprehensive medical information as well as guidelines regarding the need for medical procedures or treatment during the school day. By identifying the criteria that could qualify a child for special education services, PCPs can support caregivers by writing letters to school districts stating their findings and offering recommendations. Supporting caregivers while they navigate through the public school educational bureaucracy is critical in ensuring that the child receives the appropriate services.

PCPs can monitor a child's achievement trajectory during the annual medical check-up with discussions regarding overall school and behavioral functioning. If academic progress has been limited, the caregivers can be encouraged to request that the school district evaluate their child's eligibility for special education services. Caregivers are allowed to request educational evaluations if they are the holder of the child's educational rights. More often than not, educational rights are held by the birth parents. The formal appointment of an educational rights holder is often overlooked for youth who have experienced multiple placements and educational disruptions. The child's educational rights holder is responsible for securing the support and resources needed by a struggling student. If a foster child is having academic difficulties, the PCP can inquire whether the student has an educational advocate and ensure that this person is aware of any medical implications and barriers to academic success. If a birth parent is unavailable, school districts have a legal responsibility to appoint a surrogate parent for the student to ensure that the student's educational rights are protected [90].

Caregivers have the right to inspect and get copies of their foster child's educational records, including securing any new assessment data that are being generated for an upcoming individualized education program (IEP) meeting. When a student is found to be eligible for special education services, an IEP team meets to develop an educational plan based on the child's specific needs. The team includes the child's caregivers, teachers, and other personnel responsible for implementing the IEP. The IEP is a written document that describes any accommodations, modifications, or related services a student needs to receive an appropriate education. It also lists goals and objectives that are used to measure a student's progress and determine whether the program and placement are appropriate. Federal law provides that, before any initial IEP meeting (and at 3-year evaluations), students be assessed in their native language in all areas related to their suspected disability. If necessary, the school staff is required to provide interpretive services at IEP meetings so that caregivers can fully participate and be informed of the school's findings. PCPs can give input before the IEP assessment by providing information of any health-related issues that might adversely affect the IEP assessment, such as a diagnosis of ADHD or medication side-effects, as well as addressing any restrictions or recommendations regarding their patient's medical needs.

PCPs are in a position to make educational recommendations for their patients based on their expertise and knowledge of the patient. Suggesting intensive reading programs, summer school, and more direct instruction (teacher to student) have been effective in assisting children with educational difficulties. Tutoring, well-designed homework activities, and after school programs have also been shown to be beneficial for students struggling in school. PCPs can also contribute to the grade retention debate. Caregivers may seek out their PCP to advise whether grade retention would benefit their child. Despite evidence indicating that grade retention alone does not close the achievement gap for many foster youth, it may be beneficial in certain cases. Developmental and medical information can be factored in the decision-making process. A child with behavioral problems, developmental and academic delays, along with a height-age at the lower percentiles may benefit from repeating a grade. Some students simply need an additional year to achieve more physical, academic, and psychological development. For others, implementing an additional year of educational interventions, along with a coordinated system of comprehensive support and services designed to address the child's academic, socioemotional, behavioral, and psychological needs, may serve to promote a healthy adjustment and educational achievement.

PCPs are encouraged to take an active role in assisting the school in understanding the medical needs of foster children and the implications of the medical conditions or disabilities on their education. Supportive PCPs can encourage foster parents to become active participants in shaping the education for their foster child, promoting linkages with the school and community, and encouraging realistic, but high, educational expectations for foster youth.

MENTAL HEALTH CARE

One of the most critical and challenging of the health disparities faced by children in the child welfare system is in the area of mental health. It is estimated that 50% of children in the child welfare system have mental health needs, a rate that is higher than the national average of 1 out of 7 [91,92]. Equally concerning is that the children in the child welfare system are disproportionately from minority and low socioeconomic backgrounds [93,94]. The PCP can play an important role in the recognition and management of the mental health needs of these vulnerable youth by providing and referring for much-needed prevention and early intervention services. Because of the shortage of child psychiatrists, PCPs are often the first and only clinical contact for many children.

The multiple insults of maltreatment, family risk factors, frequent placement changes, and severe emotional and behavioral problems underscore a critical need for clinical attention to this special population of children in the child welfare system. National estimates suggest that children in child welfare settings are receiving psychotropic medications at a rate between 2 and 3 times that of children treated in the community [95]. This estimate of increased psychotropic medication use in a landscape that is already known to be chaotic and poorly coordinated further mandates that continuity of care should be emphasized and formalized.

The AAP has recently highlighted the importance of increasing the competence of PCPs in the area of child mental health given the dearth of child psychiatrists [96]. Foster youth are an especially multimorbid population with significant needs and high service utilization often persisting into adulthood. One study found that more than half (54.4%) of adults placed in foster care as children had experienced at least 1 psychiatric symptom within the preceding 12-month period, and that 25% had significant posttraumatic stress disorder (PTSD) symptoms, a rate nearly double that of US war veterans [97,98]. However, 75% of youth in the child welfare system who meet stringent diagnostic criteria often do not receive mental health care within 12 months of a child abuse and neglect investigation [92,98]. The most common disorders for foster youth are anxiety disorders (including PTSD and generalized anxiety disorder), disruptive behavior disorders (including oppositional defiant disorder [ODD], conduct disorder [CD], and ADHD), depression, learning problems, and substance abuse [99,100]. Many of these disorders occur in the setting of other biologic and environmental stressors, such as in utero exposure to substances and profound abuse and neglect. Comorbidity of these disorders tends to be the rule and not the exception, with many youth having impairment in socioemotional and academic functioning that affects their ability to have stability in their placements.

Children within the child welfare system may be subjected to trauma before entry (ie, neglect; physical, sexual, and/or emotional abuse; intimate partner violence within a dysfunctional household), on entry (ie, separation and attachment disruption) as well as during placements. PTSD symptoms may manifest in various ways according to age. Infants tend to be in placements longer, have higher rates of reentry into foster care, and may be sensitive to disrupted attachments [101]. They may experience sleeping and feeding difficulties, fearfulness, and irritability, which can be manifestations of many conditions including PTSD. Older children may display aggression, impulsivity, and sexualized behaviors, which can be a manifestation of many conditions including PTSD, ADHD, and/or sexual abuse. PTSD behaviors are stressful and can lead to disrupted placements. A careful history and evaluation may help the clinician assess whether PTSD is contributing to the foster child's symptoms.

To fully comprehend the socioemotional issues confronting foster youth, it is important to understand the potential long-term consequences of exposure to various types of maltreatment. The ACE study has brought to attention the potential cumulative effect of childhood exposure to abuse (ie, emotional, physical, and sexual abuse) and household dysfunction (ie, parental substance abuse, mental illness, incarceration, domestic violence, separation, or divorce) on future medical and psychosocial problems such as illicit drug use, depressive disorders, and attempted suicide [43,102–104]. Detection of an adverse childhood risk factor can alert the PCP to investigate for additional risk factors, which can lead to earlier recognition, intervention, and provision of support and therapeutic services. Although PCPs may not be able to provide comprehensive mental health services for foster youth, they have an important role in the identification and referral process during the course of well-child visits and other interfaces in which caseworkers may seek medical clearance for youth before or shortly following placement. During the often rushed preplacement and postplacement assessment process, many youth are only seeing the PCP and not a psychiatrist, making this interface an essential point of contact for identifying underlying mental health issues. Establishing collaborative relationships with qualified mental health specialists with expertise in this population is critical for consultation as well as referral.

The 2009 CWLA guidelines recommend that mental health screenings occur at various intervals, with the first occurring within the first 72 hours of placement to triage for acute and immediate risk following entry. This initial evaluation is critical for early identification of youth presenting with immediate risk of harm to themselves or others, who are running away, or who are in need of mental health or substance abuse services. Additional objectives are to ascertain the child's ability to function in various settings (eg, school, home, peer groups, community) [99]. If an acute risk is identified, the child should have an immediate referral to a qualified mental health provider. The acuity of the situation determines the level of care and treatment setting (eg, urgent care or outpatient setting).

The next evaluation should occur within 30 days of entry to the foster care system and should include evaluation of overall functioning and identification of children who may need ongoing services. CWLA recommends that this screening should be brief, low in cost, and simple [99]. These qualities enhance the likelihood for the screening to become part of the PCP's routine care for foster youth. Youth who have a positive screen should be referred and linked to specialty mental health services for a comprehensive mental health assessment. Given the vulnerability of children in the child welfare system and the potential for these children to be retraumatized, the American Academy of Child and Adolescent Psychiatry (AACAP), CWLA, and AAP [96,99,101] recommend ongoing periodic mental health screening and assessments whether or not they are currently receiving mental health services [99].

Even for the experienced practitioner, evaluation for emotional and behavioral problems in young children can be challenging. In addition to the PCP's face-to-face evaluation, utilization of validated screening tools can complement the general office assessment and assist in the decision-making process of referring for more specialized evaluations and interventions. The screening instrument should be easy to administer, score, and interpret for feasibility in a busy office setting. Caregivers should be able to fill out the questionnaire in a short period of time with the ease of scoring by any paraprofessional. For a listing of mental health assessment tools please refer to Ref. [105]. The following are a few examples of validated mental health screening and assessment tools that can be selected. Similar to the Ages and Stages Questionnaire (ASQ) used to screen for developmental delays, the ASQ-SE (social-emotional) tool for ages 6 to 60 months is simple to use and available in both English and Spanish. The Pediatric Symptom Checklist-35 items (PSC-35) for 4-year-olds to 16-year-olds, and the Strengths and Difficulties Questionnaire (SDQ) for 3-year-olds to 17-year-olds both screen for psychosocial problems as well as functional assessment in the area of attention. Both are available in various languages and are freely accessible. Identification of children at risk for depression can be difficult. Use of a screening tool prescored by the office staff could increase the PCP's awareness that an in-depth, sensitive interview is required during the immediate visit. An example of a depression screening tool is the Child Depression Inventory (CDI) screen, appropriate for 7-year-olds to 17-year-olds, and available in both English and Spanish [105]. Children exhibiting symptoms of significant depression with complaints of insomnia, loss of appetite, inability to function with daily activities of living definitely require urgent referral to a psychiatrist, as do those who have suicidal ideation with or without developed plans.

Disruptive behavior disorders represent a cluster of disorders that include ODD, CD, and ADHD. ADHD is a common childhood disorder affecting between 5% and 10% of school-aged children [100] and is seen more frequently among foster youth because many of them have histories of biologic and environmental risk factors. The Conner's Behavioral Checklist, which can help differentiate between the disruptive behavior disorders, is a useful screening inventory that can be sent to school to be completed by teachers.

Although some PCPs may be comfortable treating some of the more common psychiatric diagnoses, (eg, uncomplicated ADHD), given the multimorbid characteristics of the foster youth, it is recommended that those who have positive screenings receive a comprehensive mental health assessment conducted by a qualified mental health provider. In some cases it may be helpful to include the mental health provider as part of a multidisciplinary team that provides a comprehensive assessment including medical, dental, and developmental evaluations. PCPs who are not working as part of a multidisciplinary team need to collaborate with mental health partners in their community. It is critical for the PCP to use the child's caseworker and/or the agency as a source of collateral information and a partner to facilitate the referral and linkage process.

Because of the significant prevalence of mental health disorders in the foster care population, many child welfare agencies have adopted the philosophy that addressing the well-being of these children requires multimodal service plans that require partnership and collaboration with mental health partners. The pediatric provider is a key component in this process.

PSYCHOSOCIAL ISSUES

A little extra understanding and sensitivity on the part of clinicians to the unique needs of foster children and caregivers can make a big difference. The following are important areas to keep in mind and are ways of expressing your understanding of their situation.

Be sensitive to issues of loss, vulnerability, lack of control, and anxiety about the future, which are the Achilles' heels of children in foster care. Be aware that many situations that seem unrelated to a child's separation from birth parents or change in placement may trigger these uncomfortable feelings. For example, a change in teachers or schools or the loss of a pet can elicit a major emotional reaction that, in turn, can exacerbate a medical condition such as asthma. A foster child may view a hospitalization as a repeat of the abandonment by his birth family or other caregivers. Because so many foster children have low self-esteem, excessive guilt, and believe they are to blame for their situation, they may view a painful medical procedure or a hospitalization as a form of punishment. Being cognizant of these possible connections can allow the PCP to help the child and foster parents to understand the context of the child's reactions and possible manifestations of grief and loss, thereby normalizing their feelings and behaviors. Providing as much anticipatory guidance and preparing the child for medical procedures and hospitalizations with their input to the greatest extent possible helps to increase their feelings of control. Giving extra reassurance to the child that it is normal to be frightened and that they will be returning to their caregiver may help alleviate many fears.

The PCP can help caregivers understand that behaviors such as cursing, hitting, sulking, and regression in toilet training may appear during transitions that are critical periods of vulnerability as well as an opportunity for the child and new caregivers. These behaviors can be interpreted to the foster parent as normal child development in these situations. If a child's behaviors are challenging, referring for immediate intervention can help prevent escalation. Pathologizing the child's behaviors and misattributions is less likely to occur with supportive interpretations and interventions. The PCP can explain these facts to foster parents with the reassurance that, with time, consistent parenting, and appropriate mental health transition services, these behaviors are likely to diminish. Diagnosing and/or medicating a child or taking a child off psychotropic medication during transitions may be inappropriate. In the same way, visits with birth parents may evoke loyalty conflicts in the children and result in the manifestation of difficult behaviors, even exacerbation of the child's medical problems. Unless there is suspected child abuse or neglect or fear of serious harm to the child, these visits need to continue as part of the family reunification plan. Foster parents often request that the PCP write a letter to the court stating that these visits be discontinued, but caution should be exercised.

Be aware of the model of cumulative risk; that it is not any single risk factor, but the number of adverse risk factors in a child's environment that interact with one another to affect the development and behavior of children. Although foster parents cannot change certain risk factors (eg, mental illness and substance abuse of birth parents, a child's PSE, multiple past placements and/or abuse), they can be a source of protective factors for the child. They can ensure that the child receives coordinated and comprehensive medical and mental health care, consistent and nurturing care from them, and that the child's school situation is stabilized. These protective factors can interrupt the negative trajectory so often experienced by foster children. Be careful about what you say to foster parents, children's caseworkers, and school personnel, as well as what you write, because both follow the child. If you suspect a diagnosis such as FAS, ADHD, or autism, refer to specialists if you cannot rule out these diagnoses yourself. Avoid making dire predictions about the outcomes for the child based on 1 risk factor such as PSE, because not only is such a prediction inaccurate, it makes foster parents feel helpless instead of focusing on positive interventions. Using correct terminology (ie, birth parent vs real parent, children with PSE instead of drug babies) is less stigmatizing and is respectful of the child, birth parent, and foster/adoptive parent.

The foster parent

Many of the parents fostering and adopting are single parents, parents accepting transracial placements, and/or parents who are gay and lesbian, either as singles or couples. Some of the foster children themselves are lesbian, gay, bisexual, transsexual, or questioning. There are issues unique to these populations, and it is important to be familiar with them. It is also important to respect these nontraditional forms of families, and to focus on their strengths and parenting. If a PCP is uncomfortable with the family's lifestyle, then the best approach is to refer to a colleague who is willing, comfortable, and knowledgeable.

The unique and changing role of foster parents and the related stresses are often not given sufficient attention by providers, including PCPs. Foster parents traditionally have had to deal, with minimal supports, with their ambiguous and often temporary role in the child's life, as well as frequent intrusion by agency representatives. The foster family's grief reactions when a child is reunified or replaced are not given the necessary attention [106]. Concurrent planning, wherein the foster parent makes a commitment to adopt if family reunification is not successful, now poses additional challenges because so many of these families are interested in adopting, but reluctantly decide to foster as an avenue to becoming parents. If a child is reunified, the foster parents' grief may be magnified by their thwarted goal of adoption as well as prior losses such as the inability to have a birth child. Even in a brief visit, the PCP can help recognize and normalize the grieving process of foster parents and also validate the critical service they are providing to the child and the community [107]. Referrals for counseling can be made when the grief is extended; negatively affects the child and foster parent's mental and physical health and the ability of the foster parent to wish the children well as they leave; and if the foster parent's ability to attach to a subsequent placed child is impaired.

Most foster parents try hard to provide the children in their care with loving, consistent substitute parenting. However, there are always exceptions: foster parents who are indifferent, unresponsive, fail to follow through on medical appointments, abusive, mentally ill, and/or addicted. Although it is not possible for the PCP to do a comprehensive assessment of the caregiving environment, clues that there are significant problems that could be affecting the child need exploration and follow-up. Contacting the child's caseworker, referring to community resources such as public health nurses, and having the child in for more frequent follow-up are ways to provide a safety net for the foster child. However, if abuse or neglect is suspected, a child abuse report is mandated.

Cultural sensitivity

The PCP should be aware of the importance of cultural issues in approaching, assessing, and treating foster children and their caregivers. For example, there may be differences in how health and mental health treatment are viewed, how much and what kinds of information are communicated or considered private, and the ways discipline is administered. Issues related to culture and socioeconomic status enter into every aspect of life of the foster child (eg, the age at which they are toilet trained, the languages they speak, how education is viewed and educators approached). Frequently, the children may be of different cultures, races, ethnicities, socioeconomic status, and religions than the caregiver, posing some unique challenges. Although PCPs can be familiar with a variety of cultural practices and values, each family is different, and a PCP cannot become an expert about every culture. What is critical is that a PCP shows interest in and inquires nonjudgmentally about the different values and beliefs of a child and/or caregiver when an issue is affecting the child's health and functioning. The family members can then explain their viewpoints and ways of life, feel understood, and this information can be integrated into the assessment and treatment planning.

SUMMARY

Raising a foster child can be complex because of the myriad of challenges these youth present and the daunting bureaucracies the caregivers must navigate to secure appropriate services for their children. The PCP can be an important protective factor for the foster child and can provide a safety net of evaluations, services, follow-up, and referrals for specialized interventions. PCPs must take part in enrolling foster children within their busy practices even though providing care to them may be challenging and the reimbursements cannot begin to compensate for the time and effort involved. PCPs must attend to the children's needs and advocate for services within a system in which many of the children are subjected to frequent moves; changes in health care providers, teachers, and caseworkers; and lack any sustaining adult figures to stand by them while they go through this unfamiliar and frightening journey. PCPs can encourage foster parents to become active participants in shaping the development, education, and psychosocial growth for their foster child. A supportive health care provider can be a positive influence on a foster child's resiliency and future.

References

[1] The Adoption and Foster Care Reporting and Analysis System (AFCARS) Reports #10–17. Available at: http://www.acf.hhs.gov/programs/cb/stats_research/index.htm#afcars. Accessed November 17, 2010.
[2] Szilagyi M. The pediatrician and the child in foster care. Pediatr Rev 1998;19:39–50.

[3] US House of Representatives, Subcommittee on Children, Youth and Families. No place to call home: discarded children in America. Washington, DC: US Government Printing Office; 1989.
[4] The Adoption and Foster Care Reporting and Analysis System (AFCARS) Report. Trends in foster care and adoption FY 2002-FY 2009. Available at: http://www.acf.hhs.gov/programs/cb/stats_research/afcars/trends.htm. Accessed November 17, 2010.
[5] American Academy of Pediatrics. Committee on early childhood, adoption, and dependent care: health care of young children in foster care. Pediatrics 2002;109(3):536–41.
[6] The Adoption Assistance Child Welfare Act. Pub L No. 96–272 (1980). Available at: http://www.childwelfare.gov/systemwide/laws_policies/federal/index.cfm. Accessed January 21, 2011.
[7] Curtis PA, Dale G Jr, Kendall JC, editors. The foster care crisis: translating research into policy and practice. Lincoln (NE): University of Nebraska Press; 1999.
[8] US General Accounting Office. Parental substance abuse: implications for children, the child welfare system, and foster care outcomes. Washington, DC: GAO/Health, Education, and Human Services Division; 1997. p. 1–12.
[9] The NSDUH Report: children living with substance-dependent or substance-abusing parents: 2002 to 2007. Rockville (MD); 2009. Available at: http://store.samhsa.gov/product/NSDUH09-0416. Accessed November 17, 2010.
[10] Substance Abuse and Mental Health Services Administration (SAMHSA) Substance-Exposed Infants: state responses to the problem 2009;9–14. Available at: http://store.samhsa.gov/product/SMA09-4369. Accessed on November 17, 2010.
[11] May PA, Gossage JP, Kalberg W, et al. Prevalence and epidemiologic characteristics of FASD from various research methods with an emphasis on recent in-school studies. Dev Disabil Res Rev 2009;15:176–92.
[12] Abel EL, Sokol RJ. Incidence of fetal alcohol syndrome and economic impact of FAS–related anomalies. Drug Alcohol Depend 1987;19:51–70.
[13] Astley SJ. Diagnostic guide for fetal alcohol spectrum disorders: the 4-digit diagnostic code. 3rd edition. Seattle (WA): University of Washington; 2004. Available at: http://www.fasdpn.org. Accessed November 17, 2010.
[14] Astley SJ, Stachowiak J, Clarren SK, et al. Application of the FAS facial photographic screening and tool in a foster care population. J Pediatr 2002;141:712–7.
[15] Lester B, Lagasse L, Seifer R. Cocaine exposure and children. The meaning of subtle effects. Science 1998;282(5389):633–4.
[16] Bada H, Das A, Bauer C, et al. Low birth weight and preterm births: etiologic fraction attributable to prenatal drug exposure. J Perinatol 2005;25:631–7.
[17] Nguyen D, Smith L, LaGasse L, et al. Intrauterine growth of infants exposed to prenatal methamphetamine: results from the infant development, environment and lifestyle study. J Pediatr 2010;157:337–9.
[18] Miller-Loncar C, Lester B, Seifer R, et al. Predictors of motor development in children prenatally exposed to cocaine. Neurotoxicol Teratol 2005;27:213–20.
[19] Lester B, Lagasse L. Children of addicted women. J Addict Dis 2010;29:259–76.
[20] Singer L, Minnes S, Short E, et al. Cognitive outcomes of preschool children with prenatal cocaine exposure. JAMA 2004;291(20):2448–56.
[21] Hobbie C, Braddock M, Henry J. Medical assessment of children going into emergency out-of-home placement. J Pediatr Health Care 2000;14:172–9.
[22] Leslie LK, Hurlburt MS, Landsverk J, et al. Comprehensive assessments for children entering foster care: a national perspective. Pediatrics 2003;112(1):134–42.
[23] Child Welfare League of America. Standards of excellence for health care services for children in out-of-home care. revised edition. Washington, DC: Child Welfare League of America; 2007.
[24] American Academy of Pediatrics. Task force on health care for children in foster care. Fostering health, health care for children and adolescents in foster care. 2nd edition. New York: AAP District II; 2005.

[25] Steele J, Buchi K. Medical and mental health of children entering the Utah foster care system. Pediatrics 2008;122(3):e703–9.
[26] United States General Accounting Office. Foster care: health needs of many young children are unknown and unmet, 80. Washington, DC: Health, Education and Human Services Division. Child Welfare; 1995. p. 3.
[27] Simms MD, Dubowitz H, Szilagyi MA. Health care needs of children in the foster care system. Pediatrics 2000;106:909–18.
[28] Simms M. Foster children and the foster care system, part II. Impact on the child. Curr Probl Pediatr 1991;21(8):345–69.
[29] Halfon N, Mendonca A, Berkowitz G. Health status of children in foster care. The experience of the center for the vulnerable child. Arch Pediatr Adolesc Med 1995;149(4):386–92.
[30] Schor E. The foster care system and health status of foster children. Pediatrics 1982;69:521–8.
[31] Summary of Clinical Practice Guidelines. Clinical practice guideline: report of the recommendations. Hearing loss, assessment and intervention for young children (age 0–3 years). New York State Department of Health, Early Intervention Program; US Department of Education. Available at: http://www.asha.org/Members/ebp/compendium/guidelines/Clinical-Practice-Guideline–Report-of-the-Recommendations–Hearing-Loss,-Assessment-and-Intervention-for-Young-Children.htm. Accessed January 21, 2011.
[32] Takayama J, Wolfe E, Coulter K. Relationship between reason for placement and medical findings among children in foster care. Pediatrics 1998;101(2):201–7.
[33] Grubman S, Gross E, Lerner-Weiss N, et al. Older children and adolescents living with perinatally acquired human immunodeficiency virus infection. Pediatrics 1995;95:657–63.
[34] Persaud D, Chandwani S, Rigaud M, et al. Delayed recognition of human immunodeficiency virus infection in preadolescent children. Pediatrics 1992;90:688–91.
[35] Kelly DA, Hallett RJ, Saeed A, et al. Prolonged survival and late presentation of vertically transmitted HIV infection in childhood. Lancet 1987;1(8536):806–7.
[36] Espanol T, Figueras MC, Soriano V, et al. Very late presentation of vertically transmitted HIV-1 infection. Acta Paediatr 1996;85:755–7.
[37] American Academy of Pediatrics. Committee on pediatric AIDS. Identification and care of HIV-exposed and HIV-infected infants, children, and adolescents in foster care. Pediatrics 2000;106(1):149–53.
[38] Dowdell EB, Cavanaugh DJ, Burgess AW, et al. Girls in foster care: a vulnerable and high-risk group. MCN Am J Matern Child Nurs 2009;34(3):172–8.
[39] Hobbs G, Hobbs C. Abuse of children in foster and residential care. Child Abuse Negl 1999;23(12):1239–52.
[40] Black M, Oberlander S, Lewis T, et al. Sexual intercourse among adolescents maltreated before age 12: a prospective investigation. Pediatrics 2009;124:941–9.
[41] Silovksy J, Niec L. Characteristics of young children with sexual behavior problems: a pilot study. Child Maltreat 2002;7:187–97.
[42] Kellogg N. Clinical report–the evaluation of sexual behaviors in children. Pediatrics 2009;124:992–8.
[43] Felitti V, Anda R, Nordenberg D, et al. Relationship of childhood abuse and household dysfunction to many of the leading causes of death in adults: the Adverse Childhood Experiences (ACE) study. Am J Prev Med 1998;14(4):245–58.
[44] Sempik J, Ward H, Darker I. Emotional and behavioral difficulties of children and young people at entry into care. Clin Child Psychol Psychiatry 2008;13(2):221–33.
[45] Barroso U, Dultra A, Bessa J, et al. Comparative analysis of the frequency of lower urinary tract dysfunction among institutionalized and non-institutionalised children. BJU Int 2006;97:813–5.
[46] Sapi MC, Vasconcelos JS, Silva FG, et al. Assessment of domestic violence against children and adolescents with enuresis. J Pediatr 2009;85(5):433–7.

[47] Can G, Topbas M, Okten A, et al. Child abuse as a result of enuresis. Pediatr Int 2004;46(1):64–6.
[48] Joinson C, Heron J, Von Gontard A. Early childhood risk factors associated with daytime wetting and soiling in school-age children. J Pediatr Psychol 2008;33(7):739–50.
[49] Duel BP, Steinberg-Epstein R, Hill M, et al. A survey of voiding dysfunction in children with attention deficit-hyperactivity disorder. J Urol 2003;170:1521–3.
[50] Baeyens D, Roeyers H, Demeyere I, et al. Attention-deficit/hyper-activity disorder (ADHD) as a risk factor for persistent nocturnal enuresis in children: a two-year follow-up study. Acta Paediatr 2005;94:1619–25.
[51] Crimmins CR, Rathbun SR, Husmann DA. Management of urinary incontinence and nocturnal enuresis in attention-deficit hyperactivity disorder. Urology 2003;170(4):1347–50.
[52] Shreeram S, He JP, Kalaydjian A, et al. Prevalence of enuresis and its association with attention-deficit/hyperactivity disorder among U.S. children: results from a nationally representative study. J Am Acad Child Adolesc Psychiatry 2009;48:34–41.
[53] American Academy of Pediatrics. Committee on early childhood, adoption, and dependent care: developmental issues for young children in foster care. Pediatrics 2000;106(5): 1145–50.
[54] Silver J, DiLorenzo P, Zukoski M. Starting young: improving the health and developmental outcomes of infants and toddlers in the child welfare system. Child Welfare 1999;78(1): 148–65.
[55] Horwitz S, Owens P, Simms M. Specialized assessments for children in foster care. Pediatrics 2000;106:59–66.
[56] Jee S, Szilagyi M, Ovenshire C, et al. Improved detection of developmental delays among young children in foster care. Pediatrics 2010;125:282–9.
[57] 45 CFR, parts 160 and 164. Fed Regist 2003;68(34):8334. Available at: www.cms.hhs.gov/SecurityStandard/Downloads/securityfinalrule.pdf. Accessed September 22, 2010.
[58] American Academy of Pediatrics. Committee on child abuse and neglect: policy statement–child abuse, confidentiality, and the Health Insurance Portability and Accountability Act. Pediatrics 2010;125(1):197–201.
[59] Risley-Curtiss C, Kronenfeld J. Health care policies for children in out-of-home care. Child Welfare 2001;80(3):325–50.
[60] Ringeisen H, Casanueva C, Urato M, et al. Special health care needs among children in the child welfare system. Pediatrics 2008;122(1):e232–41.
[61] Pinborough-Zimmerman J, Satterfield R, Miller J, et al. Communication disorders: prevalence and comorbid intellectual disability, autism, and emotional/behavioral disorders. Am J Speech Lang Pathol 2007;16:359–67.
[62] Stock CD, Fisher PA. Language delays among foster children: implications for policy and practice. Child Welfare 2006;85(3):445–61.
[63] Shriberg LD, Tomblin JB, McSweeny JL. Prevalence of speech delay in 6 year old children and co-morbidity with language impairment. J Speech Lang Hear Res 1999;42:1461–81.
[64] Hedge MN. Introduction to communicative disorders. 2nd edition. Austin (TX): Pro-Ed; 1995.
[65] Stahmer AC, Leslie LK, Hurlbert M, et al. Developmental and behavioral needs and service use for young children in child welfare. Pediatrics 2005;116(4):891–900.
[66] Tomblin JB, Records NL, Buckwater P, et al. Prevalence of specific language impairment in kindergarten children. J Speech Lang Hear Res 1997;40:1245–60.
[67] Nelson HD, Nygren P, Walker M, et al. Screening for speech and language delay in preschool children: systematic evidence review for the US Preventative Services Task Force. Pediatrics 2006;117(2):e298–319.
[68] Cohen NJ, Davine M, Horodezsky N. Unsuspected language impairment in psychiatrically disturbed children: prevalence and language and behavioral characteristics. J Am Acad Child Adolesc Psychiatry 1993;32(3):595–603.

[69] Ely R. Language and literacy in the school years. In: Gleason JB, editor. The development of language. 6th edition. Boston (MA): Pearson Education; 2005. p. 396–443.
[70] Child welfare: poverty and families in crisis. State of America's Children. Washington, DC: Children's Defense Fund; 2005. p. 113–43.
[71] Horowitz SM, Simms MD, Farrington R. Impact of developmental problems on young children's exits from foster care. J Dev Behav Pediatr 1994;15(2):105–10.
[72] Battle D. Language development and disorders in culturally and linguistically diverse children. In: Bernstein DK, Tiegerman-Farber E, editors. Language and communication disorders in children. 5th edition. Boston (MA): Allyn and Bacon; 2002. p. 354–86.
[73] Acquiring English as a second language. What's "normal", What's not. American Speech-Language-Hearing Association. Available at: http://www.asha.org/public/speech/development/easl.htm. Accessed October 10, 2010.
[74] Culp RE, Watkins RV, Lawrence H, et al. Maltreated children's language and speech development: abused, neglected, and abused and neglected. First Lang 1991;11:377–89.
[75] Dicker S, Gordon E. Ensuring the healthy development of infants in foster care. A guide for judges, advocates, and child welfare professionals. New York (NY): Permanent Judicial Commission on Justice for Children & Zero to Three Policy Center; 2004.
[76] Child Welfare Information Gateway. Parental substance use and the child welfare system. US Department of Health and Human Services. Available at: www.childwelfare.gov/pubs/factsheets/parentalsubabuse.cfm. Accessed October 10, 2010.
[77] Malakoff ME, Mayes LC, Schottenfeld, et al. Language production of preschool children prenatally exposed to cocaine and multiple drugs and non-exposed children. J Appl Dev Psychol 1999;20:158–90.
[78] Mentis M, Ludgren K. Effects of prenatal exposure to cocaine and associated risk factors on language development. J Speech Hear Res 1995;38:1303–18.
[79] Mattson SN, Riley EP, Gramling L, et al. Neuropsychological comparison of alcohol-exposed children with or without physical features of fetal alcohol syndrome. Neuropsychology 1998;12(1):146–53.
[80] Kodituwakku PW. Defining the behavioral phenotype in children with fetal alcohol spectrum disorder: a review. Neurosci Biobehav Rev 2007;31:192–201.
[81] Thorn JC, Coggins TE, Olson HC, et al. Exploring the utility of narrative analysis in diagnostic decision making: picture-bound reference, elaboration, and fetal alcohol spectrum disorder. J Speech Lang Hear Res 2007;50:459–74.
[82] Bandstra ES, Morrow CE, Vogel AL, et al. Longitudinal influence of prenatal cocaine exposure on child language functioning. Neurotoxicol Teratol 2002;24:297–308.
[83] Lewis BA, Singer LT, Short EJ, et al. Four-year language outcomes of children exposed to cocaine in-utero. Neurotoxicol Teratol 2004;26:617–27.
[84] Morrow CE, Vogel AL, Anthony JC, et al. Expressive and receptive language functioning in preschool children with prenatal cocaine exposure. J Pediatr Psychol 2004;29(7):543–54.
[85] Zetlin A, Weinberg L, Kimm C. Improving education outcomes for children in foster care: intervention by an education liaison. J Educ Students Placed At Risk (JESPAR) 2004;9(4):421–9.
[86] Casey Family Programs. National Working Group on Foster Care and Education. Educational outcomes for children and youth in foster and out-of-home care. fact sheet: Dec 2008. Available at: http://www.casey.org/resources/publications/EducationalOutcomes.htm. Accessed December 16, 2010.
[87] American Academy of Pediatrics. Committee on children with disabilities. The pediatrician's role in the development and implementation of an individualized education plan (IEP) and/or and individual family service plan (IFSP). Pediatrics 1999;104(1):124–7.
[88] Hill K. Individuals with Disabilities Act of 2004 and the John H. Chafee Foster Care Independence Act of 1999: what are the policy implications for youth with disabilities transitioning from foster care? Child Welfare 2009;88(2):5–23.

[89] Individuals with Disabilities Improvement Education Act. 20 U.S.C. Section 1400 1400, et.seq. 2004.
[90] Stotland J, Stocco J, Darr K, et al. Special education decisions for children in foster care: everyone has a role. Child Law Practice 2007;26(2).
[91] Report of the Surgeon General's Conference on Children's Mental Health United Stated Department of Health and Human Services, 1999. Available at: http://www.surgeongeneral.gov/library/mentalhealth/toc.html#chapter3. Accessed February 10, 2011.
[92] Burns BJ, Phillips SD, Wagner HR, et al. Mental health need and access to mental health services by youths involved with child welfare: a national survey. J Am Acad Child Adolesc Psychiatry 2004;43(8):960–70.
[93] Lyons J, Rogers L, The US. Child welfare system: a de facto public behavioral health care system. J Am Acad Child Adolesc Psychiatry 2004;43(8):971–3.
[94] Masi R, Cooper JL. Children's mental health facts for policymakers: National Center for Children in Poverty, November 2006. Available at: http://nccp.org/publications/pub_687.html. Accessed February 10, 2011.
[95] Raghavan R, Zima BT, Andersen RM, et al. Psychotropic medication use in a national probability sample of children in the child welfare system. J Child Adolesc Psychopharmacol 2005;15(1):97–106.
[96] American Academy of Pediatrics. Children's Mental Health in Primary Care. Available at: http://www.aap.org/mentalhealth. Accessed February 10, 2011.
[97] Child Welfare League of America. National fact sheet 2009. Available at: http://www.cwla.org/advocacy/nationalfactsheet09.htm. Accessed February 6, 2011.
[98] Pecora P, Kessler R, Williams J, et al. Improving family foster care: findings from the Northwest foster care alumni study. Available at: http://www.casey.org/Press/MediaKit/pdf/FosterCareByTheNumbers.pdf. Accessed February 6, 2011.
[99] Jensen PJ, Hunter Romanelli L, Percora PJ, et al. Special issue: mental health practice guidelines for reform. Child Welfare 2009;88(1):1–31.
[100] McMillen JC, Zima BT, Scott LD Jr, et al. Prevalence of psychiatric disorders among older youths in the foster care system. J Am Acad Child Adolesc Psychiatry 2005;44(1):88–95.
[101] Silver J, Dicker S. Mental health assessment of infants in foster care. Child Welfare 2007;85(5):35–55.
[102] Dube S, Felitti V, Dong M, et al. Childhood abuse, neglect, and household dysfunction and the risk of illicit drug use: the Adverse Childhood Experiences study. Pediatrics 2003;111(3):564–72.
[103] Chapman D, Whitefield C, Felitti V, et al. Adverse childhood experiences and the risk of depressive disorders in adulthood. J Affect Disord 2004;82:217–25.
[104] Dube S, Anda R, Felitti V, et al. Childhood abuse, household dysfunction, and the risk of attempted suicide throughout the life span. JAMA 2001;286(24):3089–96.
[105] Addressing mental health concerns in primary care: a clinician's toolkit. Mental health screening and assessment tools for primary care. Pediatrics 2010;125(Suppl 3):S173–192.
[106] Edelstein SB. When foster children leave: helping parents to grieve. Child Welfare 1981;60(7):467–73.
[107] Edelstein SB, Burge D, Waterman J. Helping foster parents cope with separation, loss, and grief. Child Welfare 2001;80(1):5–26.

Advances in Pediatrics 58 (2011) 113–121

ADVANCES IN PEDIATRICS

School-Based Health Centers: A Model for the Provision of Adolescent Primary Care

Steven G. Federico, MD[a,b,*], Wanda Marshall, MS, CPNP[a], Paul Melinkovich, MD[b,c]

[a]School-Based Health Centers, Denver Health, Denver, CO, USA
[b]University of Colorado School of Medicine, Aurora, CO, USA
[c]Community Health, Denver Health, Denver, CO, USA

CASE STUDY

Annie (identity disguised) is a student at one of the public high schools where a school-based health clinic (SBHC) is located in the building. Annie is called to the clinic during school to receive her second human papilloma virus (HPV4) vaccination. The medical assistant checking her into the clinic noticed that she has lost quite a bit of weight. When questioned further, Annie stated that she was not trying to lose weight. The medical assistant had her see the primary care provider in the clinic instead of only vaccinating her and sending her back to class. After a history and physical examination were obtained, the clinician notes that Annie has experienced polyuria and polydipsia. A urinalysis in the clinic displays glucosuria and ketonuria. Fortunately, she was not severely acidotic at this time. Ultimately, Annie was referred to endocrinology and diagnosed as having Type I diabetes.

Health care of adolescents can be challenging for a primary health care provider in a typical clinic or office setting. Adolescents are the least likely group of patients to seek health care in traditional clinic settings [1]. Many of the health needs of this age group are unique in nature related to risky health behaviors, such as unprotected sex, substance abuse, and violence. Traditional health care settings are often not adequate and primary health care providers in these settings do not have the time to delve into the risky behaviors of this patient population. Although this case study does not highlight one of these risky behaviors, it does illustrate an advantage of having a clinic in a setting that is convenient for at-risk youth. It is likely that because of barriers faced by this teenager, her presentation as a new diabetic would have been more severe had it not been for the clinic located in her school.

*Corresponding author. School-Based Health Centers, Denver Health, Denver, CO. *E-mail address:* steve.federico@dhha.org

0065-3101/11/$ – see front matter
doi:10.1016/j.yapd.2011.03.003

It is difficult for children to attend school and learn if they are sick. Illness for the adolescent may come in the form of either physical health or mental health. These illnesses may commonly be chronic and need follow-up care. Learning is affected by high absenteeism rates associated with chronic illness and disciplinary actions related to behavior and mental health issues. Delay or failure of high school graduation is also affected by teen pregnancy rates [2].

The major focus of Healthy People 2010 was access to quality health care for every person [1]. Access to care for adolescents remains an issue despite improvements in health care access for the general United States population. Adolescents have an average of 2 visits to a health care provider each year, fewer than any other age group with the exception of young adults [3]. Lack of health insurance, convenience, confidentiality, and cost are all factors that may affect teenagers' ability to access health care.

The objective of this article is to describe the evolving models of SBHCs in the United States. To date, peer-reviewed studies have documented the success of SBHCs in decreasing emergency room use and improving access to preventive services, such as immunizations. The authors highlight the long-standing comprehensive model located in Denver.

SCHOOL-BASED HEALTH CENTERS

School-based health centers present a solution to some of the barriers by adolescents related to access to care, school absenteeism, and their unique health care needs. Comprehensive services offered in the place where adolescents spend their days has become an alternative to traditional primary health care for this age group. Although this model has existed for decades, generally knowledge of SBHCs among health care workers remains limited.

History

School-based health centers originated to provide health care to underserved children in urban areas. With the support of the Community Access to Child Health program, a part of the American Academy of Pediatrics, the first school-based health centers opened in the late 1960s and early 1970s. The first centers opened in Cambridge, Massachusetts and were organized by Philip J. Porter, a local pediatrician. More centers followed in Minneapolis and Dallas. The Robert Wood Johnson Foundation supplied funding for several new centers in 1978. State level funding assisted the further growth of school-based health centers throughout the country. In 1995, federal funding came from the Health Resource and Service Administration in the form of Healthy Schools-Healthy Communities grants to build more school-based health centers [1].

As of November, 2009, more than 1900 school-based health centers existed across the United States, including those centers that are school linked and mobile. The majority of the centers are based in high schools (33.3%) but with the increase in centers, more are found in middle schools, elementary schools, and combination schools. More than half of the school-based health centers have been open for at least 10 years. The concentration of school-based health centers remains in urban areas, having more than 50%, but there has been an increase in rural centers. A variety of ethnic backgrounds are found in the student populations served with 36.8% Hispanic, 29.5% white, and 26.2% African American [4].

The growing popularity of this model has lead to the creation of a national organization representing school-based health centers. The National Assembly of School-Based Health Care (NASBHC) located in Washington, DC states that its mission is to improve the health status of children and youth by advancing and advocating for school-based health care. NASBHC reported 16 different state affiliates in 2010. In its 2009 annual report, NASBHC reported that the number of SBHCs had doubled from 1000 to more than 2000 since 1995 [5]. Aside from growth and organizational structure, SBHCs have also received recent validation through federal language in both the Children's Health Plan reauthorization and the Patient Protection and Affordability Act. Both acts of Congress establish SBHCs as sites for comprehensive primary care, which enhance opportunities for billing and federal funding.

Models of care

The majority of school-based health centers are built based on a primary care model with the primary care provided by a nurse practitioner, a physician's assistant, or physician. There are 3 variations of this model: primary care, primary care and mental health, or primary care and mental health plus. The primary care model may have medical assistants, registered nurses, or licensed practical nurses that complement and support the services offered by the primary care provider. This model does not include mental health services. The primary care and mental health model combines the services of a primary care provider with the those of a mental health provider who is either a licensed clinical social worker, psychologist, or substance abuse counselor. The primary care and mental health plus model have expanded services that may be dental, health education, or case management services [4].

Services

There are a variety of services that may be offered at any of the school-based health centers. The most common services include comprehensive health assessments, acute minor illness care, health screenings, chronic illness care (eg, asthma), immunizations, and anticipatory guidance. Many centers provide medications for treatment of acute minor illnesses and chronic care. These medications are dispensed on-site and taken home. Laboratory testing and referral to specialty services are also included in the care [4].

Reproductive health services are a component of the primary care services in school-based health centers. Many centers offer testing and treatment for sexually transmitted infections, pregnancy testing, family planning counseling, and referral for contraceptive methods. However, local school and community policies may limit such testing and the delivery of services for related health topics [6]. For example, despite the fact that most centers provide some form of reproductive health service, the percentage of those who offer contraception is difficult to estimate because it ranges drastically by region [7]. The majority of centers refer to other health care facilities for the actual acquisition of the contraceptive methods [4].

Although all centers screen for mental health needs, not all provide therapeutic services on-site. Of those that do, services vary from individual to group and family therapy. Therapists care for anxiety disorders, posttraumatic stress disorders, depression, and adolescent adjustment disorder. The counselors are able to screen for depression, provide grief therapy, report abuse, case manage, and maintain confidentiality [1]. Psychiatric consultation is available in some centers along with mental health medication management [4]. Substance abuse counseling separate from mental health care is offered by some centers [1].

Prevention and early intervention are a major focus of school-based health center care. Besides the preventative care offered by the primary care provider, a health educator may work with students emphasizing such topics as pregnancy prevention or nutrition. These educators meet individually with students to give counseling and classroom instruction in these areas.

Dental services, such as dental screenings, cleaning, and sealants, are provided as part of the services in approximately 10% to 25% of the centers [8]. The availability of space and cost of equipment limit the expansion of this service. Primary care providers in many centers report providing oral health education and referral to various dental facilities as possible.

Follow-up care is a vital component of the care in school-based health centers. Primary care providers in traditional settings experience the limitations of access, cost, and compliance when following patients with chronic illnesses, such as asthma. School-based health centers have the distinct advantage of being located in the same building as their patients. They often have ubiquitous access to the students. Thus, school-based health centers eliminate many of the traditional barriers that make follow-up care difficult. Cooperation between medical home providers and the staff of these centers enhance the long-term successful care of students with chronic illness.

Collaboration

Although located in a school facility, most school-based health centers are financially supported and managed by outside facilities. The most common model is to have a primary care provider, medical assistants, mental health therapists, and other health care providers employed by a health care sponsor. School personnel, such as the school nurse, school psychologist, and school social worker, are considered team members of the school-based health center but are usually employed by the educational system. This interdisciplinary team approach with regular in-school follow-up is the hallmark of comprehensive services offered in this setting [1].

School nurses are not replaced by the school-based health center. Besides fulfilling the legal and public health requirements of the school, the school nurse has an essential role of triage in the effective use of the school-based health center. School nurses are a vital component of the multidisciplinary team colocated within a successful school-based health center.

Financing

The two most common financial sponsors of school-based health centers are currently health systems and public health departments. Other sponsors of centers include community health centers, nonprofit health organizations, school systems, and medical or nursing schools. Large health systems with integrated delivery systems may benefit from sponsoring school-based health centers. The centers serve as portals of entry for adolescents into their health care system. The affiliation also provides an alternative site for education of health care professionals [1].

Most school-based health centers are funded from a variety of sources. Some states provide grant support to school-based health centers. Additionally, many sponsoring agencies have developed the ability to bill Medicaid and the Children's Health Insurance Program. Caused in part by limited public funds and growing interest in expansion of the model, centers have also sought support from nonprofit agencies [9]. As school-based health centers serve largely uninsured and underinsured children, insurance revenues are much lower than what is needed for sustainability [10].

Quality initiatives

School-based health centers adhere to nationally recognized standards of care as evidenced in the census reports gathered by the National Assembly of School-Based Health Centers. More than three-quarters of the centers use Early Periodic Screening and Treatment standards. Almost half use some form of the Adolescent Preventive Services guidelines set by the American Medical Association. Many adhere to both the American Academy of Pediatrics clinical standards and the federal Maternal and Child Health Bureau's Bright Futures [10]. Those that are sponsored by health systems are part of the Joint Commission Accreditation for health care organizations. Many centers report the use of staff credentialing, chart audits, patient surveys, and the Clinical Laboratory Improvement Act Certification [10].

Outcomes

Several studies have documented the impact of school-based health centers. Specifically, improvements have been reported in access to care for adolescents, including decreased emergency room use and improved immunization rates [11,12], and an ability to address unique health needs of adolescents (eg, use of mental health and substance abuse services and family planning) [13–15]. However, the literature is sparse relative to the impact of school-based health centers on pediatric health outcomes. Robert Wood Johnson grantees found significance in improving access to care but did not demonstrate significance in changing health status or health behaviors [3].

A meta-analysis published in 2004 reported that school-based health centers may influence absenteeism, attendance, graduation rates, and suspension rates [16].

However, these indicators, along with academic performance overall, have not been shown to have significant changes as a result of the use of a school-based health center. Academic performance is multifactorial and assessing the significance of school-based health center impact is difficult. Other indicators that may be more readily measurable include seat time and teacher and student satisfaction [16].

Despite the difficulty of associating school-based health centers with individual student success, data focused on health and health care use has been more promising. Primary care has been a consistent focus of school-based health centers. Their unique location and consistent access to patients makes them ideal for immunization delivery. A national survey of school-based health centers documented the frequency and barriers of SBHC vaccine administration [17]. Several studies have documented the success of school-based health centers and improved immunization rates among adolescents [11,12,18]. This success has become increasingly important with the evolution of new vaccines, new recommendations, and adolescent vaccine series. In at least one study, school-based health centers were shown to improve the completion rates of immunization series (specifically HPV4) as compared with a traditional community health center setting [12].

DENVER SCHOOL-BASED HEALTH CENTERS: A CASE STUDY

The Denver School-Based Health Centers were started in 1987. The 13 centers are sponsored and managed by Denver Health and Hospital Authority as part of their Federally Qualified Health Center Community Health Services program. Services are provided in collaboration with the Denver Public School system. There are centers in 7 of the Denver Public School's high schools and 6 in middle schools or combination schools. Each center follows the model of primary care and mental health plus (Box 1).

Box 1: Services offered at Denver Health School-Based Health Centers

- Immunizations
- Sports and other physical examinations
- Mental and behavioral health counseling
- Acute illness care
- Chronic illness care
- Sexually transmitted infection testing and treatment
- Pregnancy testing
- Reproductive health education counseling
- Laboratory screening and testing
- Insurance outreach and enrollment services
- Limited formulary medication dispensing

Currently, 10 nurse practitioners and 3 physician's assistants are the primary care providers in the 13 clinics. Each clinic has a Denver Health attending pediatrician who is responsible for 2 to 4 school-based health centers. There is a full-time medical assistant in each clinic that has clerical and medical responsibilities. A full-time mental health therapist is located within each center. Denver Health collaborates with the Mental Health Center of Denver (MHCD) to share the mental health services. Eight centers have therapists from MHCD and 5 centers have Denver Health therapists. Another collaborating partner is Arapahoe House who offers limited substance abuse counseling in the schools.

Each center has either a part-time or full-time health educator who is part of an overarching pregnancy prevention program. Most high school centers have full-time health educators with middle schools and smaller high schools sharing a health educator with another center. Based on the success of the health educator teen pregnancy prevention program, a similar health educator model to focus on obesity is in a pilot phase at 2 sites.

Since their inception, the Denver Health clinics have had an emphasis on underserved populations. In order to enhance the service model for this population, the Denver School-Based Health Centers have also incorporated an insurance outreach program. This model includes a community health advisor who works with uninsured families to provide support and to seek enrollment in a health insurance plan for the entire family. This model enhances not only the family's ability to seek health care for all the children in the family but assists in the financial stability as more students are covered under Medicaid or the Children's Insurance Plan. The community health advisor identifies families who are eligible for public health plans and guides the family through the enrollment process. Once all of the necessary documentation is obtained, families are enrolled on-site by a designated enrollment specialist. This process, which has been in place in its current format for 4 years, has decreased the percentage of Denver School-Based Health Center patients from 50% to less than 30%.

Each center collaborates with the host school's health team of nurses, social workers, and psychologists. The health center clinician coordinates the team in routine meetings to provide the comprehensive care that is the benefit of this type of care. Providing services to this vulnerable population where they spend time (in school) and regardless of their ability to pay has proven to be an effective way to ensure greater use of needed services. The provision of preventive services in this setting may in fact be easier than in traditional settings. Providing an integrated model that combines all services (medical, mental, and oral health) certainly better meets the health needs of an at-risk population. In the event that a student needs additional or specialized care, the model allows for referrals into the integrated Denver Health system and all of its associated clinics. Since the inception of Denver Health's SBHC program, more than 96,600 students have received care in one of the school-based health centers. Currently half of all Denver Health adolescent primary care users receive care in a school-based health center.

The centers are involved in formal education of medical residents, medical students, nurse practitioner students, and physician assistant students. They collaborate with the Denver Health Community Health Centers to provide services, such as contraceptive care and specialty care, that cannot be provided through the school-based health center.

Because of their location in schools, school-based health centers are in a unique position to offer primary care to adolescents. The goal of universal access to health care is complemented by this source of primary care. Preventive and chronic care can both be accentuated in this type of setting. Policy makers, school administrators, and health professionals should continue to work collaboratively to promote this successful model of care.

References

[1] Gustafson E. History and overview of school-based health center in the United States. Nurs Clin North Am 2005;40:595–606.
[2] Friedrich M. 23 years of school-based health centers. JAMA 1999;281(9):781–2.
[3] Britto M, Klostermann B, Bonny A, et al. Impact of a school-based intervention on access to healthcare for underserved youth. J Adolesc Health 2001;29:116–24.
[4] National census: school year 2007–2008. Report of the national assembly of school-based health Centers. National Assembly on School-Based Heath Care; 2008. Available at: http://ww2.nasbhc.org/NASBHCCensusReport07-08.pdf. Accessed May, 2011.
[5] National assembly on school-based heath care (2008–09 Annual Report). Available at: http://www.nasbhc.org/atf/cf/%7Bcd9949f2-2761-42fb-bc7a-cee165c701d9%7D/NASBHC%20ANNUAL%20REPORT%2008-09%20FINAL.PDF. Accessed December 15, 2010.
[6] Juszczak L, Schlitt J, Moore A. School-based health centers: national census school year 2004–05. Washington, DC: National Assembly on School-Based Heath Care; 2007.
[7] Fothergill K, Feijoo A. Family planning services at school-based health centers: findings form a national survey. J Adolesc Health 2000;27(3):166–9.
[8] National assembly of school-based health centers. Policy brief: October 2010. Oral Health Opportunities in School-based Heatlh Centers. Available at: http://www.nasbhc.org/atf/cf/{cd9949f2-2761-42fb-bc7a-cee165c701d9}/ORAL%20HEALTH%20OPPORTUNITIES%20IN%20SBHCS%20ISSUE%20BRIEF%2011-10.PDF. Accessed December 15, 2010.
[9] Lear J. School-based health centers a long road to travel. Arch Pediatr Adolesc Med 2003;157:118–9.
[10] Brindis C, Klein J, Schlitt J, et al. School-based health centers: accessibility and accountability. J Adolesc Health 2003;325:98–107.
[11] Allison MA, Crane LA, Beaty BL, et al. School-based health centers: improving access and quality of care for low-income adolescents. Pediatrics 2007;120(4):e887–94.
[12] Federico S, Abrams L, Jagunich C, et al. Overcoming immunization disparities: a retrospective analysis of school-based health center immunization delivery. Am J Public Health 2010;100(9):1630–4.
[13] Anlin TM, Naylor KE, Kaplan DW. Comprehensive school-based health care: high school students' use of medical, mental health, and substance abuse services. Pediatrics 1996;97:318–30.
[14] Juszczak L, Melinkovich P, Kaplan D. Use of health and mental health services by adolescents across multiple delivery sites. J Adolesc Health 2003;32(6):108–18.
[15] Klein JD, Handwerker L, Sesselberg TS, et al. Measuring quality of adolescent preventive services of health plan enrollees and school-based health center users. J Adolesc Health 2007;41(2):153–60.

[16] Geierstanger S, Amaral G, Mansour M, et al. School-Based Health Centers and Academic Performance: Research, Challenges, and Recommendations. J Sch Health 2004;74(9): 347–52.
[17] Daley MF, Curtis CR, Pyrzanowski J, et al. Adolescent immunization delivery in school-based health centers: a national survey. J Adolesc Health 2009;45(5):445–52.
[18] Deuson RR, Hoekstra EJ, Sedjo R, et al. The Denver school-based adolescent hepatitis B vaccination program: a cost analysis with risk simulation. Am J Public Health 1999; 89(11):1722–7.

Advances in Pediatrics 58 (2011) 123–151

ADVANCES IN PEDIATRICS

The Past Decade in Pediatric Education: Progress, Concerns, and Questions

Kenneth B. Roberts, MD[a,b,*]

[a]The University of North Carolina School of Medicine, Chapel Hill, Greensboro, NC 27599, USA
[b]Moses Cone Health System, Greensboro, NC 27401, USA

The 1990s ended optimistically for the United States and for pediatric education: the country had accumulated a financial surplus, the pediatrics community had come together to deliberate the Future of Pediatric Education II, and medical education had a new paradigm (the Outcome Project). The past decade has been a tumultuous one, and optimism is now tempered by concerns and questions. Any attempt to discuss medical education needs to take into account the societal forces that affect health care, which is the context for medical education. Of the 10 issues addressed in this article, the first 5 are societal factors with implications for education; the last 5 are issues within medical education, with emphasis on pediatric education. The 10 are discussed individually but clearly interact and overlap. The order in which they are discussed is not intended to convey a rank of importance.

SOCIETAL FACTORS WITH IMPLICATIONS FOR MEDICAL EDUCATION

1. Focus on patient safety

At the close of 1999, the Institute of Medicine (IOM) released its landmark report *To Err is Human: Building a Safer Health System* [1]. The report received widespread exposure and drew public attention to the need to reduce medical errors and increase patient safety, a need the IOM termed urgent. Public concern about the safety of care rendered by trainees has led to efforts to reduce the effect of fatigue on trainees by limiting the consecutive number of hours they are permitted to care for patients and to increase supervision by faculty.

Implications for education: graduate medical education work hour regulations

Consideration of the effect of resident fatigue on the care of patients largely stems from the death of 18-year-old Libby Zion in 1986. She was admitted to New York Hospital with fever, agitation, and abdominal pain. She did not reveal that she was taking a monoamine oxidase (MAO) inhibitor, phenelzine,

*3005 Bramblewood Drive, Mebane, NC 27302. *E-mail address*: kenrobertsmd@gmail.com

0065-3101/11/$ – see front matter
doi:10.1016/j.yapd.2011.03.007

prescribed by her psychiatrist. A resident on duty in the early hours of the morning prescribed meperidine to assuage her pain, and the combination of meperidine with the MAO inhibitor resulted in the young woman's death. Sidney Zion, Libby's father, a newspaper columnist and attorney, was convinced that the hospital was responsible for the death of his daughter. In the aftermath of Libby Zion's death, a commission was formed, with Bertrand Bell as its leader. The Bell Commission identified both faculty supervision and resident fatigue from long work hours as issues that needed to be addressed. The resulting New York 405 Rules limited continuous work hours for residents to 24 with an additional 3 hours of nonpatient care activity permitted for education and to ensure adequate transfer of responsibility to another physician [2]. Hospitals that did not adhere to the Rules were subject to a fine, imposed daily until compliance was attained. In October, 2002, 13 years after the implementation of the 405 Rules, 75 of the 118 residency programs (64%) were found to be out of compliance [3], evidence of the inability of the profession to address what was publicly perceived to be a dangerous patient care situation.

In 2001, Representative Conyers proposed legislative action in the form of the Patient and Physician Safety Act, and Senator Corzine sponsored the act in the Senate in 2002. The Accreditation Council for Graduate Medical Education (ACGME) responded by developing work hour regulations that went into effect on July 1, 2003, forestalling federal legislation [4]. Continuous work hours were limited to 24 as in the 405 Rules, but an additional 6 hours were permitted for education and patient transfer, rather than 3. The total number of hours a resident could work per week was capped at 80, averaged over 4 weeks. A minimum of 10 hours was required between shifts (rather than 8 in the 405 Rules), and 1 day (24 continuous hours) free of clinical responsibility had to be provided per week, averaged over 4 weeks [2].

Although not a surprise to medical educators, a restriction in work hours did not result in a sharp decrease in mortality, and patient harm remained "common, with little evidence of widespread improvement" [5]. Some studies reported that residents were getting more sleep but felt no less stressed by the responsibilities of residency [6]; a study of residents in 3 large pediatric residency programs documented increased sleep and decreased rates of resident burnout but no change in medication errors, resident depression, or resident injuries [7]. Three potential reasons were proposed to explain the lack of consistent improvements: (1) work hours were still too long; (2) Compliance with the standard was lacking; (3) benefits from reduced fatigue might be offset by worsened continuity of care and inadequate handovers [8].

Evidence began to accumulate that a further reduction of work hours was associated with fewer medical errors and injuries [9–11]. Congress continued to apply pressure. The IOM responded by convening a panel and issuing *Resident Duty Hours: Enhancing Sleep, Supervision, and Safety* in December, 2008 [12]. Recommendations included keeping the 80 hours per week cap but without the flexibility to average over 4 weeks as in the 2003 ACGME regulations. The key changes were limiting shifts to no more than 16 hours unless 5 hours of protected sleep were provided and not permitting more than 4 night shifts in a row. Also included was the recommendation that interns be supervised by senior residents or faculty, not junior residents.

To assess public opinion regarding resident work hours, a national survey between November, 2009, and January, 2010, polled individuals from a sample designed to reflect the US Census estimates by region, gender, age, and race [13]. Of the 1200 respondents, only 1% approved of shifts lasting more than 24 hours. Respondents believed the maximum shift duration should be 10.9 hours and the maximum work week 50 hours; 81% believed that reducing resident work hours would be "very" or "somewhat" effective in reducing medical errors. A total of 81% believed patients should be informed if a treating resident had been working for more than 24 hours; 80% would then want a different doctor.

In response to the IOM report, the ACGME convened its own panel and issued regulations in 2010 [14]. The ACGME regulations were clearly influenced by the IOM recommendations but included some differences: flexibility to average the 80 hours per week cap over 4 weeks was maintained; the maximum number of night shifts in a row was set at 6, rather than 4. The most dramatic change recommended by the IOM (limiting shifts to a maximum of 16 hours) was adopted for interns, although residents beyond internship were still permitted 24-hour shifts, as in the 2003 regulations, but 4 hours for education and transfer of patient care rather than 6. The new ACGME regulations become effective on July 1, 2011. As of this writing, residency program directors are working to devise schedules that satisfy the new requirements [15].

Concerns and questions

Concern was raised in 2003 that an increased number of transitions of care (variably referred to as handovers, handoffs, signovers, or signouts) might offset any benefit to patients from being cared for by less fatigued residents. In the past 5 years, there has been more literature on the subject of handovers than in the previous 25 years, but the conclusion in 2010 is that "the 'perfect' handoff process does not yet exist" [16]. One proposed framework for handovers uses the mnemonic TEAM to identify 4 major domains: time, elements, anticipatory management, and mutual trust [16]. Several mnemonics have been developed to ensure that the necessary elements of handovers are addressed, but they can only ensure structure, not quality. As Philibert notes: "Much of the work to improve patient handoffs has focused on enhancing communication and access to data. Yet the handoff is first and foremost a clinical task that relies on participants' ability to discern and interpret information about the patient's condition, including the likelihood that it will worsen and the warning signs that this is occurring. Development of clinical acumen is critical to the emergence of this aspect of handoff skills that allows residents to convey this information when they are in the role as the outgoing physician and to understand it when they are the recipient" [17].

The ACGME Common Program Requirements for 2011 address the need to ensure effective transitions of care ("Sponsoring institutions and programs must ensure and monitor effective, structured handover processes to facilitate both continuity of care and patient safety") but paradoxically state "Programs must design clinical assignments to minimize the number of transitions in patient care" *and* reduce work hours, inevitably creating more transitions [18].

It is not clear whether the reduced hours benefit patient care, as shown in studies and simulation [19], or whether more handovers increase errors. In addition, the effect on education is unknown. Will the reduced hours during internship make the transition from intern to supervising resident more difficult? Might a crisis of coverage prompt more than an exercise in rescheduling, resulting in a creative reengineering of how residents' time is spent? Concerns about the effect on professionalism and the promotion of a shift mentality are being voiced again, as they were when the 2003 ACGME Requirements were instituted [4].

Implications for education: increased faculty supervision and direct involvement in patient care

Although increased supervision of residents was a major thrust of the Bell Commission and was reiterated by the IOM and the ACGME, the concern was largely lost in the tumult caused by the recommendations for reduced work hours. Direct involvement of teaching faculty in patient care has increased markedly in the past few decades (more because of reimbursement issues than because of concerns for patient safety or the quality improvement movement). In 1996, the Health Care Financing Administration (currently named the Centers for Medicare and Medicaid Services) issued Intermediary Letter 372 (IL-372), which prohibited teaching physicians from submitting bills to Medicare unless they personally provided services to the patient beyond supervising a resident and documented their services in the medical record [20]. Because academic departments have become increasingly dependent on clinical revenue (and test cases showed the resolve of the government to recover Medicare payments when documentation did not confirm the personal provision of services by faculty [21,22]), pressure was brought to bear on teaching physicians to be more directly involved in the care of patients. In recent years, additional factors may have resulted in increased direct care by teaching faculty: reduced resident presence (from restricted work hours and additional responsibilities such as continuity clinic); caps on the number of patients residents are permitted to admit; and the increasing number of hospitalists.

Concerns and questions

As trainee work hours are shortened and teaching physicians assume more direct responsibility for patient care, it becomes more challenging to ensure sufficient decision-making opportunities to prepare interns to become senior residents and to prepare senior residents for independent practice. Residents and faculty differ in their assessments of the degree of independence that should be permitted in various situations [23]. Trying to achieve and maintain a balance between supervision and autonomy "is among the greatest challenges in medical education. The 'hidden curriculum' that overvalues physician autonomy must be put aside for an explicit curriculum of safety, quality, and humility. Master clinician-educators at the bedside must provide 'supervised autonomy'" [24]. Babbott refers to the process as "watching closely at a distance" [25].

A prospective study in 1 large residency program before the 2003 ACGME work hour restrictions showed that the introduction of a hospitalist program was associated with decreases in senior resident reports of their decision-making abilities and autonomy in the first few years of the program; the ratings then returned to the levels recorded before the hospitalist program [26]. The investigators speculate that the dip in ratings might have represented resident dissatisfaction with change, inexperienced hospitalists, or statistical fluctuation; they speculate further that the return to baseline levels may be because of the newer senior residents' lack of awareness of the previous system or the learning curve of hospitalists. The data do not address the objective outcome of decision making when the senior residents graduated and were expected to function independently. Outcome data are the critical piece regarding preparation for practice, and are lacking.

2. The quality improvement movement

In 2001, 2 years after releasing *To Err is Human: Building a Safer Health System* [1], the IOM followed up with *Crossing the Quality Chasm: A New Health System for the 21st Century* [27]. Increasingly, the public, particularly payers, wanted to know what they were getting for their money, and report cards created awareness within health care systems of a higher level of accountability than previously.

Implications for education: ACGME Outcome Project identification of practice-based learning improvement and systems-based practice as core competencies

The education community was involved in quality improvement at the same time as the IOM reports. In 1999, the ACGME launched the Outcome Project (see number 6, later discussion) [28]. In conjunction with the American Board of Medical Specialties (ABMS) and its 24 Member Boards, the Project delineated 6 General Competencies, among which were 2 new ones: practice-based learning and improvement and systems-based practice. Both relate to quality improvement. The important distinction between the two is that practice-based learning applies to the improvements individuals can make in their own practice; systems-based practice involves making changes in a system of care. The requirement for practice-based learning and improvement was stated as follows: "Residents must be able to investigate and evaluate their patient care practices, appraise and assimilate scientific evidence, and improve their patient care practices. Residents are expected to: analyze practice experience and perform practice-based improvement activities using a systematic methodology; locate, appraise, and assimilate evidence from scientific studies related to their patients' health problems; obtain and use information about their own population of patients and the larger population from which their patients are drawn; apply knowledge of study designs and statistical methods to the appraisal of clinical studies and other information on diagnostic and therapeutic effectiveness; use information technology to manage information, access online medical information, and support their own education; and facilitate the learning of students and other health care professionals."

The ABMS and its 24 Member Boards embraced practice-based improvement as part of a transition from recertification to a more continuous maintenance of certification (MOC) process [29]. Part IV of MOC requires that physicians show that they can assess the quality of care they render and improve that care using follow-up measurements. During the past decade, the Accreditation Council for Continuing Medical Education (ACCME) has aligned its goals with those of the ACGME and ABMS MOC to require an assessment of the outcome of continuing medical education (CME) activities (ie, how they improve patient care) [30]. The move is away from random lectures and toward a process that begins with identifying gaps in care and what practitioners need to address such gaps. Evaluation of CME activities previously was generally limited to assessments of the speaker; now, the key question is whether clinical practice changes as a result of the activity.

Concerns and questions

The potential for the movement to improve quality has been shown in multiple individual projects, but it is not yet clear what the effect will be on the quality of care rendered by individual practitioners or the health of the public. Moreover, because report cards and related activities have increased the competitiveness of hospitals regarding quality outcomes, pressures on supervising physicians can affect education at all levels, not just the autonomy of senior residents discussed earlier. For example, formerly, the attending could teach, and the students and residents would do the charting: a trade-off in terms of time; now, the attending is required to document personally and extensively, resulting in less time available for teaching. As stated by Irby and Wilkerson, "Teaching–a time-intensive and largely unsponsored activity–has been slowly crowded out of the schedules of both full-time and voluntary medical school faculty members" [31]. Ludmerer suggests that we are returning to the pre-Flexner era, in which hospitals, rather than universities, directed medical education [32].

3. Advances in technology

Technology has advanced so rapidly that it is difficult to recall the era before the widespread access to the Internet, the ubiquitous use of cell phones, and affordable fast computer processors coupled with memory of sufficient capacity to enable complex activities such as simulation to be commonplace. It is difficult to overestimate the effect that advances in technology have had on daily life.

Implications for education

Electronic health records (EHRs) permit ready review of patient records for multiple purposes, including education and research. For example, practice-based learning is greatly facilitated by easily being able to identify patients with a particular condition and retrieve their records. Drug interactions can be identified as prescriptions are being written and as part of computerized physician order entry (CPOE) in hospitals. Programs that provide information when key words are clicked or that offer assistance with diagnoses can be incorporated in EHRs. This just-in-time education is valuable for patient care, patient safety, and education. Students and residents who receive training in an environment rich in technology resources and then move to institutions with less sophisticated technology perceive the latter as having lower "quality of care in many domains surveyed, including safety, efficiency, and system learning. Of considerable note, this group reported having less confidence in their knowledge about drug interactions and drug management than they did during their training, even months after changing institutions. Additionally, many respondents felt weakened in their ability to prescribe medications safely" [33].

The term e-learning comprises all forms of electronically supported learning and teaching, including distance learning and computer-assisted instruction [34]. Modules and entire courses can be accessed electronically. Relevant examples range from medical school courses that permit students to be widely dispersed, CME offerings in Web sites such as the American Academy of Pediatrics (AAP) PediaLink, and CME Master's Programs in Medical Education [35]. The transition from books to electronic access has even permitted many medical libraries to go bookless, a cure for the increasing problem of finding space for the ever-increasing number of journals and books. Moreover, live webcasts can be interactive, and telemedicine instruction and consultation are becoming more widespread [36]. Software that can reduce or accelerate speech without altering pitch permits learners to process lectures at their own pace, improving both efficiency and effectiveness.

Simulation, of one sort or another, is currently used by all medical schools in the United States and Canada [37]. "The power of simulation," as noted by Satava, "is that it gives 'permission to fail' in a safe environment (the laboratory setting), so students learn from their mistakes. Until now, whenever an error was committed, the patient suffered" [38]. The use of mannequins and software of ever-increasing sophistication permits the acquisition of competence under conditions that are controlled and can be altered to achieve specific learning objectives. The ability to simulate medical crises is particularly important for the training of pediatricians, because crises are rare events in children, making mastery of the skills and decision-making difficult to teach, to learn, and to assess. The difficulty is compounded by the unique features of neonates and children that limit the ability to transfer directly the skills acquired during the care of adults.

Computerized cases combine the benefits of simulation and e-learning. Educational objective 2 (ED-2) of the accrediting body for medical schools, the Liaison Committee for Medical Education (LCME), requires that faculty define "the types of patients and clinical conditions that students must encounter" and that "if a student does not encounter patients with a particular clinical condition (eg, because it is seasonal), the student should be able to remedy the gap by a simulated experience (such as standardized patient experiences, online or paper cases, etc.), or in another clerkship" [39]. Because many common conditions in pediatrics are seasonal (eg, respiratory syncytial virus infection) and others are important but not of such frequency as to ensure a clinical encounter during the brief period of a clerkship, computer-based cases have come into widespread use. In a 2005 survey, 83% of clerkships were using computer simulations, such as CLIPP (Computer-assisted Learning in Pediatrics Program), to meet ED-2 [40]. CLIPP consists of 32 cases designed to encompass the learning objectives of the Council on Medical Student Education in Pediatrics (COMSEP) curriculum [41]. Cases address child care at different ages and such situations as a newborn with respiratory distress, a 6-day-old with jaundice, a 2-week-old with lethargy, a 6-month-old with fever, a 10-month-old with a cough, an 18-month-old with congestion, a 16-month-old with a first seizure, and others. The cases include images, sound (eg, murmurs), and progressively revealed data, with frequent questions posed (and answered) along the way. In a study of CLIPP use and integration in pediatric clerkships, students spent an average of 17 hours using CLIPP and assessed it as being more valuable and effective than traditional learning methods; "reduction or elimination of redundant teaching activities such as required textbook reading or other unrelated assignments," to make time for CLIPP, was associated with increased perception of integration, greater satisfaction, and increased perceived learning [42].

Searching the medical literature used to require visiting a medical library and flipping through countless pages of *Index Medicus.* Now, with programs such as PubMed, the medical literature can be searched anywhere a user has a computer (or handheld device) with Internet access.

Handheld devices with cameras and software enable physical findings to be captured and shared, references to be queried instantly, and communication to occur without having to return to an office. Trainees and practitioners stymied by a rash can capture its appearance digitally and solicit consultation without delay; they can become familiar with drugs their patients are taking, without having to leave the room and find a reference book; they can ensure that drug interactions do not occur before prescribing; and the list goes on. In 1 study, 70% of medical residents reported using a personal digital assistant (PDA) daily, most commonly for referencing medication-prescribing guides, medical textbooks, patient documentation programs, or medical calculators [43]. PDAs have also been shown to increase entries in patient logs by medical students when compared with paper logs, facilitating not only documentation but reflection and learning [44].

Concerns and questions

Implementing an EHR system is associated with decreased physician productivity because of the increased time required to record information. In 1 study spanning 2003 to 2006, the initial decrease in productivity was 25% to 33%, compared with data collected before the introduction of the EHR. In subsequent months, productivity by internists increased but neither pediatricians nor family physicians were able to return to their original productivity levels [45]. It is possible that more current EHR systems may be more user friendly and have less of a deleterious effect on productivity, but that remains to be shown. Many pediatricians are also concerned that attention to an inputting device draws attention away from the patient and family and may have a deleterious effect on rapport and the doctor-patient relationship. A creative solution for both productivity and rapport has been the use of scribes to enter information into the EHR [46]. There may be value not only for physicians but also for the scribes; undergraduates interested in medicine or preclinical medicine students can gain exposure to clinical encounters and become familiar with the questions used in the medical history and the findings elicited during physician examination.

The introduction of EHRs and CPOE in teaching hospitals has been accompanied by prohibition of students writing in the medical record in many hospitals [47,48]. The effect on learning and on developing a sense of responsibility for the patient (ownership) is concerning [47].

Although searching the medical literature has never been easier, it requires skill to avoid being overwhelmed by a long list of articles. The result may be reliance on the first page of references, which may not include the most useful article. If the journal article is not readily available on line, the abstract may be used as evidence, without recognition of the limitations of the study. Another alternative to a skillful search is to obtain a quick response from a generic search engine or online encyclopedia, the accuracy of which cannot always be verified.

Simulation is resource intensive, and the effect of medical school simulation training on later performance has not been well characterized. The Millennium Conference 2007 on Education Research identified studying the effect of simulation as the highest rated priority for education research [49]. Also, the role of computer-assisted instruction needs to be maintained as a complement to interaction with physician-instructors and real patient encounters, rather than as a replacement [42].

A growing concern relates to social networking and professional boundaries [50]. What may be considered humorous when whispered in the hospital may be considered offensive and unprofessional by the public. Students and physicians who use social networking sites may make a distinction between their personal life and their professional life, but such a distinction may not be made by the public, including their patients. The following is a case in point: "A patient's family member requested a change in resident physician because of questionable behavior exhibited on a resident's personal MySpace page. Such anecdotal reports continue to increase in frequency" [50].

4. Recognition of a need for more physicians

The public has been made aware that the aging of baby boomers will be associated with a shortage of physicians. By increasing the number of individuals who can access health care, health care reform legislation is expected to exacerbate the looming shortage. The Association of American Medical Colleges (AAMC) Center for Workforce Studies estimated in June, 2010, that the physician shortage in all specialties would reach 91,500 in 2020 and 130,600 in 2025 [51].

Implications for education: new medical schools, increased class sizes

In 2006, the AAMC recommended a 30% increase in US medical school enrollment by 2015 [52]. Compared with the first-year enrollment in 2002 (16,488), this recommendation would require an increase of 4946 students per year (to 21,434). One new medical school was authorized in 2000, after more than 2 decades in which no new allopathic medical schools were established [53]. Between 2006 and 2010, 15 institutions notified the LCME of their intent to start a new medical school; of these, 6 have received preliminary accreditation and 2 have suspended plans. New osteopathic schools have also been established or are in planning stages. In addition, 82% of the 125 medical schools accredited in 2002 have expanded their enrollment, and satellite training sites are now common. The most current projection is that first-year medical school enrollment in 2014 will be 20,281, a 23% increase over 2002. The 30% targeted increase is projected to be reached by 2018 [54].

Meeting the needs of a greatly increased number of medical students requires using facilities outside the medical school and its primary hospital, but there is also good reason to engage these sites. In 1999, the federal Council on Graduate Medical Education (COGME) recommended that "clinical education should occur in settings that are representative of the environment in which graduates will eventually practice. Medical schools and residency training programs should develop or acquire clinical teaching sites that offer the best learning opportunities and the highest standards of clinical practice" [55]. An additional hope of using community and rural sites is that familiarity and comfort in such settings might attract graduates and, thereby, help address the shortage of primary care physicians and the geographic maldistribution of primary care for children [56]. Previous attempts to attract physicians to primary care by simply providing more time in ambulatory settings have shown that dysfunction settings can discourage trainees from entering primary care [57]. Well-functioning community practices afford the opportunity to expose learners to optimal real-world primary care environments and achieve desired outcomes. Programs designed to increase the rural physician supply through a focused admissions process or extended rural clinical curriculum have been successful, with a rate of graduates practicing in rural areas of 53% to 64% [58]. Students in regional settings have scores on standardized tests at the end of clerkships comparable with students in tertiary settings but rate the experience more highly [59]. Pediatric residents whose continuity experience was in community practices have been shown to be particularly well prepared for primary care practice [60,61].

Concerns and questions

As noted earlier, the LCME requires that clerkship rotations at different sites be comparable and that experiences with types and numbers of patients be equivalent. Technology has been a valuable tool for meeting this requirement, but concerns about adequate space, faculty, community faculty development, staff, time, and finances remain. In the most recent AAMC survey, 73% of medical schools expressed concern with their supply of qualified preceptors, and 58% were concerned with the number of clinical training sites. Twelve schools indicated plans to reduce enrollment, mainly because of fiscal pressures [54]. As Mallon points out, the previous expansion in medical school enrollment in the 1960s and 1970s was fueled by a large influx of federal funding; such financial support "does not appear on today's horizon" [62].

Concerns are also expressed about maintaining the quality of medical school applicants [63]. One ready source might be the US citizens who would otherwise attend international medical schools (USIMGs). However, these candidates score less well on various measures than graduates of US medical school and non-US international medical graduates [63]. Of the USIMGs who graduated from medical school between 1980 and 2000 and applied for certification by the Education Commission for Foreign Medical Graduates, 30% had not achieved certification by 2005 [63].

Perhaps most important, increasing the number of medical school graduates does not address the looming shortage of practicing physicians without a corresponding increase in the number of residency positions [64]. Teaching hospitals are already grappling with what reduced work hours for interns will mean for staffing costs in the immediate future. The Affordable Care Act (Health Care Reform) includes $168 million for training more than 500 new primary care physicians by 2015 [65]. Still, in the present financial climate, it is not clear that the number of graduate medical education positions will parallel the increase in medical school graduates (or address a looming physician shortage) any time soon.

5. The current generation

Generations at Work, published in 2000, was one of the seminal publications at the start of the decade that brought differences among generations into pop culture [66]. The investigators characterized 4 generations, which they dubbed the "veterans" (born before 1943), the "boomers" (born between 1943 and 1960), "generation Xers" (born between 1960 and 1980), and "nexters" (born between 1980 and 2000). Other investigators have applied different labels (eg, the "silent generation" instead of "veterans"; "millennials" or "generation Y" instead of "nexters") and slightly different years of birth (using 20-year increments starting in 1945), but the general concepts have been widely acknowledged.

Implications for education

The subtitle of *Generations at Work* is worth noting: "Managing the clash of veterans, boomers, Xers, and nexters in your workplace" [66]. Present-day learners are "technology natives" (compared with faculty, who are "technology immigrants"), meaning that they have grown up with technology and are more facile than the members of previous generations who have to adapt to use current technology. Students (and, increasingly, residents) prefer their computer or handheld device to books or the library as a central source of information. Search engines, such as Google, and online sources, including Wikipedia, have largely replaced standard textbooks and the regular review of peer-reviewed journals. The current generation of learners is also characterized as more interested in learning in groups than previous generations.

The attempt to achieve work-life balance is more overt and active. For example, during the past decade, the rate of pediatricians working part-time progressively increased from 15% in 2000 to 20% in 2003 and 23% in 2006, a 53% relative increase in 6 years; in pediatricians younger than 40 years, the rate increased from 18% to 29% [67]. Although there is no evidence that trainees and young pediatricians are less committed to patients or dedicated to their profession, they clearly are more likely to seek and expect shorter, better-defined hours than a generation or 2 ago (as reflected in the percentage who choose part-time work, for example). The night-call burden on practitioners has been ameliorated in many areas by the availability of nurse call-in services and relieved further by the presence of hospitalists on inpatient services. The desire of trainees and young pediatricians for increased control over their schedules is a reflection of generational changes that extend to the community at large.

Concerns and questions

As awareness of work-life balance has heightened the difficulty of achieving such balance has become more apparent and more readily expressed. In an AAP Annual Survey, fewer than half of the 1020 respondents identified themselves as satisfied with time with their children, time with spouse/partner, time with elderly parents, time for personal interests, or hours worked per week [67]. The quest for balance may account in part for reduced participation in professional activities, such as membership of the AAP, despite the AAP attempt to attract young pediatricians by creating a Section specifically for them in 2000. It seems paradoxic that the current generation is characterized as preferring to learn in groups and work in teams yet chooses not to join organizations or attend meetings as previous generations of pediatricians did; it may be that electronic social networking has efficiently and effectively replaced the social function of professional meetings. The implications for the other function of meetings (CME) are not clear.

ISSUES WITHIN MEDICAL EDUCATION

6. The ACGME outcome project

In 1999, the ACGME acknowledged that accreditation of residency programs was based on structure and process components, what Hodges calls the "tea-steeping" model "in which the student 'steeps' in an educational program for a historically determined fixed time period to become a successful practitioner" [68]. The Outcome Project proposed a paradigm shift, designed to move to an assessment of accomplishments [28]. For example, instead of requiring programs simply to have written goals and objectives, the Outcome Project also required programs to assess whether residents were achieving the learning objectives and to provide supportive evidence. The ACGME, in conjunction with the ABMS and its Member Boards, solicited input to identify core competencies expected of all physicians, regardless of specialty. The Outcome Project Advisory Group reviewed the list of 86 statements that were proposed and drew from them 6 General Competencies: patient care; medical knowledge; interpersonal and communication skills; practice-based learning and improvement; professionalism; and systems-based practice.

The Outcome Project was designed to be implemented in 4 phases:

- Phase 1 (July, 2001–June, 2002): forming an initial response to changes in requirements
- Phase 2 (July, 2002–June , 2006): sharpening the focus and definition of the competencies and assessment tools
- Phase 3 (July, 2006–June, 2011): full integration of the competencies and their assessment with learning and clinical care
- Phase 4 (July, 2011 and beyond): expansion of the competencies and their assessment to develop models of excellence.

In 2009, the ACGME and the American Board of Pediatrics (ABP) launched the Pediatrics Milestone Project to further define the 6 competencies as they apply in pediatrics and to identify by what point in the continuum of education and training the milestones should be achieved [69]. The third goal of the project is to identify meaningful tools to assess performance.

The 6 Competencies have been accepted not only in graduate medical education but in continuing education as well. In 1996, 3 years before the Outcome Project, the AAMC launched the Medical Student Objectives Project (MSOP) [70]. Rather than specify competencies, the MSOP identified 4 attributes that medical students should possess when they graduate and defined 6 or 7 objectives to guide the attainment of the attributes: physicians must be altruistic; physicians must be knowledgeable; physicians must be skillful; and physicians must be dutiful. That this is a more meaningful approach for undergraduate medical education than the Competencies was reaffirmed in 2004 [71]. However, as medical students look ahead to residency, they become mindful of the ACGME Competencies. The Pediatric Subinternship Curriculum developed for fourth-year medical students by the curriculum task forces of COMSEP and the Association of Pediatric Program Directors (APPD) is organized according to the ACGME Competencies [72]. So it is fair to say that the ACGME influence has extended throughout medical education.

Concerns and questions

During the first few years after the launch of the Outcome Project, residency program directors learned the new language of the ACGME and accommodated by reclassifying observations by Competency rather than by transforming education to assess the outcome of training [73]. One major concern raised about the Competencies is whether the whole equals the sum of its parts; that is, whether achieving each Competency adds up to being a competent physician [73,74]: "Documenting that a graduating resident has mastered, at some predetermined level, the knowledge, skills, and attitudes associated with each of the core competencies, while informative, does not ensure that the individual is a competent physician. Something more is needed: graduating residents must be able to *translate and integrate* their knowledge, skills, and attitudes so they can perform the complex tasks required to deliver high-quality medical care" [75]. A conceptual framework to bridge the gap, proposed by ten Cate and colleagues [76], is based on the assessment of the "critical activities that constitute a specialty–all the elements that society and experts consider to belong to that profession, the activities of which we would all agree should be only performed by a trained specialist"; ten Cate labels these activities "Entrustable Professional Activities (EPAs)." These EPAs map back to Competencies and may be a fruitful direction for assessing the outcome of training [77].

The critical assessment as to whether training has been completed successfully remains the opinion of the program director, as was the case before the Outcome Project; although this opinion may be better informed than previously, critics point out that there is no standardized examination of performance required to graduate from residencies, only tests of medical knowledge. Assessment of performance in the first months after residency by a senior physician (rather than self-assessment of preparation) would reflect the thrust of the Outcome Project; however, few examples exist [60].

7. Assessment of performance

The ACGME recognized when the Outcome Project was launched that the key to moving from a time-served model to identifying whether training objectives were achieved was improved assessment of performance. Carraccio and Englander [78] proposed 4 requisites of assessment: (1) the tasks being evaluated should be authentic and directly observed; (2) the evaluation should be criterion based rather than norm based; (3) feedback should be given to aid improvement; and (4) a breadth of tools should be used to encompass the 6 Competencies. They also proposed the use of a portfolio containing a reflective component as well as the quantitative assessments of performance.

The infrequency with which students and residents are directly observed by faculty has long been recognized as a problem in medical education. One barrier has been faculty time. An approach to addressing this is the structured clinical observation method, introduced as a "feasible, inexpensive, qualitatively effective method of teaching clinical skills" [79]. Faculty were trained in a 2-hour session to use standardized observation forms to assess history-taking, physical-examination and information-giving skills on brief segments of encounters. Because the observation process took only 5 minutes, many more direct observations of performance were made in each clinic session than formerly. Although proposed as a teaching tool, faculty also reported an effect on assessment, changing their opinions of two-thirds of the students, generally in a more positive direction. Of the students 12% reported inconsistencies in the feedback, which could represent the limited generalizability of 5-minute observations. Multistation objective structured clinical examinations can assess a broader array of skills in a controlled environment, but are resource intensive [80]. Trained, standardized patients (SPs) are now widely accepted for both training and assessment; students identify that a particular benefit from SPs is feedback from the patient perspective [81].

To illustrate the importance of criterion-based rather than norm-based assessment, Carraccio and Englander [80] point out: "It makes little difference to have one candidate score better than another, and potentially allow the better-scoring one to pass, when neither reach baseline competency for independent practice". The absence of benchmarks at various stages of training to determine whether performance is at the level expected for a trainee at that stage remains a major obstacle to applying criterion-based assessment. The Pediatric Milestone Project is attempting to address this [69,82].

For the breadth of tools needed to encompass the 6 Competencies, the ACGME developed a tool box and required programs to specify the tools used to assess performance [83]. Terms like "360° assessment" became part of the medical education lexicon to indicate the inclusion in the evaluation of trainees of multiple individuals who interacted with the trainee, including individuals from various disciplines and patients, in addition to supervising physicians. In 2007 to 2008, the ACGME convened an Advisory Committee on Educational Outcome Assessment to identify high-quality assessment methods for use by all programs in a specialty [84]. The committee considered the following characteristics: reliability; validity; ease of use; resources required; ease of interpretation; and educational effect. Of current assessment methods, 9 with published evidence were selected for review and classification according to the following scheme:

- Class 1: the assessment method is recommended as a core component of the evaluation system of the program.
- Class 2: the assessment method can be considered for use as 1 component of the evaluation system of the program.
- Class 3: the assessment method can be used provisionally as a component of the evaluation system of the program.

Of the methods reviewed, no class 1 methods were identified.

Concerns and questions

The traditional basis for assessing clinical performance, the observations of supervising faculty, has many shortcomings. Supervising faculty may have few direct observations on which to base their assessment, and the observations in 1 setting or clinical situation may not be representative. Moreover, faculty interpret observations differently, based on several factors, one of which is their level of expectation [85], which may, in turn, be affected by their own degree of clinical skill [86]. Another confounder is the learner's social skills; affective, nonverbal behaviors have been shown to account for nearly half the variance in medical student grades [87]. Affective skills are clearly important, but the possibility of a halo effect extending to the assessment of other skills and knowledge exists. And although criterion-based assessment is clearly preferable to norm-based assessment, even the latter may be difficult for faculty without years of experience and an extensive mental database from which to draw comparisons and apply an expected level of performance to match the learner's stage of training.

The reliability and validity of current assessment tools have been questioned [88]. As noted earlier, the ACGME Advisory Committee on Educational Outcome Assessment was unable to identify a class 1 method [84]. In addition to the limitations of the tools is the "inconsistent use and interpretation of such instruments by unskilled faculty" [89]. What is clear is that robust, psychometrically sound, standardized assessment tools and defined benchmarks for performance at different levels of trainees are needed, with faculty development to promote reliable implementation.

8. Faculty development and educational scholarship

Faculty development, as applied to medical educators, includes programs to improve activities such as teaching, evaluation of learners, curriculum building, and educational scholarship. Mentoring, a long-established method by which senior physicians aid the development of junior physicians, is a form of faculty development that has received increased interest during the past decade [90,91]. Organizations have created awards to acknowledge the value of mentorship, including the APPD Robert S. Holm Award and the Academic Pediatric Association (APA) Miller-Sarkin Mentorship Award. In addition to traditional dyadic mentoring is "facilitated peer group mentoring," in which a group of junior peers works as a team with a senior mentor as facilitator. An example involving the Associate Program Directors in the APPD identifies the importance of a common project/goal and planned, regular communication; as a result of the facilitated peer-group mentoring, "the group participants expanded their efforts, forming a professional network that has resulted in a community of scholars who provide mutual support, rewarding collaboration, opportunities for scholarly projects, as well as offering additional leadership opportunities" [92].

Particular attention has been directed to voluntary community-based faculty, considered a priority in the 1999 COGME report cited earlier [55]. The federal agency that convened COGME, the Bureau of Health Professions in the Health Resources and Services Administration (HRSA), had been awarding Title VII faculty development grants for 2 decades but was concerned that the funding had benefitted only individual programs rather than having a national effect. In response to this concern, the APA developed a program to train individuals from all 10 APA regions to conduct faculty development activities locally, in their regions, and nationally, creating the first national network of faculty development in pediatrics [93]. The HRSA/APA Faculty Development Scholars Program consisted of 3 tracks: community teaching, educational scholarship, and executive leadership. Two cohorts of pediatric faculty, totaling 112 scholars, participated in train-the-trainer workshops for a 2-year period, enabling them to conduct their own faculty development workshops: Even before the last session of the program was convened, the scholars had presented 438 local workshops and 161 regional/national workshops to a total of 7989 participants. HRSA/APA Faculty Development Scholars Program graduates assumed leadership roles in pediatric education, such as the presidency of organizations (COMSEP, APPD) and created the APA Educational Scholars Program (see "Educational scholarship," later discussion) [94]. Although other national faculty development programs preceded the HRSA/APA Faculty Development Scholars Program (and a new one has been announced as recently as December, 2010 [95]), the HRSA/APA Program is singled out because it remains the only one for pediatric faculty exclusively.

Faculty development programs to improve the quality of teaching have largely been voluntary. Participants express satisfaction and perceive their teaching is better; evidence of improved outcomes (eg, gains by learners) is limited but generally positive [96]. One benefit commonly voiced by participants is the creation of a community, echoed by participants of facilitated peer-group mentoring. During the past decade, medical schools have increasingly built on this idea of community by creating academies of educators. Irby and colleagues [97] describe 4 defining characteristics of academies:

- "A mission that advances and supports educators, provides faculty development, promotes curriculum improvement, advances educational scholarship, and offers protected faculty time for education;
- a membership composed of distinguished educators who are selected through a rigorous peer review process that assesses contributions to teaching, mentoring, curriculum development and leadership, and educational scholarship;
- a formal school-wide organizational structure with designated leadership; and
- dedicated resources that fund mission-related initiatives."

The intent of academies goes beyond developing individual faculty and seeks to "transform the basic culture of academic medicine" and "place education at the center of academic medicine" by creating a critical mass [95]. If academies are to succeed in their mission, the key piece is likely to be educational scholarship.

By the end of the 1990s, educational scholarship was coming into its own in medical education generally [98] and in pediatrics specifically. Examples of the latter are the educational scholarship track in the HRSA/APA National Faculty Development Scholars Program; the revision of ABP criteria for eligibility to be certified in a subspecialty, broadening the definition of "accomplishment in research" to include educational scholarship [99]; and the launch of the APA Educational Scholars Program to "assist pediatric educators in developing themselves as productive, advancing and fulfilled faculty members and to increase the quality, status and visibility of pediatric educators in academia" [94]. The 3-year curriculum of the Educational Scholars Program includes didactic sessions, participation in and review of workshops, and a mentored project. The program is offered to members of the Pediatric Academic Societies, and successful completion is acknowledged with a Certificate of Excellence in Educational Scholarship. Since its inception, the program has awarded Certificates to 31 scholars, and another 40 are currently enrolled.

To distinguish the scholarship of teaching from scholarly teaching, 3 criteria have been proposed: the work must be made public; the work must be available for peer review and critique according to accepted standards; and the work must be able to be reproduced and built on by other scholars [98]. Opportunities to accomplish these 3 standards have increased markedly in the past decade. In addition to journals devoted to medical education, general pediatrics journals have members of their editorial boards seeking articles related to education. The AAMC, in conjunction with the American Dental Education Association, created MedEdPORTAL as a "a free online peer-reviewed publication service … designed to promote educational collaboration by facilitating the open exchange of peer-reviewed teaching resources such as tutorials, virtual patients, simulation cases, lab guides, videos, podcasts, assessment tools, etc." [100]. MedEdPORTAL enables medical educators to disseminate their ideas (and show scholarship) for their educational innovations. The APPD has created a "share warehouse" with similar intent [101]. In addition, APPD has launched a new Longitudinal Education Assessment Research Network (LEARN) to "provide an infrastructure for multi-centered, collaborative research projects and a centralized data collection system" [102]. LEARN is intended to "facilitate programs coming together to address an assessment question, test instruments, test curricula, and ultimately share these products with other programs and help shape future program accreditation."

Concerns and questions

Research in medical education is complicated and difficult [103]. In the 3 cohorts of fellows who have completed fellowship since the revision of the ABP acceptance of educational scholarship to satisfy the requirement for scholarly activity during fellowship, fewer than 2% of candidates have taken advantage of the opportunity. Attempts at creating a critical mass of educational scholars locally (eg, academies) and nationally (eg, the Educational Scholars Program) may succeed, but only time will tell if the current enthusiasm is sustainable or succumbs to financial pressures and the demand for ever-increasing clinical productivity. The lowest rated priority topic by participants of the Millennium Conference 2007 on Educational Research was "related to the essential elements or impact of faculty development about adult learning theory" [49].

9. Pediatric initiatives to improve education

In 1976, a Task Force on the Future of Pediatric Education was formed with representatives from 10 collaborating societies [104]. In its report, the Task Force recommended, among other things, that residency be extended to 3 years and that more emphasis be placed on behavioral and development issues, adolescent medicine, ambulatory care, and working in teams with other health professionals. Nearly a quarter of a century later, a second Task Force was convened, comprised again of leaders from various organizations, to meet 3 overarching goals: "To evaluate the 1978 Report with respect to its relevancy to the education of pediatricians and others providing health care to children in the 21st century; to provide direction for the improvement of pediatric education, with special emphasis on workforce requirements, new instructional methodologies, and the financing of pediatric education; and to recommend essential changes in the educational process to meet the current and future health care needs of all infants, children, adolescents, and young adults" [105]. To achieve the 3 goals, 5 Workgroups were formed: the Pediatric Generalists of the Future Workgroup; the Pediatric Subspecialists of the Future Workgroup; the Pediatric Workforce Workgroup; the Financing of Pediatric Education Workgroup; and the Education of the Pediatrician Workgroup. Through surveys, interviews, questionnaires, literature reviews, and deliberations, each Workgroup developed a report. The Task Force addressed the changing pediatric practice environment, recognizing changing demographics, biomedical advances, technological advances, changes in health care delivery, changing patterns of morbidity, and changes in the pediatric workforce. In its final, extensive (149 pages, 99 references) report in 2000, the Task Force issued 34 recommendations and reaffirmed 19 fundamental educational principles, concepts, and recommendations from the original 1978 Future of Pediatric Education report.

The leaders of the Task Force identified that a major limitation of the effect of the original Future of Pediatric Education report was the lack of a body with the responsibility and authority to implement the recommendations. They addressed this as follows: "The FOPE II Task Force recommends that the oversight for implementation of the recommendations in this report be vested in the Federation of Pediatric Organizations (FOPO). The Task Force further suggests that FOPO hire an Executive Director and appropriate staff to coordinate implementation. Additionally, FOPO should consider delegating recommendations from this report to various, appropriate organizations within the pediatric community for implementation and monitoring" [105] (Recommendation 34). FOPO, formed in the late 1980s, consists of 7 member organizations: APA, AAP, ABP, American Pediatric Society, Association of Medical School Pediatric Department Chairs (AMSPDC), APPD, and the Society for Pediatric Research [106]. Representatives of the 7 organizations had been meeting semiannually, largely for information sharing. A few FOPO Statements had been developed, but the process was arduous, because FOPO's bylaws required all decisions of the group to be unanimous. FOPO accepted the recommendations of the Task Force, including the hiring of an Executive Director (Richard Behrman) and staff. It took the additional step of establishing a Pediatric Education Steering Committee (PESC), comprised of the 7 FOPO organizations plus the Council on Medical Student Education in Pediatrics. Decisions made by the PESC did not have to be unanimous, but approval was required by FOPO, in essence retaining the unanimity standard. As suggested in Recommendation 34, the constituent organizations that comprise FOPO were invited to identify which Task Force recommendations they were positioned to address. Some key areas (such as improving the financing of graduate medical education) were not under the control of any of the organizations.

In 2000, the APA responded to the paradigm shift at the ACGME and the need for pediatric residency programs to have specified goals and objectives to meet the 6 general competencies by initiating a revision of its Educational Guidelines for Residency Training in General Pediatrics [107]. To accomplish the task, the pediatrics community was engaged by the creation of an Advisory Board, with representatives from 7 organizations, and by the inclusion of 50 contributors and reviewers [108]. To enhance the availability and usefulness of the final Guidelines, the format was Web-based, with search capability and the opportunity to download and modify the content for local application. Since the Guidelines were posted on the APA Web site in 2004, 97% of residency programs have used them [109].

In 2005, the Residency Review and Redesign Project (R3P) was begun, with the desire initially to provide the specific blueprint for graduate education that had not been furnished by the FOPE II Task Force [110]. The R3P leadership committee consisted of 13 pediatricians; 34 individuals served as the Project Group. Three colloquia were conducted to inform the process: I. The future of pediatric health care delivery and education; II. The theory and practice of graduate medical education; and III. Challenges for pediatric graduate medical education and how to meet them. Input was also derived from resident, subspecialty fellow, and practitioner surveys. It became apparent that one size does not fit all residency programs and that a single blueprint was more likely to stifle progress than to advance it. After extensive deliberation, the conclusion of the Project was that "children, adolescents, and young adults would be best served by a process of deliberate, careful experimentation across residency programs, which would allow for examination of new ways to organize resident learning experiences and different ways of assessing learning outcomes" [110].

Based on the R3P's conclusion, the Initiative for Innovation in Pediatric Education (IIPE) was developed [111]. The IIPE Mission Statement mirrors the R3P conclusion: "To initiate, facilitate and oversee innovative change in pediatric residency education through carefully monitored, outcome-directed experimentation." The aim of the IIPE is "to support high-quality research in medical education through its call for proposals, Innovation/Improvement Plans (I-Plans), and promote the development of evidence-based medical education." Governance is provided by an Oversight Committee, consisting of 2 representatives each from the ABP, AMSPDC, APPD, and the AAP Section on Medical Students, Residents, and Fellowship Trainees. The Oversight Committee also has 1 liaison representative each from the ABP and the ACGME. The IIPE does not directly fund experimental initiatives in residency programs but provides valuable assistance to programs identified through a competitive application process. In its first year (2009), IIPE approved 4 applications, 2 addressing handovers, 1 assessing structured extended career-centered block time, and 1 creating a rigorous faculty development program. In year 2 (2010), IIPE approved 1 application, a longitudinal curriculum to improve residents' self-evaluation and self-improvement. A third cycle is planned.

Concerns and questions

The R3P project "challenged the pediatric community to confront the need for change but, importantly, declined to prescribe solutions" [112]. Those words, written by the chair of the R3P Committee in 2010, echo what Abraham Flexner wrote 100 years earlier: "The endeavor to improve medical education through iron-clad prescription of curriculum or hours is a wholly mistaken effort" [113]. The pediatrics community has been engaged in identifying the challenge; the question now is whether it is able to meet the challenge in an era of increased regulation and limited financial resources.

10. Collaboration

FOPE, FOPE II, R3P, and the revision of the APA Educational Guidelines are examples of engaging the pediatrics community under the leadership of one of the pediatric organizations. During the past decade, collaboration among the organizations has begun to flourish. For example, the APPD established a Task Force structure that parallels that of COMSEP, enabling the 2 organizations to work together in areas of common interest: curriculum, evaluation, faculty and professional development, learning technology, and research. One product of this collaboration is the Pediatric Subinternship Curriculum, launched in 2009 [72]. Also in 2009, COMSEP and APPD held their annual meetings together for the first time [73], and a second joint meeting is scheduled for 2013.

In 1998, the ABP established a Program Directors Committee. Through the work of the Committee this past decade, the ABP and APPD have produced a guide for program directors on teaching and assessing professionalism [114] and are working on a general assessment guide.

The APA, COMSEP, and APPD jointly sponsored a Pediatric Educational Excellence Across the Continuum meeting in 2009, in conjunction with the Council of Pediatric Subspecialties (CoPS). The creation of CoPS is itself a case study of collaboration [115]. CoPS addresses the difficulties of communication across pediatric subspecialties and even within individual pediatric subspecialties; for example, within pediatric endocrinology, there is the Lawson Wilkins Pediatric Endocrinology Society, the AAP Section on Endocrinology, and the ABP Pediatric Endocrinology Sub-board Committee. Multiple organizations faced the frustration of communicating with the numerous entities that were not linked to respond with a single voice, such as when the ABP sought to revise its requirements for subspecialty training programs and desired input from subspecialty groups; when the APPD sought to reach out to subspecialty fellowship program directors; when the AAP Resident Section wanted a uniform application process for fellowships; and when FOPO desired to implement its Policy Statement on the Fellowship Application Process in Pediatrics. In 2006, a planning group developed an organizational model and obtained sponsorship from AMSPDC and APPD. The first meeting of CoPS was held in 2006, with 34 participants representing 17 pediatric subspecialties and related specialties and 6 pediatric organizations; 21 potential issues were identified to be addressed by the organization, including several that relate to education, such as fellowship training; workforce and pipeline; faculty development; development and sharing a core curriculum for subspecialty training; development and sharing evaluations of the core competencies; and subspecialty-specific CME courses.

Two other key organizations that have agreed to collaborate on a pediatrics project are AAMC and ACGME. The Pediatric Redesign Pilot Project will integrate the educational path for selected medical students from undergraduate medical education through residency.

Concerns and questions

Undergraduate, graduate, and continuing education are often spoken of as a continuum of medical education, yet it is clear that they are more discrete than continuous (Table 1) [116]. We are beginning to see collaboration of the major organizations in undergraduate and graduate education (eg, the Pediatric Redesign Pilot Project). A redefinition of the fourth year of medical school would certainly be fertile ground for collaboration. The COMSEP-APPD Subinternship Curriculum is a start, but there is little consensus about the most beneficial use of the remainder of the fourth year [117].

Within the pediatrics community, organizations such as COMSEP, APPD, and the APA are comprised of volunteers, who frequently refer to their organization as their home. What will be necessary to achieve full synergy is for these homes to become neighborhoods. The annual meetings of the 3 organizations are now separate, but the leaders recognize the value and importance of collaboration, an ongoing work in progress.

Table 1
Noncontinuum of education at different levels: different accrediting bodies, credentialing bodies, and educator organizations

	Accrediting body	Credentialing body	Educator organization
Medical school	LCME	USMLE	COMSEP
Residency	ACGME	ABP	APPD
Continuing education	ACCME	State licensing boards; ABP	

Abbreviation: USMLE, United States Medical Licensure Examination.

Reproduced from Roberts KB. 2009 Joseph W. St Geme Jr Leadership Award Address: The whole and the sum of its parts. Pediatrics 2010;125:174; with permission.

NOW AND THE FUTURE

As noted at the beginning of this article, the past decade has been a time of great activity, but it can be questioned whether major change has occurred. The Carnegie Foundation for the Advancement of Education, which sponsored the Flexner Report, has supported a 100-year follow-up study. The authors of the current report characterize the current situation in medical education as follows: "As we reflect on medical education in the United States at the beginning of the 21st century, we find, like our famous forbearer, that it is lacking. Medical training is inflexible, overly long, and not learner-centered. Clinical education for both students and residents excessively emphasizes mastery of facts, inpatient clinical experience, teaching by residents, supervision by clinical faculty who have less and less time to teach, and hospitals with marginal capacity or willingness to support the teaching mission. We observed poor connections between formal knowledge and experiential learning and inadequate attention to patient populations, health care delivery, patient safety, and quality improvement. Learners lack a holistic view of patient experience and poorly understand the broader civic and advocacy roles of physicians. Finally, the pace and commercial nature of health care often impede the inculcation of fundamental values of the profession" [118].

With all the concerns and questions, should we be pessimistic? I, for one, am not. Noting that 15 major US and Canadian reports that have been written in the past decade, all calling for significant change in medical education, Skochelak notes: "We are experiencing the 100-year echo of 1901–1910, the decade of medical education reform that culminated in the Carnegie Foundation report by Abraham Flexner" [119], implying that the coming decade may be a momentous one. In her review, Skochelak found "remarkable congruence" in the recommendations of the 15 reports and concludes "We can be assured that we don't need to keep asking 'What should we do?' but rather 'How do we get there?'" The pediatrics community is getting there by coming together, collaborating, and supporting 2 key projects: the Pediatrics Milestone Project and IIPE. In addition, a third project, the Pediatric Redesign Pilot Project, has the potential to inform efforts to create a true continuum of preparation for a career in pediatrics. The pediatrician leader of all 3 efforts is Carol Carraccio, so it seems fitting to allow her the final word: "This is an exciting time in medical education. Many of the national initiatives are beginning to connect and provide synergy for each other. If we continue on this current trajectory, we will have the opportunity to make transformative change in pediatric medical education and training" [120].

Acknowledgments

The author gratefully acknowledges the valuable assistance of the following valued colleagues: to create and consolidate a top ten list, Drs Carol Carraccio, Larrie Greenberg, Stephen Ludwig, Robert Perelman, and Christopher White; to suggest valuable references, Drs Kevin Johnson and Joseph Lopreiato; to confirm facts, Drs Gail McGuinness, Daniel Rauch, and Steven Shelov,

Ms Jean Bartholomew (ABP), Ms Julie Raymond (AAP), and Mr Kenneth Slaw (AAP).

References

[1] Institute of Medicine. To err is human: building a safer health system. Washington, DC: Institute of Medicine, National Academies Press; 1999.
[2] IPRO. ACGME-NYS 405 regulations resident work limits comparison guideline. Available at: http://www.docstoc.com/docs/17820605/ACGME-NYS-405-comparison-resident-work-llimits. Accessed December 20, 2010.
[3] Johnson T. Limitations on residents' working hours at New York teaching hospitals: a status report. Acad Med 2003;78:3–8.
[4] Philibert I. The 2003 common duty hour limits: process, outcome, and lessons learned. J Grad Med Educ 2009;1:334–7.
[5] Landrigan C, Parry G, Bones C, et al. Temporal trends in rates of patient harm resulting from medical care. N Engl J Med 2010;363:2124–34.
[6] Ludmerer K. Resident burnout: working hours or working environment? J Grad Med Educ 2009;1:169–71.
[7] Landrigan CP, Fahrenkopf A, Lewin D, et al. Effects of the accreditation council for graduate medical education duty hour limits on sleep, work hours, and safety. Pediatrics 2008;122:250–8.
[8] Volpp K, Landrigan C. Building physician work hour regulations from first principles and best evidence. JAMA 2008;300:1197–9.
[9] Landrigan C, Rothschild J, Cronin J, et al. Effect of reducing interns' work hours on serious medical errors in intensive care units. N Engl J Med 2004;351:1838–48.
[10] Lockley S, Cronin J, Evans E, et al. Effect of reducing interns' weekly work hours on sleep and attentional failures. N Engl J Med 2004;351:1829–37.
[11] Levine A, Adusumilli J, Landrigan C. Effects of reducing or eliminating resident work shifts over 16 hours: a systematic review. Sleep 2010;33(8):1043–53.
[12] Institute of Medicine. Resident duty hours: enhancing sleep, supervision, and safety. Washington, DC: Institute of Medicine, National Academies Press; 2008.
[13] Blum A, Raiszadeh R, Shea S, et al. US public opinion regarding proposed limits on resident physician work hours. BMC Med 2010;8:33–44.
[14] Accreditation Council for Graduate Medical Education. Information Related to the ACGME's Effort to Address Resident Duty Hours and Other Relevant Resource Materials. Available at: http://www.acgme.org/DutyHours/dutyHrs_Index.asp. Accessed December 21, 2010.
[15] Burke A, Rushton J, Guralnick S, et al. Resident work hour requirements: medical educators' perspectives. Acad Pediatr 2010;10:369–71.
[16] Logio L, Djuricich A. Handoffs in teaching hospitals: situation, background, assessment, and recommendation. Am J Med 2010;123:563–7.
[17] Philibert I. Supervision, preoccupation with failure, and the cultural shift in patient handover. J Grad Med Educ 2010;2:144–5.
[18] Accreditation Council for Graduate Medical Education. Common Program Requirements VIB. Available at: http://www.acgme.org/acWebsite/home/Common_Program_Requirements_07012011.pdf. Accessed December 21, 2010.
[19] Gordon J, Alexander E, Lockley S, et al. Does simulator-based clinical performance correlate with actual hospital behavior? The effect of extended work hours on patient care provided by medical interns. Acad Med 2010;85:1583–8.
[20] Cohen J, Dickler R. Auditing the Medicare-billing practices of teaching physicians–welcome accountability, unfair approach. N Engl J Med 1997;336:1317–20.
[21] Association of American Medical Colleges. AAMC-Physicians at Teaching Hospitals (PATH) audits. Available at: https://www.aamc.org/advocacy/teachphys/73578/teachphys_phys0040.html. Accessed December 21, 2010.

[22] Medicare fraud case settled for $30 million. Healthc Financ Manag February 1996.
[23] Sterkenburg A, Barach P, Kalkman C, et al. When do supervising physicians decide to entrust residents with unsupervised tasks? Acad Med 2010;85:1408–17.
[24] Bush R. Supervision in medical education: logical fallacies and clear choices. J Grad Med Educ 2010;2:141–3.
[25] Babbott S. Watching closely at a distance: key tensions in supervising resident physicians. Acad Med 2010;85:1399–400.
[26] Landrigan C, Muret-Wagstaff S, Chiang V, et al. Senior resident autonomy in a pediatric hospitalist system. Arch Pediatr Adolesc Med 2003;157:206–7.
[27] Institute of Medicine. Crossing the quality chasm: a new health system for the 21st century. Washington, DC: Institute of Medicine, National Academies Press; 2001.
[28] Accreditation Council for Graduate Medical Education. The outcome project. Available at: http://www.acgme.org/outcome/. Accessed December 21, 2010.
[29] American Board of Medical Specialties. Maintenance of certification. Available at: http://www.abms.org/Maintenance_of_Certification/ABMS_MOC.aspx. Accessed December 21, 2010.
[30] Accreditation Council for Continuing Medical Education. 2006 Updated decision-making criteria relevant to the essential areas and elements. Available at: http://www.accme.org/dir_docs/doc_upload/f4ee5075-9574-4231-8876-5e21723c0c82_uploaddocument.pdf. Accessed December 21, 2010. p. 2–3.
[31] Irby D, Wilkerson L. Educational innovations in academic medicine and environmental trends. J Gen Intern Med 2003;18:370–6.
[32] Ludmerer K. Time to heal. New York: Oxford University Press; 1999.
[33] Johnson K, Chark D, Chen Q, et al. Performing without a net: transitioning away from a health information technology-rich training environment. Acad Med 2008;83:1179–86.
[34] Ruiz J, Mintzer M, Leipzig R. The impact of e-learning in medical education. Acad Med 2006;81:207–12.
[35] Baker R, Lewis K. Online master's degree in education for healthcare professionals: early outcomes of a new program. Med Teach 2007;29:987–9.
[36] Spooner S, Gotlieg E. Steering Committee on Clinical Information Technology and Committee on Medical Liability. American Academy of Pediatrics Technical Report. Telemedicine: pediatric applications. Pediatrics 2004;113:e639–43.
[37] Anderson M, Kanter S. Medical education in the United States and Canada, 2010. Acad Med 2010;85(Suppl 9):S2–18.
[38] Satava R. The revolution in medical education–the role of simulation. J Grad Med Educ 2009;1:172–5.
[39] Liaison Committee on Medical Education. Functions and structure of a medical school. Available at: http://www.lcme.org/functions2010jun.pdf. Accessed December 22, 2010. p. 6–7.
[40] Li S, Smith S, Gigante J. A national survey of pediatric clerkship directors' approaches to meeting the LCME ED-2 requirement for quantified patient criteria for medical students. Teach Learn Med 2007;19:352–6.
[41] CLIPP. Available at: http://www.med-u.org/virtual_patient_cases/clipp. Accessed December 22, 2010.
[42] Berman N, Fall L, Smith S, et al. Integration strategies for using virtual patients in clinical clerkships. Acad Med 2009;84:942–9.
[43] Tempelhof M. Personal digital assistants: a review of current and potential utilization among medical residents. Teach Learn Med 2009;21:100–4.
[44] Ho K, Lauscher H, Broudo M, et al. The impact of a personal digital assistant (PDA) case log in a medical student clerkship. Teach Learn Med 2009;21:318–26.
[45] Conn J. EHRs have varying effects on productivity: UC Davis study. Modern healthcare Posted December 17, 2010. Available at: http://www.modernhealthcare.com/article/20101217/NEWS/312179998. Accessed December 22, 2010.

[46] Scribes, EMR please docs, save $600,000. ED Manag 2009;21:117–8.
[47] Friedman E, Sainte M, Fallar R. Taking note of the perceived value and impact of medical student chart documentation on education and patient care. Acad Med 2010;85:1440–4.
[48] Mintz M, Narvarte H, O'Brien K, et al. Use of electronic medical records by physicians and students in academic internal medicine settings. Acad Med 2009;84:1698–704.
[49] Fincher R-M, White C, Huang G, et al. Toward hypothesis-driven medical education research: task force report from the Millennium Conference 2007 on Educational Research. Acad Med 2010;85:821–8.
[50] Farnan J, Paro J, Higa J, et al. The relationship of digital media and professionalism: it's complicated. Acad Med 2009;84:1479–81.
[51] Association of American Medical Colleges. Physician shortages to worsen without increases in residency training. Available at: http://www.communityoncology.org/wp-content/uploads/AAMC-MD-Shortage.pdf. Accessed December 22, 2010.
[52] Association of American Medical Colleges. AAMC Statement on the Physician Workforce. Available at: https://www.aamc.org/download/55458/data/workforceposition.pdf. Accessed December 22, 2010.
[53] Whitcomb M. New medical schools in the United States. N Engl J Med 2010;362: 1255–8.
[54] Association of American Medical Colleges. Results of the 2009 Medical School Enrollment Survey. Center for Workforce Studies. March 2010. Available at: https://www.aamc.org/download/124780/data/enrollment2010.pdf.pdf. Accessed December 22, 2010.
[55] Council on Graduate Medical Education. Thirteenth report: physician education for a changing health care environment. Bethesda (MD): US Department of Health and Human Services, Bureau of Health Professions, Health Care Resources and Services Administration; 1999.
[56] Shipman S, Lan J, Chang C, et al. Pediatrics In press (published online December 20, 2010), Available at: http://pediatrics.aappublications.org/papbyrecent.dtl. Accessed December 22, 2010.
[57] Keirns C, Bosk C. The unintended consequences of training residents in dysfunctional outpatient settings. Acad Med 2008;83:498–502.
[58] Rabinowitz H, Diamond J, Markham F, et al. Medical school programs to increase the rural physician supply: a systematic review and projected impact of widespread replication. Acad Med 2008;83:235–43.
[59] Stein R, Johnston I, Bannister S. Students completing a pediatric clinical clerkship in a regional center perform as well as their peers training at a university teaching hospital-...and they liked it better. Teach Learn Med 2009;212:225–8.
[60] Roberts K, Starr S, DeWitt T. The UMMC office-based continuity experience: are we preparing pediatrics residents for primary care practice? Pediatrics 1997;100(4):e2.
[61] Roberts K, Starr S, DeWitt T. Resident preparedness for practice: a longitudinal cohort study. Ambul Pediatr 2002;2:132–5.
[62] Mallon W. Medical school expansion: déjà vu all over again? Acad Med 2007;82: 1121–5.
[63] Bonaminio G, Leapman S, Norcini J, et al. The educational realities of increasing medical school class size. Acad Med 2008;83(Suppl 10):S101–4.
[64] Whitcomb M. Physician supply revisited. Acad Med 2007;82:825–6.
[65] Fact sheet: creating jobs and increasing the number of primary care providers. Available at: www.healthreform.gov/newsroom/primarycareworkforce.html. Accessed December 22, 2010.
[66] Zemke R, Raines C, Filipczak B. Generations at work. Managing the clash of veterans, boomers, Xers, and nexters in your workplace. New York: American Management Association; 2000.
[67] Cull W, O'Connor K, Olson L. Part-time work among pediatricians expands. Pediatrics 2010;125:152–7.

[68] Hodges B. A tea-steeping or i-Doc model for medical education? Acad Med 2010;85(Suppl 9):S34–44.
[69] Hicks P, Schumacher D, Benson B, et al. The pediatrics milestones: conceptual framework, guiding principles, and approach to development. J Grad Med Educ 2010;2:410–8.
[70] The Medical School Objectives Writing Group. Learning objectives for medical student education–guidelines for medical schools: report I of the Medical School Objectives Project. Acad Med 1999;74:13–8.
[71] Whitcomb M. More on competency-based education. Acad Med 2004;79:493–4.
[72] COMSEP Curriculum Task Force, APPD Curriculum Task Force. COMSEP and APPD Pediatric Subinternship Curriculum. Available at: http://www.comsep.org/Curriculum/pdfs/COMSEP-APPDF.pdf. Accessed December 21, 2010.
[73] Roberts K. 2009 Miller-Sarkin Lecture. Outcome and process in medical education: does the whole equal the sum of the parts? Acad Med 2010;10:1–6.
[74] Huddle T, Heudebert G. Taking apart the art: the risk of anatomizing clinical competence. Acad Med 2007;82:536–41.
[75] Whitcomb M. Redirecting the assessment of clinical competence. Acad Med 2007;82: 527–8.
[76] ten Cate O, Scheele F. Competency-based postgraduate training: can we bridge the gap between theory and clinical practice? Acad Med 2007;82:542–7.
[77] Carraccio C, Burke A. Beyond competencies and milestones: adding meaning through context. J Grad Med Educ 2010;2:419–22.
[78] Carraccio C, Englander R. Evaluating competence using a portfolio: a literature review and web-based application to the ACGME Competencies. Teach Learn Med 2004;16: 381–7.
[79] Lane J, Gottlieb R. Structured clinical observations: a method to teach clinical skills with limited time and financial resources. Pediatrics 2000;105:973–7.
[80] Carraccio C, Englander R. The objective structured clinical examination. A step in the direction of competency-based evaluation. Arch Pediatr Adolesc Med 2000;154: 736–41.
[81] Bokken L, Rethans J, Jobsis Q, et al. Instructiveness of real patients and simulated patients in undergraduate medical education: a randomized experiment. Acad Med 2010;85: 148–54.
[82] Hicks P, Englander R, Schumacher D, et al. Pediatrics milestone project: next steps toward meaningful assessment. J Grad Med Ed 2010;2:577–84.
[83] Accreditation Council for Graduate Medical Education. Toolbox of assessment methods. Available at: http://www.acgme.org/Outcome/assess/Toolbox.pdf. Accessed December 22, 2010.
[84] Swing S, Clyman S, Holmboe E, et al. ACGME Advisory Committee on Educational Outcome Assessment. Advancing resident assessment in graduate medical education. J Grad Med Educ 2009;1:278–86.
[85] Carraccio C, Englander R, Adams D, et al. Is there a gap between program directors' expectations and residents' performance? Comparing predictions with outcomes for competence in patient care. Acad Med 2010;85:1152–6.
[86] Kogan J, Hess B, Conforti L, et al. What drives faculty ratings of residents' clinical skills? The impact of faculty's own clinical skills. Acad Med 2010;85(Suppl 10):S25–8.
[87] Rosenblum N, Wetzel M, Platt O, et al. Predicting medical student success in a clinical clerkship by rating students' nonverbal behavior. Arch Pediatr Adolesc Med 1994;148: 213–9.
[88] Lurie S, Mooney C, Lyness J. Measurement of the general competencies of the accreditation council for graduate medical education: a systematic review. Acad Med 2009;84:301–9.
[89] Green M, Holmboe E. The ACGME toolbox: half empty or half full? Acad Med 2010;85: 787–90.
[90] Ludwig S, Stein R. Anatomy of mentoring. J Pediatr 2008;152:151–2.

[91] Gusic M, Zenni E, Ludwig S, et al. Strategies to design an effective mentoring program. J Pediatr 2010;156:173.e1–174.e1.
[92] Spector N, Mann K, Anderson M, et al. Facilitated peer group mentoring: a case study of creating leadership skills among the associate program directors of the APPD. Acad Pediatr 2010;10:161–4.
[93] Osborn L, Roberts K, Greenberg L, et al. APA/HRSA Faculty Development Scholars Program. Ambul Pediatr 2004;4(Suppl 1):83–128.
[94] Academic Pediatric Association. APA Educational Scholars Program. Available at: http://www.academicpeds.org/education/education_scholars_program.cfm. Accessed December 23, 2010.
[95] Macy J Jr. Foundation Faculty Scholars Program. Available at: http://www.josiahmacyfoundation.org/docs/macy_pubs/JMF_FacultyScholars_Brochure_final.pdf. Accessed December 23, 2010.
[96] Steinert Y, Mann K, Centeno A, et al. A systematic review of faculty development initiatives designed to improve teaching effectiveness in medical education: BEME guide No. 8. Med Teach 2006;28:497–526.
[97] Irby D, Cooke M, Lowenstein D, et al. The academy movement: a structural approach to reinvigorating the educational mission. Acad Med 2004;79:729–36.
[98] Glassick C. Boyer's expanded definitions of scholarship, the standards for assessing scholarship, and the elusiveness of the scholarship of teaching. Acad Med 2000;75:877–80.
[99] American Board of Pediatrics. Training requirements for subspecialty certification. Available at: https://www.abp.org/abpwebsite/publicat/trainingrequirements.pdf. Accessed December 23, 2010.
[100] Association of American Medical Colleges. MedEdPORTAL. Available at: http://www.aamc.org/mededportal. Accessed December 21, 2010.
[101] Association of Pediatric Program Directors. Share Warehouse Available on Members Only Section of APPD website at, Available at: http://www.appd.org/ed_res/share_warehouse.cfm?frommem=true. Accessed December 23, 2010.
[102] Association of Pediatric Program Directors. LEARN. Available at: http://www.appd.org/ed_res/LEARN.cfm. Accessed on December 23, 2010.
[103] Regehr G. It's not rocket science: rethinking our metaphors for research in health professions education. Med Educ 2010;44:31–9.
[104] Task Force on Pediatric Education. The future of pediatric education. Evanston (IL): American Academy of Pediatrics; 1979.
[105] The Future of Pediatric Education II: organizing pediatric education to meet the needs of infants, children, adolescents, and young adults in the 21st century. Pediatrics 2000;105:163–212.
[106] Federation of Pediatric Organizations. Available at: http://www.fopo.org. Accessed December 23, 2010.
[107] Academic Pediatric Association. Educational Guidelines for Pediatric Residency. Available at: www.academicpeds.org/education/education_guidelines.cfm. Accessed December 23, 2010.
[108] Kittredge D, Baldwin C, Bar-on M, et al. One specialty's approach to competency-based education: collaborative development of customizable curricular tools. Acad Med 2009;84:1262–8.
[109] Beach P, Bar-on M, Baldwin C, et al. Use of an interactive, online resource for competency-based curriculum development. Acad Med 2009;84:1269–75.
[110] Jones M, Leslie L, McGuinness G. Residency review and redesign in pediatrics: new (and old) questions. Pediatrics 2009;123:S1–60.
[111] Initiative for Innovation in Pediatric Education. Available at: http://www.innovatepedsgme.org. Accessed December 23, 2010.
[112] Jones M. Innovation in residency education and evolving pediatric health needs. Pediatrics 2010;125:1–3.

[113] Flexner A. Medical Education in the United States and Canada: a report to the Carnegie Foundation for the Advancement of Teaching. Cited by Ludmerer K. Understanding the Flexner Report. Acad Med 2010;85:193–6.
[114] American Board of Pediatrics and Association of Pediatric Program Directors. Teaching and assessing professionalism: a program director's guide. Available at: https://www.abp.org/abpwebsite/publicat/professionalism.pdf. Accessed December 23, 2010.
[115] Sectish T, Stapleton F, Schnaper W, et al. The creation of the Council of Pediatric Subspecialties: addressing the needs of the subspecialties and subspecialists. J Pediatr 2007;151:105–6.
[116] Roberts K. 2009 Joseph W. St Geme Jr Leadership Award address: the whole and the sum of its parts. Pediatrics 2010;125:173–7.
[117] Kanter S. How to win an argument about the senior year of medical school. Acad Med 2009;84:815–6.
[118] Irby D, Cooke M, O'Brien B. Calls for reform of medical education by the Carnegie Foundation for the Advancement of Teaching: 1910 and 2010. Acad Med 2010;85:220–7.
[119] Skochelak S. A decade of reports calling for change in medical education: what do they say? Acad Med 2010;85(Suppl 9):S26–33.
[120] Carraccio C. Fall 2010 update on the initiative for innovation in pediatric education. APPD Newsletter. Available at: http://www.appd.org/Newsletter/Fall2010/iu.cfm. Accessed December 23, 2010.

Advances in Pediatrics 58 (2011) 153–179

ADVANCES IN PEDIATRICS

Controversies Surrounding Pediatric Psychopharmacology

Robin Steinberg-Epstein, MD[a,b,c,*],
Teri Book, RN, MSN, CPNP[c], Sharon B. Wigal, PhD[d]

[a]Division of Developmental-Behavioral Pediatrics, USA
[b]University of California, Irvine School of Medicine, USA
[c]For OC Kids Neurodevelopmental Center, 1915 West Orangewood Avenue, Suite 200, Orange, CA 92686, USA
[d]Department of Pediatrics, Child Development Center, University of California, 19722 MacArthur Boulevard, Irvine, CA 92612, USA

The past several decades have witnessed an increased awareness of mental health disorders and neurobehavioral problems in children [1]. These behavioral issues now represent a growing portion of pediatric visits. Addressing and appropriately managing early-onset disorders may improve quality of life while providing hope that adult morbidity may be attenuated [2]. Given the shortage of mental health providers and the concept of the pediatric practice as "medical home," many pediatricians are poised to receive this population. Caring for this population of children is riddled with systemic obstacles. Lack of time, training, support, and compensation, together with poor integration of collaboration with mental health resources, all contribute to this challenge. Children's mental health has become a priority issue for the American Academy of Pediatrics [3].

A better understanding of the magnitude of mental health issues facing children was highlighted by the recently completed National Comorbidity Study, which examined the prevalence of psychiatric disorders in a sample of more than 10,000 children between the ages of 13 and 18 years. The investigators found that almost 50% of adolescents would have had enough symptoms at some point in their life to meet criteria for a psychiatric disorder by 18 years of age [1]. Twenty-two percent were found to have significant

Disclosures: Dr Robin Steinberg-Epstein is a consultant for McNeil; has received grant/research support from Addrenex, Eli Lilly & Co., McNeil, Next Wave Pharmaceuticals, Otsuka, Psychogenics, Quintiles, Shionogi Pharm., Shire, and the NIMH; is on the speaker or advisory boards for McNeil. Ms. Book has nothing to disclose. Dr Sharon B. Wigal is a consultant for Abbott, McNeil, NuTec, Shire, Taisho, and the NIMH; has received grant/research support from Addrenex, Eli Lilly & Co., McNeil, Next Wave Pharmaceuticals, Otsuka, Psychogenics, Quintiles, Shionogi Pharm., Shire, NICHD, and the NIMH; is on the speaker or advisory boards for Eli Lilly & Co., McNeil, Shionogi Pharm., and Shire.

*Corresponding author. *E-mail address*: rsteinb@uci.edu

0065-3101/11/$ – see front matter
doi:10.1016/j.yapd.2011.03.002

impairment as a result of their symptomatology. These numbers are alarming. The fact that there are fewer than 8000 child psychiatrists and fewer than 600 developmental behavioral pediatricians in the United States to care for these children highlights the tremendous shortage of subspecialty providers, and compounds the problem of providing adequate care.

In response to the imbalance between the number of patients and providers, the American Academy of Pediatrics (AAP) Committee of Psychosocial Aspect of Child and Family Health and Task Force on Mental Health has set a goal for pediatricians to be competent in the use of medications to treat attention-deficit/hyperactivity disorder (ADHD), major depressive disorder, and anxiety [4]. The AAP has created several valuable tools in the area of mental health (Addressing Mental Health Concerns in Primary Care: A Clinician's Toolkit, Autism Toolkit, ADHD Toolkit) to support pediatricians in assessment, decision-making, management, coding, and so forth, and these are now available for purchase. These tools are helpful, but it will be important for clinicians to familiarize themselves with current research and the medications used to treat these common problems.

At present there seems to be an overdependence on psychotropic medication solutions for the treatment of mental health disorders. This situation is influenced by many issues. Our understanding of the neurobiological basis of psychiatric illness has greatly advanced over the past two decades, with even more emphasis on the role of medication as a viable treatment. Furthermore, there now is an understanding that these psychiatric conditions that were thought to only affect adults often originate in childhood. This convergence of ideas, together with a lack of community resources to support children suffering from psychiatric conditions, has contributed to this tendency to resort to medication. In addition, clinicians may be influenced by nonpediatric psychopharmacology research or their anecdotal prescribing experience as well as the experience of colleagues. The popular media and the pharmaceutical industry also play a role in providing sensationalized appeals or biased opinions that may influence even the most critically minded physician and parent.

The goal of this article is to bring up-to-date information regarding advances in medical psychopharmacology research to general pediatricians. The article identifies the common psychiatric disorders in children, pivotal research shaping treatment recommendations, and some of the controversies surrounding the use of psychotropic medication in children. Care providers can thereby develop an informed approach to management of psychotropic medication.

The National Comorbidity Study found that the top 3 pediatric mental health disorders in decreasing frequency are anxiety (specific phobia at 19.3%, social phobia at 9.1%), depression (11.7%), and ADHD (8.7%). This finding is consistent with previous studies [5,6]. Although autism is not considered among the most common disorders (frequency of 1:110) [7], it is considered to be the fastest-growing developmental disability [8]. Therefore, autism and its pharmacotherapy are also described in this article.

EMPIRICALLY DRIVEN TREATMENT MODELS

Management of many common disorders in medicine often relies on treatment models that are based on a comprehensive base of research and observed clinical outcomes in adult patients. Until recently, most medication interventions in pediatric mental health were extrapolated from adult treatment patterns and used in an off-label fashion [9,10]. However, research over the past two decades has led to the emergence of pediatric-specific practice parameters for several common conditions, including some neurobehavioral disorders. Psychopharmacologic agents are now being used with greater frequency than ever before. The use of second-generation antipsychotics has more than doubled in the past decade [11–13]. Almost one-third of psychotropic medications are prescribed by non–mental health providers [14].

Both anecdotal experience and empirical clinical data suggest that medication can play an important role in managing behavioral disorders in children. Only recently have large and well-designed treatment studies been conducted for childhood mental health disorders. These studies help to inform the medical community on the application of evidence-based interventions. While these studies are far from comprehensive, they are a step toward creating treatment algorithms that incorporate the dual priorities of safety and efficacy in the care of children with psychiatric disorders. Before examining the specific classes of medications, it is important to be aware of these seminal research works guiding treatment for children. Familiarizing oneself with these studies will help the practitioner to understand best-practice medication and therapeutic alternatives.

Anxiety

The Surgeon General estimates that more than 13% of children have an anxiety disorder, which includes specific phobia, social phobia, obsessive-compulsive disorder (OCD), and generalized anxiety disorder [15]. A recent large multisite study, the Child/Adolescent Multimodal Study (CAMS), reported the effects of anxiety treatments on a randomly assigned group of 488 children. Children aged 7 to 17 years were given 1 of 4 treatments for 12 weeks: sertraline alone, cognitive-behavioral therapy (CBT) alone, combination sertraline and CBT, or control. The results showed that 81% in the combination group showed significant improvement, 60% of those in the CBT-only group, 55% in the antidepressant group (sertraline), and 24% in the placebo group. This study suggests that first-line treatment for anxiety disorders should include CBT. In addition, this study found that the sertraline group had no more side effects than the placebo group, suggesting safety and tolerability [16].

Obsessive thoughts and compulsive behaviors are important presentations of childhood anxiety. The large multisite Pediatric Obsessive Compulsive Treatment Study II (POTS) focused specifically on OCD. One hundred and twelve children with OCD, aged 7 to 17 years, entered 1 of 4 study arms: CBT alone, sertraline alone, combination sertraline and CBT, or placebo, over 12 weeks. In this study combination therapy proved to be the superior treatment, followed by CBT or sertraline (neither of which showed superiority to one another). All active treatments were superior to placebo. These results support the use of combination treatment for children with OCD, and identify the lesser impact of CBT or sertraline used alone [17].

It should be noted that these studies looked at CBT and not play therapy, talk therapy, or other therapies. However, many therapists are not trained in this therapeutic method, which highlights 3 common challenges for the pediatrician: identification of patients who might benefit from nonpharmacologic mental health treatment, locating community resources that can apply best-practice mental health treatments (in this case CBT) with children, and circumventing financial barriers that limit access [18].

Depression

Depression is another common pediatric mental health disorder. Childhood depression can have very serious consequences. In 2005, 16.9% of United States high school students reported seriously considering suicide during the 12 months preceding the survey. More than 8% of students reported that they had actually attempted suicide one or more times during the same period [19]. Many adult physicians treat depression with antidepressants, such as selective serotonin reuptake inhibitors (SSRIs). However, until recently limited pediatric data were available to support an evidence-based approach for the management of depression in children. The Treatment for Adolescent Depression Study (TADS) study examined 327 adolescents with depression in 1 of 4 treatment groups: fluoxetine, CBT, combination of fluoxetine and CBT, or placebo. The results of this important study showed that all 3 treatment groups showed improvement over placebo (Fig. 1). In the first few weeks all 4 groups improved. By 6 weeks post intervention the 3 active treatments were superior to placebo, with the combination treatment group and fluoxetine group showing the greatest changes. Surprisingly, this difference dissipates over time and all 3 treatment groups show significant and equivalent benefits over placebo by 3 to 6 months (see Fig. 1). Therefore, if symptoms require rapid amelioration, such as when depression is severe or associated with significant suicidality, medication should be used in conjunction with CBT [20]. However, in patients with mild to moderate symptoms of depression and taking into account the potential side effects of a medication, CBT is an appropriate first option for families who can access this treatment with an appropriate pediatric CBT provider. Follow-up of the cohort revealed that those children who continued to receive intervention, regardless of the treatment, fared better. This finding would support the idea that ongoing support is helpful in maintaining a positive outcome. The length of this ongoing support is not clear. Interpretation of studies examining antidepressant response in children must be interpreted carefully and replicated, as there is a known high placebo response rate.

Attention-deficit/hyperactivity disorder

Epidemiologic studies revealed prevalence rates for ADHD generally ranging from 4% to 12% in the general population of 6- to 12-year-olds [5,6]. ADHD

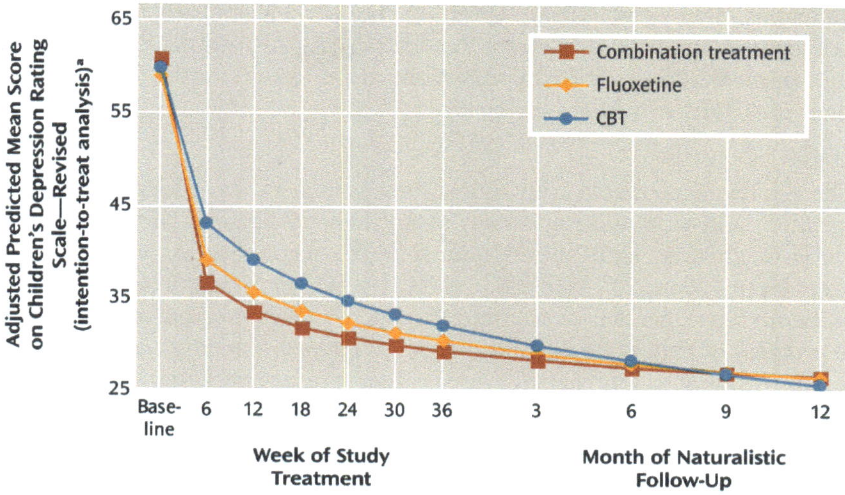

Fig. 1. Depression scores from baseline to end of naturalistic follow-up of 327 adolescents with major depressive disorder treated with fluoxetine, CBT, or combination. (*From* Treatment for Adolescents with Depression Study (TADS) team. The Treatment for Adolescents with Depression Study (TADS): Outcomes over 1 year of naturalistic follow-up. Am J Psychiatry 2009;166:1141–9; with permission from *American Journal of Psychiatry* (Copyright © 2008), American Psychiatric Association.)

is characterized by inattention and/or hyperactivity and impulsivity. Many Americans question the very existence of ADHD, and feel that ADHD treatment is unjustified. However, decades of detailed analysis validate the presence, prevalence, morbidity, progression, and scientific validity of this mental health disorder. Until the 1990s there was considerable debate over the management ADHD. In 1995 the Multimodal Treatment Study of children with ADHD (MTA) explored a variety of treatment options. The MTA is the largest study to systematically examine the role of behavioral interventions and/or medication in the treatment of disruptive behavior in children. This study examined 579 children with combined-type ADHD, aged 7.9 to 9.9 years, over a 14-month period. There were 4 treatment arms: treatment with stimulant medication, behavioral intervention, combination of medication and behavioral treatment, and control. The results showed the medicine and medicine plus behavior groups experienced the largest reductions in ADHD symptoms, and the responses were considered superior to those seen by children receiving behavioral treatment alone or in the control group. Furthermore, the behavior plus medication did not show superiority to medication alone in ADHD symptoms [21]. There are limitations to the study, but the overall message is clear. Medication can be an important component of a successful short- to medium-duration intervention for children with ADHD. Behavioral interventions are important tools for the treatment of ADHD symptoms and for children with ADHD and common comorbid conditions. This seminal study led to practice parameters from the American Academy of Child and Adolescent Psychiatry (AACAP) and AAP recommending that medication, specifically stimulants, are an option for the first-line treatment of ADHD in school-aged children [22,23].

Autism

The behaviors associated with autism such as anxiety, hyperkinetic behavior, agitation, and aggression are often severe and debilitating. More than two-thirds of children with autism ultimately try medication to manage these behavior problems [24]. Medication is NOT a treatment for the core symptoms of autism but rather is used to control secondary behaviors that create barriers to progress or danger for patients or others. There are no large or multimodal studies guiding comprehensive medication management for autism. The primary treatment is a multimodal treatment program that incorporates intensive therapy such as applied behavioral analysis, language therapy, occupational therapy, social cognition interventions, and cognitive support [25]. Only when a child fails to respond to interventions or when behaviors are extremely disruptive should medications be considered.

PSYCHOPHARMACOLOGY

In addition to understanding the major research that influences medication treatment, physicians should understand the nuances of psychopharmacologic agents. The decision to use medication to treat a behavioral disorder is not a decision that parents take lightly. Parents commonly consult friends, family, and the internet before making a decision with their child's physician. Thus, in this "electronic age," physicians need to be ultra-prepared to anticipate questions and to provide reassurance about the risks and benefits associated with each of the major classes of medications for pediatric patients. What follows is a discussion addressing commonly expressed concerns regarding the most frequently used psychopharmacologic agents used in pediatrics: antidepressants, stimulants and stimulant alternatives, and antipsychotics. This discourse will arm the pediatrician with information to educate parents and guide medication choice and treatment.

Selective serotonin reuptake inhibitors

SSRIs are a class of compounds typically used in the treatment of depression and anxiety disorders. SSRIs are among the most commonly prescribed antidepressant drugs on the market today. The use of SSRIs in the treatment of behavioral disorders in children is based on the assumption that abnormalities exist in the serotonergic activity of the brain. The primary action of SSRIs is to block the action of the presynaptic serotonin reuptake pump, thereby increasing the level of serotonin in the synaptic gap. Thus the postsynaptic neuron is exposed to more serotonin to treat what is suspected as the cause of many emotional and behavioral disorders [26].

There are 6 SSRIs currently being regularly prescribed in the United States: fluoxetine, sertraline, fluvoxamine, paroxetine, citalopram, and escitalopram.

Of the 6, fluoxetine (Prozac) is one of only two SSRIs approved for use by the Food and Drug Administration (FDA) for the treatment of children and adolescents aged 8 to 17 years who suffer from depression. It is also approved for the treatment of OCD in children 7 to 17 years of age. Fluoxetine has the longest half-life (between 4 and 7 days) of all the SSRIs. It also takes the longest time to achieve steady state, between 2 and 4 weeks. Its long half-life decreases the symptoms associated with the abrupt discontinuation of therapy, which is a major advantage in regulating treatment and limiting side effects from accidental noncompliance [27]. Fluoxetine tends to be the most activating of the SSRIs. Sertaline (Zoloft) is licensed by the FDA for treatment of children from 12 to 17 years of age who are diagnosed with OCD. Paroxetine (Paxil) is not licensed by the FDA for treatment of children with depression or anxiety. Fluvoxamine (Luvox) is the least activating of all the SSRIs, but interacts with many common medications. It is approved for use in children older than 8 years who are diagnosed with OCD, but has not been approved for treatment of depression in children in the United States. Fluvoxamine has the shortest half-life of all SSRIs, at 15 hours [27]. Because of its pharmokinetics, citalopram (Celexa) is thought to be the SSRI with the fewest drug-to-drug interactions. Escitalopram (Lexapro) is the *S*-stereoisomer of citalopram. It is typically twice as potent as the racemic version citalopram. Escitalopram is FDA-approved for the treatment of depression in adolescents aged 12 to 17 years [28].

When measured in adults, all of the SSRIs have similar efficacy and side-effect profiles. Studies of their effectiveness in treating depression in children are limited. The different pharmacodynamic properties of the SSRIs, especially their drug-drug interaction potential, should be considered when selecting a distinct SSRI for treatment. The following sections highlight some of the controversies surrounding SSRI use in children.

Suicidal ideation

There is ongoing debate about the risk of SSRIs and other antidepressants increasing the chance of suicidal behavior in children and adolescents. Evidence for and against the association of suicidal risk with antidepressant therapy emerged from several randomized trials on adolescents and children [20,29]. In addition, observational studies and population-based studies were reviewed, and the rates of suicide during treatment with antidepressants compared. No clear-cut causal relationship was identified between the use of antidepressants and suicide. This uncertainty led to the creation of an FDA advisory panel to study the issue in more depth. The panel's meta-analysis determined that there was a small but real increased risk of suicidal thought or behaviors in children and adolescents on SSRIs when compared with placebo. There were no completed suicides in the subjects participating in the studies. The review also found that the time for highest risk of suicidal ideation was in the period of initiation of treatment with antidepressants [30–32]. This finding mirrors the adult treatment experience with SSRIs. It is generally accepted that in the adult population the greatest risk for suicide attempt occurs directly after starting antidepressant therapy. One theory is that the first symptom to improve after initiation of an antidepressant is the patient's low energy level. This activation may enable a still depressed adult to act on their thoughts. Alternatively, the medication may depress mood or raise anxiety or distress in a minority of treated individuals. The findings of the FDA meta-analysis led the FDA in 2004 to ask the manufacturers of all antidepressant medication to change their labeling to inform patients and families about the issue. The "Black Box" warning states that the use of antidepressants may increase the risk of suicidal ideation and behavior in adolescents and children. In addition, all pharmacies were instructed to provide a patient medication guide along with each prescription. This guide highlights important safety issues and warnings, and is required when families receive any antidepressant [33,34].

Subsequent studies seemed to support that the Black Box warning was necessary [20]. On the other hand, other studies have not supported the need for these warnings. In 2004 the American College of Neuropsychopharmacology (ACNP) Task Force on SSRI and Suicidal Behavior in Youth included published and unpublished evidence for 15 trials regarding the safety and effectiveness of 5 different SSRI medications (citlopram, fluoxetine, paroxetine, sertraline, venlafaxine). There were no completed suicides and the rate of suicidal behavior was no different between treatment and placebo groups in the studies examined. In addition, the investigators found that only fluoxetine had strong statistical evidence of efficacy [32].

By 2003 there was genuine concern that the Black Box warning may have scared providers, and prescribing rates of these very important medications declined. Olfson and colleagues [34] found that in the decade before the Black Box warning, adolescent suicide rates were declining at rates comparable to the increase in prescribing rates of antidepressant medications. This trend stopped after the Black Box warning was introduced. An increase in suicides and behavior was noted (Fig. 2). New evidence for studies that assessed the effect of the resulting Black Box warning began to emerge. Gibbons and colleagues [35] found that the suicide rates were lower in counties with higher SSRI prescribing rates. These studies have resulted in a shift in opinion about the use of SSRI to treat major depression in adolescents and children. Many clinicians now have accepted a view that the potential benefits of antidepressants outweigh the suicide risk.

Many of the pivotal pediatric studies (TADS, CAMS, POTS) support a consideration of medication in the treatment algorithms for childhood mental health disorders [16,17,20]. These studies all support the combined use of medications along with other modalities. The risk of suicide most often seems to emerge primarily from the depression itself. A decision to not treat a major depressive episode with medication may at times be a bigger risk than the risk of using SSRIs. Clinicians must consider the severity of illness, the availability of nonmedication therapies, and the literature on antidepressants and suicide risk when choosing a path for treatment of their individual patients.

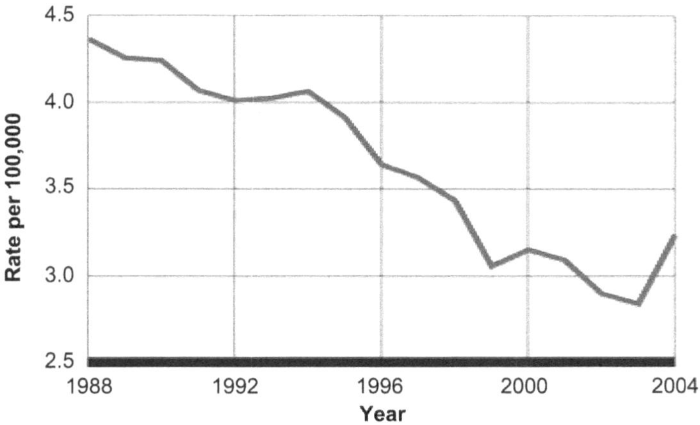

Fig. 2. Suicide rate among youth leaps from 2003 to 2004. After a steady decline since 1988 in suicide among youth aged 5 to 19 years, the number jumped suddenly in 2004, to a rate of 3.23 per 100,000, back to where it was in the mid-1990s. The shift in suicide rate in youth corresponds to a shift in opinion of SSRI use. (*From* Gibbons RD, Brown CH, Hur K, et al. Early evidence on the effects of regulators' suicidality warnings on SSRI prescriptions and suicide in children and adolescents. Am J Psychiatry 2007;164:1356–63; with permission from *American Journal of Psychiatry* (Copyright © 2007), American Psychiatric Association.)

Monitoring

The FDA Black Box warning led to an additional recommendation for a follow-up schedule to monitor children started on SSRI medications. This procedure was extremely restrictive, suggesting weekly visits for 4 weeks, then every other week for 4 weeks, and so forth. These recommendations were found to be unrealistic and were not followed by practicing providers for obvious reasons. The new recommendations for monitoring children and adolescents started on SSRI state that they "...should be monitored and observed carefully by mental health providers and family members" [36,37]. Monitoring should include the watching for a worsening of depression or the onset of suicidal ideation. Also important in the initiation phase of intervention is the need to pay attention to potential side effects of SSRIs. This change in monitoring recommendation allows practitioners to develop an individualized approach that includes in-person visits combined with telephone follow-up monitor a patient's response to medication. There is no recommendation to check laboratory tests or electrocardiogram (ECG) when using SSRIs.

Other adverse effects

SSRIs are generally well tolerated. The recognized side effects of SSRI include headache, abdominal pain, nausea, diarrhea, sleep changes, jitteriness or agitation, diaphoresis, and change in sexual function. As with all antidepressants there is the possibility of an induced manic or hypomanic episode, particularly in individuals with a predisposition to bipolar disorder. Anecdotally, some children and adolescents are very sensitive to even low doses of SSRIs. Common behavioral side effects of even low-dose SSRIs include agitation, an escalation in anxiety, and an increase in impulsiveness or disinhibition [38]. The possibility of these negative side effects makes it imperative to monitor carefully, especially in vulnerable populations such as those with autism, traumatic brain injury, or cognitive deficiency.

Serotonin syndrome

The use of SSRIs is also associated with a small risk of serotonin syndrome. Sometimes the cause is idiopathic or metabolic in nature, but also may be the result of drug-to-drug interaction or overdose [39]. Serotonin syndrome is the consequence of flooding the central nervous system with serotonin. The symptoms emerge suddenly and may include a change in mental status: anxiety, agitated delirium, restlessness, or disorientation. Physical manifestations can include autonomic effects such as diaphoresis, tachycardia, hyperthermia, hypertension, vomiting, and diarrhea, and neuromuscular hyperactivity such as tremor, muscle rigidity, myoclonus, and hyperreflexia [40]. Serotonin syndrome can be life threatening.

Dosage

The recommended dosage ranges that are currently published in the literature are controversial, and may reflect more the historical ranges that are recommended for adults. Primary care pediatric providers are best served by a much more conservative approach. Adjusting the adult dosage in the table downward to between one-half to one-third of the adult dosage is a common approach [38]. For example, fluoxetine might start at 4 mg in a preadolescent. Although it may sound like an oversimplification, many practitioners ascribe to the "common lore" of "start low and go slow."

"SSRI addiction"

The abrupt termination of SSRI usage by patients has been recognized as a major issue. This withdrawal syndrome has lent credence to the idea that SSRIs are addictive. There is no evidence to support this idea, but abrupt cessation of these medications can trigger a cascade of uncomfortable symptoms, which can be avoided if the medications are tapered over a period of weeks. The symptoms of serotonin withdrawal syndrome are disequilibrium, nausea and vomiting, fatigue and lethargy, myalgia, tremor, insomnia, migraine-like auras, agitation, anxiety, crying spells, irritability, low mood, and vivid dreams. Some medications have a much higher likelihood of causing this problem. The medications with shorter half-lives have a significantly higher chance of causing withdrawal symptoms. Fluoxetine is the least likely to cause severe symptoms of withdrawal, and paroxetine or fluvoxamine the most likely to cause discontinuation symptoms [41]. Some consideration could be given to switching from a short-acting SSRI to fluoxetine as a tool for tapering, with a reduced chance of causing distress.

Fetal exposure

The use of SSRIs in treating moderate to severe depression during pregnancy has escalated since their introduction in 1988. There is a growing awareness of the need to determine the effects, if any, of this use on the developing fetus. At present there are no reliable data on the short-term or long-term effects on the developing child's neurodevelopment. Neonates born with antenatal exposure in the third trimester can experience symptoms similar to adults with SSRI discontinuation syndrome [42]. Neonates can experience either a single symptom or a constellation of symptoms including jitteriness, tremors, diarrhea, emesis, irritability, agitation, hypoglycemia, hyperreflexia, hypotonia or hypertonia, respiratory distress, excessive crying, difficulty with feeding, sleep disturbances, and seizures. It is important to bear in mind that the actual incidence of neonatal behavioral syndrome in the exposure of SSRI use has not been established [43,44]. Long-term antenatal exposure to SSRI has also been implicated in disorders such as persistent pulmonary hypertension, low birth weight, and being small for gestational age [45].

Autism

The use of SSRI medication for the treatment of comorbidity associated with autism has become commonplace in both pediatric and psychiatric practice. It is well known that children on the autism spectrum can suffer with anxiety and depression as well as obsessive-compulsive behaviors. In 2010 a Cochrane review by Williams and colleagues [46] evaluated 7 different studies with 271 subjects to determine whether SSRI medications (1) improve the core features of autism; (2) improve other noncore behaviors such as self-abusive behaviors; (3) improve the quality of life of the children and their caregivers; (4) has short-term and long-term effects on outcome; and (5) causes harm. Four SSRIs were evaluated: fluoxetine, fluvoxamine, fenfluramine, and citalopram. The subjects of these studies were both children and adults with autism [46]. One of the larger studies in children found no benefit in the treatment of stereotypies in autism [47]. Two small studies in adults showed positive outcomes for the Clinical Global Impression (CGI) and obsessive-compulsive behavior (OCB). One study showed improvement in aggression and another improvement in anxiety. The investigators concluded that there is only limited evidence on the effectiveness of SSRIs in adults and children with autism. There was no evidence of harm found in any of the studies.

On the surface, the results of this review would suggest that the use of SSRI medications in the treatment of autistic individuals is without merit. However, it would be a mistake to base clinical practice on this limited number of studies with such a small number of subjects. Common sense suggests that the use of SSRIs, because of their low incidence of side effects, is a preferable choice to the use of antipsychotic medications with their multitude of negative side effects. Antidotal evidence in clinical practice suggests that the use of subclinical doses of SSRI can sometimes improve anxiety levels that might not be well captured on the existing clinical assessment scales. Managing the often difficult behaviors of autistic people makes it essential that more comprehensive studies be done in an effort to determine what, if any, benefit SSRIs can provide for this population.

Stimulants/stimulant alternatives

Psychostimulants are very well studied, with initial reports of significant efficacy by Bradley dating back to 1937 in the *American Journal of Psychiatry* [48]. These medications are used to treat hyperactivity, inattention, and impulsivity as seen in ADHD, or are used off-label for disturbances of attention in other disorders such as autism, traumatic brain injury, or depression. Stimulants act by blocking dopamine and norepinephrine reuptake transporters, stimulating release of dopamine from the presynaptic storage vesicles, and weakly stimulating the release of norepinephrine.

In evaluating treatment options for children, clinicians must consider both functional impairments and risks/benefits. Several controversies exist regarding the use of these treatments, including growth effects, tics, sudden cardiac death, substance abuse potential, and the potential for early intervention in preschoolers. Each of these areas is addressed here.

Growth effects

The most common short-term effects of stimulant use on children are appetite suppression and weight loss, which leads to parental concern regarding stunted growth. Spencer and colleagues [49] have reported the absence of stimulant-related growth suppression. Findings from the MTA study indicate that long-term side effects of mild growth suppression are likely to occur and accumulate over the initial 3 years of treatment, with little or no rebound before puberty [50,51]. However, Biederman and colleagues [52] recently completed a 10-year case-controlled, longitudinal study following 124 children without ADHD compared with 137 children with ADHD on and off medication. The investigators found no relationship between height, weight, ADHD, or ADHD medication status in the long term. Many of the studies, including the Biederman study, showed growth inhibition in the first year of medication use, which appears to dissipate with time [52,53]. The current message to clinicians is that while these medications do not appear to have a long-term effect on growth, there is enough data on either side of the issue to continue the debate. Larger studies will need to be conducted to further assess this issue. It is important to monitor height, weight, and body mass index (BMI) biannually as a means of surveillance. If a child shows a significant change in height, drug holidays or altered dosages should be considered [23].

Tics

There is long-standing concern regarding the possibility that stimulants may cause tics. ADHD is common in children with tics [54]. Often the onset of ADHD symptoms predates the onset of tics, whether or not they have been exposed to medication. Therefore, is it sometimes difficult to ascribe cause. The literature suggests that 15% to 30% of children develop tics while on stimulants, most of which are transient [22]. The withdrawal of methylphenidate can result in a decrease in severity and frequency of tics, with an increase when reinstated [55]. The literature suggests that a similar number of children develop tics whether they are on medication or not [54,56].

Children with preexisting tics or tic disorders commonly have ADHD and disruptive behavior disorders. The use of stimulants in this population is another area for debate. The Physicians' Desk Reference guided by the FDA lists tics or a family history of tics as a contraindication for the use of stimulants. There are now good alternatives to stimulants, but there are times when these medications fail or are not tolerated and where a stimulant may still be beneficial. A preponderance of the evidence suggests that the use of stimulants in the treatment of ADHD and co-occurring tics is both safe and effective [57–59]. While many children with a tic disorder show a lessening of tics over time on medication, there is a minority of children with a tic disorder who do appear to show at least a temporary worsening of symptoms [58,59]. One interesting study conducted by the Tourette Syndrome Study group, which examined 136 children with ADHD and a tic disorder, showed that stimulants at a low dose can be used to treat ADHD effectively without exacerbating the tic disorder in 75% of the children studied, with only a slight increase in the remaining 25% [60]. Although there are nonstimulant alternatives available that are not associated with increased tic generation, stimulants should still play a role as a treatment consideration in a child with a tic disorder.

Hematologic findings

It is not necessary to order routine laboratory tests as part of safety monitoring unless there are other medical comorbidities that suggest a medical necessity. The cost and discomfort of blood sampling during short-term or long-term stimulant use outweighs the potential benefit, as no clinically significant effects on blood biochemistry in general, and on hematologic findings in particular, are found [61,62].

Sudden cardiac death

In 2005 Health Canada suspended sales of mixed amphetamine salts (Adderall) based on postmarketing reports of 12 children and adolescent deaths in the United States over a 4-year period (1999–2003), but without full investigation. Half of the deaths had underlying serious heart conditions that were not detected prior to death. Those that died had aberrant origins of coronary arteries, bicuspid aortic valves, cardiomyopathy, toxic levels from overuse, family history of ventricular arrhythmias, extreme exercise, and dehydration, with numbers slightly higher in the amphetamine group than in the methylphenidate group [63]. Later that year, Health Canada determined that the incidence of sudden unexplained death was similar to, and even lower than, that which occurred in the general population. The risk for such an event was calculated by the FDA to be between 1.0 and 8.5 per 100,000 [64]. Regardless, such medications were labeled by the FDA to warn against the use of stimulants in children with existing cardiac symptoms, and to use caution regarding use in children with prior cardiac disease or significant family history.

Previous studies looking at the effects of stimulants have shown increases of 3 to 6 beats/min in heart rate and 2 to 4 mm Hg in systolic/diastolic blood pressure [65–67]. Although statistically significant, these numbers are not clinically relevant. There has been debate regarding the need for prior ECGs and/or echocardiograms before initiating medications. At this time, the AAP and AACAP are not recommending an ECG or echocardiogram before starting stimulants or a serotonin norepinephrine reuptake inhibitor (SNRI) [22,23]. Instead, a thorough cardiac family history (arrhythmia, sudden unexpected death, hypertrophic cardiomyopathy, or Marfan syndrome) and personal cardiac history (palpitations, syncope, chest pain, prior surgeries, congenital heart conditions, murmur, or arrhythmia) should be obtained. Examination would also include blood pressure and auscultation. These components are an important part of the ADHD evaluation [68–70]. A positive cardiac history or concerning findings on physical examination necessitates further evaluation with ECG, echocardiogram, and/or cardiology referral [71]. Prior cardiac history does not preclude stimulant use, but necessitates appropriate assessment of potential benefit and acknowledgment of the FDA warning.

Substance abuse potential

ADHD in childhood is a risk factor for later substance abuse. This risk is present regardless of exposure to stimulant medication. Stimulant treatment does not appear to increase the risk of substance abuse [72–74]. The association between ADHD and substance abuse is more closely linked to whether a young adult develops conduct disorder than to whether they have ADHD [75].

Claims that childhood treatment with stimulants *decreases* the danger of future substance abuse [72] were not supported as "protective" either by the recent publications of long-term follow-up of these cohorts or by the MTA study [74,76]. The hypothesis that taking medications during adolescence is protective against substance abuse should be addressed by a prospective, longitudinal study of children with ADHD on and off medication and matched controls, from treatment onset into adulthood.

Preschoolers

ADHD historically has been viewed as a disorder of elementary school-aged children. Increasingly, ADHD has become one of the most commonly recognized behavioral disorders in preschoolers. The startling increase in stimulant prescriptions written for this age group along with the lack of diagnostic and treatment consensus for these children, led to the Preschool ADHD Treatment Study (PATS), a 6-site study funded by the National Institute of Mental Health (NIMH). Because the lowest age approved for use of methylphenidate by FDA guidelines is 6 years, one of the primary aims of the study was to investigate its safety and efficacy in 3- to 5.5-year-olds (at screening).

Multiple publications have emerged from the PATS. A pharmacokinetic substudy is highlighted here. The pharmacokinetic substudy demonstrated slower clearance in preschoolers than in school-aged children with ADHD. Thus, preschoolers respond differently to stimulants than do school-aged children, even when weight is controlled, accounting for a different volume of distribution from older children [77].

Overall, the PATS study has helped to validate the diagnosis of ADHD in preschoolers and to contribute a guide to assessment in this age group [78]. The initial findings of this study suggest that stimulants are safe and effective for preschoolers. It was also noted that preschoolers are more sensitive to side effects and have a small dosage window of therapeutic effect, which make the planning of treatment more challenging. Taken together, the main message to clinicians is to proceed cautiously with the use of stimulants in very young children. Nonmedication interventions were used prior to medication treatment in the PATS. Clinicians should seek behavioral treatment for their patients before turning to stimulant medications in this age group.

Monitoring stimulants

Children started on stimulants should be seen after the first month to follow progress and review for side effects. Children can then be followed at regular intervals. Seeing children every 3 months on a stable dose helps to ensure safe management and monitoring of emergent side effects of treatment. Rating scales should be used to ensure optimal treatment. One should watch for mood alterations, explore social and family relations, and encourage a structured, positive behavior system. Laboratory surveillance is not indicated [23].

Stimulant alternatives

This discussion is not inclusive of all alternative medication options. The goal is to focus on the most commonly used medications.

Atomoxetine

Atomoxetine belongs to the class of drugs known as the SNRIs. It is the first nonstimulant approved by the FDA for the treatment of ADHD in children. It has a very low abuse potential. While it is considered a first-line treatment for ADHD, it has a lower effect size of about 0.6 [79], suggesting moderate effectiveness; this is less than the reported effect sizes for traditional stimulants (0.8) [79], suggesting their stronger effectiveness. As an alternative to the stimulants, atomoxetine may offer the benefit of longer activity and lower abuse potential. Originally explored as an antidepressant, it seems to have some additional benefit in the area of anxiety, but this has not been clearly corroborated by empiric data. Atomoxetine has a long onset to therapeutic benefit (2–6 weeks). Its side-effect profile is similar to the stimulants with the exception of tics (atomoxetine is not associated with exacerbation of tics), but it carries additional side effects such as cough, dizziness, and an idiosyncratic hepatotoxicity risk. In 2005, the FDA added a Black Box warning suggesting a small but real risk of increased suicidal behavior (the same as for SSRIs). There are "long-term" studies at 4.8 years that show no change in growth and ECG, and no unexpected new adverse events [80]. This medication should be considered for a child with ADHD and anxiety or a tic disorder, or for a child who needs medication with a longer duration of action. Although not studied, atomoxetine is often used adjunctively with stimulants.

α2-Adrenergic agonists

Despite having been used for years, neither immediate-release clonidine nor guanfacine are approved by the FDA for the treatment of ADHD. These agents seem to have their best effect on the hyperactive/impulsive part of this disorder by dampening the norepinephrine-mediated arousal system. These drugs have also been shown to reduce tic production and improve working memory, planning, and behavioral inhibition. Guanfacine XR has been FDA-approved for the treatment of ADHD and clonidine LA is the first drug to be approved for use adjunctively to stimulants. Some of the noted side effects include sedation, which appears to lessen over the first 2 to 4 weeks, hypotension, bradycardia, constipation, dry mouth, and increased appetite. α2-Adrenergic agonists are likely to play a role as second-line treatment agents for ADHD.

Neurofeedback

While obviously not a medication, biofeedback has emerged as an important and controversial treatment for ADHD. Limited randomized controlled trials (RCTs) are available examining its effectiveness. In 2005 Loo and Barkley [81] published an analysis of available neurofeedback studies, and concluded that electroencephalographic feedback is not well established as a treatment or adjunct to medication in the treatment of ADHD. However, they did not address some promising studies. A recent small, but controlled study shows a modest effect on ADHD symptoms, with an effect size of 0.71 [82,83]. Although this effect size is still lower than that often reported for stimulant medications used to treat ADHD, there appears to be a significant positive effect on the disorder in this study. Neurofeedback has not yet been accepted by most physicians as a component of treatment for ADHD, but this topic deserves more investigation. Biofeedback should be factored into the comprehensive understanding of treatment alternatives.

Antipsychotics

Antipsychotics are the subset of psychopharmacologic agents that historically have been used to treat schizophrenia and psychotic disorders. Over the years their applications have been broadened to treat bipolar disorder, agitation in autism, tics, anxiety, impulsivity, sleep, and aggression. These medications are not part of the typical repertoire generally prescribed by pediatricians. However, they are discussed here because they are increasingly part of the psychopharmacologic landscape. Their very use in children creates great controversy secondary to their significant side-effect profile. These medications are often necessary to treat severe behavior disturbance in children. After stimulants and SSRIs, they are now among the psychotropic medications most frequently used to treat childhood psychiatric disorders. Great caution must be used when prescribing antipsychotic medications to children and adolescents.

The traditional antipsychotics such as haloperidol, pimozide, and thorazine have been replaced by what was perceived to be the safer atypical or second-generation antipsychotics (SGAs). These alternatives were supposed to have higher efficacy and fewer side effects. However, they may have merely switched one set of side effects, such as extrapyrimidal side effects (EPS), for metabolic syndrome including weight gain, elevated lipid profile, and insulin resistance.

Thus far, only a few of the SGAs have received approval from the FDA for pediatric indications. Risperidone and aripiprazole are approved for the treatment of schizophrenia in children older than 13 years, bipolar disorder, mania, or mixed episodes in children 10 years and older. SGAs are also approved for the treatment of irritability associated with autism for children between 5 and 17 years of age. It should be noted that the FDA originally refused the application for risperidone because of its significant side effects. However, given additional studies and the severity of the untreated conditions, the benefits of treatment with SGAs were determined to ultimately outweigh the risks in enough cases to warrant FDA approval for children, with warnings.

Despite these relatively few recommended indications, antipsychotic use in children is on the increase. The number of prescriptions for the SGAs in the pediatric population rose 160% in the United States between 1990 and 2000 [84]. This trend continues, with an additional 22% increase in the prescriptions of atypical antipsychotics between 2004 and 2008 for children younger than 17 years [12,13,85]. The majority of the prescriptions were written by psychiatrists for mood disorders. The most popular medication was risperidone [86]. A study in the United States found that antipsychotics are often used to treat ADHD and hyperactivity despite no empirical evidence supporting their use for this indication [12,87].

Mechanism

The mechanism of action among the older and newer antipsychotics differ somewhat. The traditional antipsychotics such as haloperidol strongly block dopamine (DA2) receptors while having more minor effects on other neuroreceptors to differing degrees. The atypical or newer antipsychotics are known as serotonin dopamine antagonists (SDAs), again with slightly differing activity profiles based on effects at other neuroreceptor sites. The associated potencies and side effects are determined by the neuroreceptors affected by a particular antipsychotic. For example, if drug X has the strongest affinity for the dopamine receptor it will have both the strongest antidopamine potency and side effects. This profile determines a medication's action and its side effects (Table 1).

Side effects

It is not the intention to cover all side effects associated with antipsychotics. What follows is a discussion of some of the more concerning side effects that

Table 1
Depression - response to treatment

Neuroreceptor	Effect	Example (Strongest Effect)
Dopamine blockade	Extrapyramidal signs (EPS), tardive dyskinesia (TD), prolactin stimulation (improves positive symptoms)	Haloperidol
Serotonin stimulation	Anti-EPS, sexual dysfunction, antidepressant activity, gastric upset	Aripiprazole
α-Adrenergic blockade	Postural hypotension, dizziness, syncope	Thioridazine
Muscarinic blockade	Memory, cognition, urinary retention, constipation	Olanzepine, chlorpromazine
Histamine blockade	Sedation, weight gain, protective against EPS (improve negative symptoms)	Olanzepine, seroquel

influence the decision to use these medications, which should be included in any discussion of informed consent.

Extrapyramidal side effects. It was originally thought that EPS were not ascribed to the atypical antipsychotics, but were commonly associated primarily with the traditional antipsychotics. EPS comprise a set of involuntary movement disorders such as dystonia, tardive dyskinesia, akathesia, or parkinsonian-like movements. This response is attributable to D2 blockade in the basal ganglia, which is strongest with the typical antipsychotics. The newer medications still have an effect at the D2 receptor and thus can also cause EPS, albeit to a lesser extent [88–91]. Some of these movement disorders, such as tardive dyskinesia, are irreversible.

Blood dyscrasias. A variety of blood dyscrasias have been reported in children on atypical antipsychotics. These effects have been mostly in anecdotal and case reports, but have occurred with enough frequency to warrant obtaining a complete blood count (CBC) at regular intervals, perhaps after 3 months then annually.

Prolactin. Prolactin levels are also affected by both the older and newer antipsychotics. The effect seems to be greater with the older antipsychotics but also occurs with the newer ones. Several studies show a transient increase in prolactin, and a few others show a more sustained increase in almost a quarter of children on antipsychotics [91–93]. The effect of the increase is unclear. However, altered menstrual cycles are a common phenomenon, and suggest the need to lower the dose or consider a change of medication. This type of endocrine abnormality brings into play fertility, breast tissue development in males, and nipple discharge.

Metabolic syndrome. Metabolic syndrome is probably the most significant issue facing this newer class of medications. By 2004 these medications were clearly linked to weight gain and altered glucose levels [92]. Out of concern for cardiometabolic effects, the FDA issued a warning. The evidence continued to mount as the use of these medications continued to escalate. In the Second-Generation Antipsychotic Treatment Indications, Effectiveness and Tolerability in Youth (SATIETY) study, Correll and colleagues [94,95] corroborated the move by the FDA. This study found that 10% to 36% of 272 patients between 4 and 19 years of age who were antipsychotic medication–naïve became overweight or obese during the 11-week study. There was minimal weight change in the control group who did not take the medications. The study monitored treatment with aripiprazole, olanzapine, quetiapine, or risperidone to treat psychosis, mood disorder, aggression, or spectrum disorders in children. The greatest weight gain was seen with olanzepine (8.5 kg) and the least with aripiprazole (4.4 kg). It must be borne in mind that this is 8.5 kg in only 11 weeks. Adverse changes in levels of total cholesterol, triglycerides, and non–high-density lipoprotein (HDL), and in the ratio of triglycerides to HDL cholesterol were also noted.

Weiss and colleagues [87] further corroborate these findings in a retrospective study of emergency room admissions in Canada. This study found that children treated with atypical antipsychotics were much more likely (27%) than unexposed controls (2.9%) to exhibit metabolic syndrome or associated features. Furthermore, children were much more likely than adults to exhibit metabolic syndrome. These studies suggest that the benefits of atypicals must be balanced with the cardio-metabolic risks suggested by the research. These findings portray significant risks.

Traditional versus newer antipsychotics

As discussed, there are several side effects associated with these medications. Atypical antipsychotics were billed as safer, better alternatives to the traditional antipsychotics. The atypical antipsychotics are similar to the classic antipsychotics in terms of reducing psychotic symptoms, but there does not appear to be superiority, with the exception of clozapine. Clozapine (the first atypical) has shown efficacy in patients for whom other medications have failed [96,97].

There are some benefits to these newer medications, which are used at a frequency of 9:1 over the traditional medications. The atypical antipsychotics seem to offer some treatment benefits over the traditional medications with improved depression, less energy suppression, and a less flattened affect. An adult study was initiated to investigate this question. The Clinical Antipsychotic Trials of Intervention Effectiveness (CATIE) by the NIMH set out to compare atypical to traditional antipsychotics. In this multicenter study, adults with schizophrenia were randomized to receive olanzapine, perphenazine, quetiapine, risperidone, and ziprasidone [98]. The outcome showed that olanzapine appeared to be more effective than the other drugs studied, but it also showed the highest weight gain and changes in hemoglobin A1c, cholesterol, and triglycerides. There did not appear to be any difference in efficacy between the remaining traditional or atypical medications. Although the study does not examine the pediatric population, it is important to reconsider the notion that the atypical antipsychotics are safer than the traditional antipsychotics. Instead, this study emphasizes judicious use of all antipsychotic medication.

A study in 2008 had similar findings in children. Sikich and colleagues [99], in the Treatment of the Early Onset Schizophrenia Spectrum Study (TEOSS study), compared a typical antipsychotic to 2 SGAs in the treatment of schizophrenia in 119 children. This study did not show any superiority of the SGAs. Furthermore, each medication had its own profile of side effects. Risperidone had the greatest increase in prolactin; olanzepine led to greatest weight gain, and increase in insulin and cholesterol. This result would suggest that the SGAs may not be superior in benefit and seem to have substantial, albeit different, side effects as compared with the typical antipsychotics.

Antipsychotics in the treatment of autism

One of the more pivotal studies related to autism examined the use of risperidone in the treatment of agitation or other serious behaviors in children with autism by the Research Units on Pediatric Psychopharmacology [100]. In this multicenter study, 101 children aged 7 to 17 years received either risperidone or placebo. Sixty-nine percent of those receiving risperidone were rated by clinicians as improved or very much improved compared with 19% in the placebo group. This study had the most robust outcome for any study in autism to date. However, this study also showed that risperidone is not benign, with side effects including significant weight gain.

Brief summary of antipsychotics

Clozapine has shown superiority over other antipsychotics, but has a significant risk of weight gain and metabolic syndrome. It is the only antipsychotic that requires regular CBC monitoring, due to the small but life-threatening risk of agranulocytosis. Olanzepine has shown genuine benefit over some of the other medications in adults but has also showed the greatest weight gain and sedation. Risperidone is the most commonly used medication in children. It has FDA approval for the treatment of pediatric schizophrenia, bipolar disorder, mania, and autism. Of the newer medications it has a higher tendency toward prolactin abnormalities, EPS, and weight gain. Ziprasidone is the only medication associated with QTc prolongation and therefore necessitates an ECG. Quetiapine may cause significant sedation and weight gain. Aripiprazole tends to be the most weight neutral, among the least EPS generating, and may show the most qualitative improvement in depressive symptoms. Quetiapine has FDA approval for childhood schizophrenia, mania, bipolar disorder, and autism.

Table 2
Monitoring strategies in children and adolescents treated with antipsychotic agents: antipsychotic medication and receptor impact

Assessment	Routine Follow-Up
Personal and family medical history	Annually
Lifestyle behaviors	Each visit
Sedation/somnolence	Each visit
Sexual/reproductive dysfunction	During titration, then every 3 months
Parkinsonism, akathisia	During titration, at 3 months, then annually
Height, weight, body mass index	Each visit
Blood pressure and pulse	At 3 months and annually
Electrolytes, blood count, renal and liver function	Annually
Fasting blood glucose and lipids	At 3 months, then every 6 months
Liver function tests	At 3 months, then annually
Prolactin	Only if symptomatic
Electrocardiography	Only if taking ziprasidone

From Correll CU, Kratochvil CJ, Antipsychotic use in children and adolescents: minimizing adverse affects to maximize outcomes. J Am Acad Child Adolesc Psychiatry 2008;47(1):9–20; with permission.

Monitoring

Despite the recognition of significant and potentially harmful side effects, most patients placed on antipsychotics are not appropriately screened and monitored. A study in the *American Journal of Psychiatry* showed that the younger the patient was, the less likely they were to be screened [101]. While a psychiatrist may prescribe these medications, it may be necessary for the primary care physician to help monitor for side effects. Traditional medical visits can be used to monitor personal and medical history, pulse, blood pressure, height, weight, and BMI. Each visit should include a review of systems addressing potential side effects such as akathisia, dystonias, sedation, and reproductive dysfunction. After 3 months laboratory studies should be obtained, including a CBC, fasting blood glucose, lipids, and liver function tests. Blood glucose, lipids, and perhaps hemoglobin A1c should be reviewed every 6 months thereafter. Comprehensive chemistry panels should be repeated annually for children who continue to receive these medications. Prolactin levels should be checked if the child is symptomatic, and an ECG should be done if a child is taking ziprasidone [102] (Table 2).

SUMMARY

Mental health conditions are some of the most significant and chronic concerns for children and adolescents. Parents and some physicians are often reluctant to consider a potentially long-term psychotropic medication treatment for these children. Pediatricians can serve a vital role by helping families sift through the vast amount of information on psychotropic medication to help them make informed decisions regarding their child. Despite all of the aforementioned controversy regarding the use of psychotropic medications, they can be invaluable for children whose well-diagnosed conditions are not responsive to other interventions. Although the risks are undeniable, there are valid and important reasons to use these medications. Depression, impulsivity, inattention, psychosis, agitation, and mood lability can all profoundly affect daily living, independence, and the well-being of children. Untreated, these disorders negatively affect relationships with parents, family members, teachers, and peers. Physicians who can help children and families weigh risks and benefits of treatment, inform, and monitor appropriately, can provide important care for their patients with neurobehavioral disorders.

There is a growing understanding that the subspecialty health care system is not able to accommodate the vast numbers of children with the most common mental health issues: anxiety, depression, and ADHD. The AAP is emphasizing the need for pediatricians to play a major role in the identification, assessment, and management of this population. There is clearly a role for both behavioral treatments and medication in that care. The ability to integrate the research presented will be important in creating comprehensive treatment pathways.

This movement toward a broader scope of practice is admittedly daunting for many who were not trained to provide this care. It necessitates pediatricians to deepen their knowledge in the area of behavioral health. It also emphasizes the need for system-wide change incorporating more collaboration and shared care between psychiatrists, pediatricians, psychologists, and other behavioral support services [103]. Understanding the roles of behavior and medicine in the care of children with common mental health conditions is an important step toward this goal.

References

[1] Merikangas KR, He Jp, Burstein M, et al. Lifetime prevalence of mental disorders in US adolescents: results from the National Comorbidity Survey Replication (NCS-A). J Am Acad Child Adolesc Psychiatry 2010;49(10):980–9.

[2] Arango C, Parellada M, Moreno DM. Clinical effectiveness of new generation antipsychotics in adolescent patients. Eur Neuropsychopharmacol 2004;14:471–9.

[3] Foy JM, Duncan P, Frankowski B, et al. American Academy of Pediatrics Task Force on Mental Health. Enhancing pediatric mental health care: report from the American Academy of Pediatrics Task Force on Mental Health. Introduction. Pediatrics 2010;125(Suppl 3):S69–74.

[4] Coleman WL, Dobbins MI, Garner AS, et al. Committee on Psychosocial Aspects of Child and Family Health and Task Force on Mental Health. The future of pediatrics: mental health competencies for pediatric primary care. Pediatrics 2009;124:410–21.

[5] Brown RT, Freeman WS, Perrin JM, et al. Prevalence and assessment of attention-deficit/hyperactivity disorder in primary care settings. Pediatrics 2000;107(3):e43.

[6] Costello EJ, Angold A, Burns J, et al. The great smoky mountains study of youth. goals, design, methods, and the prevalence of DSM-III-R disorders. Arch Gen Psychiatry 1996;53(12):1129–36.

[7] Rice C, et al. Prevalence of autism spectrum disorders—autism and developmental disabilities monitoring network, United States, 2006. Mobid Mortal Week Rep 2009; 58(Suppl 10):1–20.

[8] Cavagnaro AT. Autistic spectrum disorders: changes in the California caseload, an update June 1987-June 2007: California Health and Human Services Agency. State of California 2003 survey of developmental disabilities. Available at: http://www.dds.ca.gov/autism/docs/AutismReport_2007.pdf. Accessed December 5, 2011.
[9] Radley DC, Finkelstein SN, Stafford RS. Off-label prescribing among office-based physicians. Arch Intern Med 2006;166:1021–6 [psychiatric drugs].
[10] Zito JM, Derivan AT, Kratochvil CJ, et al. Off-label psychopharmacologic prescribing for children: history supports close clinical monitoring. Child Adolesc Psychiatry Ment Health 2008;2:24.
[11] Cooper WO, Hickson GB, Fuchs DC, et al. New users of antipsychotic medication among children enrolled in TennCare. Arch Pediatr Adolesc Med 2004;158(8):753–9.
[12] Cascade E, Kalali A, Findling R. Use of antipsychotics in children. Psychiatry (Edgmont) 2009;6(6):21–3.
[13] Patel NC, Sanchez RJ, Johnsrud MT, et al. Trends in antipsychotic use in a Texas Medicaid population of children and adolescents: 1996 to 2000. J Child Adolesc Psychopharmacol 2002;12(3):221–9.
[14] Cooper WO, Arbogast PG, Ding H, et al. Trends in prescribing of antipsychotic medications for US children. Ambul Pediatr 2006;6(2):79–83.
[15] Available at: http://www.surgeongeneral.gov/library/mentalhealth/chapter3/sec6.html. Accessed December 5, 2011.
[16] Walkup JT, Albano AM, Piacentini J, et al. Cognitive-behavioral therapy, sertraline and their combination for children and adolescents with anxiety disorders: acute phase efficacy and safety. N Engl J Med 2008;359(17):2753–66.
[17] Franklin M, Foa E, March J. Pediatric obsessive-compulsive disorder treatment Study. J Am Acad Child Adolesc Psychiatry 2004;292:1969–76.
[18] Foy JM, Perrin J, American Academy of Pediatrics Task Force on Mental Health. Enhancing pediatric mental health care: strategies for preparing a community. Pediatrics 2010;125:S75–86.
[19] Eaton DK, Kann L, Kinchen SA, et al. Youth risk behavior surveillance—United States, 2005. MMWR Surveill Summ 2006;55(Suppl 5):1–108.
[20] March J, Silva S, Curry J, et al. Treatment for adolescents with Depression Study (TADS): long-term effectiveness and safety. Arch Gen Psychiatry 2007;64(10):1132–43.
[21] The MTA Cooperative Group: a 14-month randomized clinical trial of treatment strategies for attention-deficit/hyperactivity disorder. Arch Gen Psychiatry 1999;56:1073–86.
[22] American Academy of Pediatrics. Subcommittee on Attention-Deficit/Hyperactivity Disorder and Committee on Quality Improvement. Clinical practice guideline: treatment of the school-aged child with attention-deficit/hyperactivity disorder. Pediatrics 2001;108(4):1033–44.
[23] Pliszka S, AACAP Work Group. Practice parameters for the assessment and treatment of children and adolescents with attention-deficit/hyperactivity disorder. J Am Acad Child Adolesc Psychiatry 2007;46(7):894–921.
[24] Oswald DP, Sonenklar NA. Medication use among children with autism spectrum disorders. J Child Adolesc Psychopharmacol 2007;l17(3):348–55.
[25] Available at: www.Nationalautismcenter.org. Study Accessed December 5, 2011.
[26] Preskorn SH. Clinically relevant pharmacology of selective serotonin reuptake inhibitors: an overview with emphasis on drug metabolism. Clinical Pharmacokinet 1997;32:1–21.
[27] DeVane CL. Pharmacokinetics of the selective serotonin reuptake inhibitors. J Clin Psychiatry 1992;53:13–20.
[28] Leslie LK, Newman TB, Chesney PJ, et al. The Food and Drug Administration's deliberations on antidepressants use in pediatric patients. Pediatrics 2005;116:195–201.
[29] Khan A, Khan S, Kolts R, et al. Suicide rates in clinical trials of SSRIs other antidepressants and placebo: analysis of FDA reports. Am J Psychiatry 2003;160:790–2.
[30] Hammad TA, Laughren T, Racoosin J. Suicidality in pediatric patients treated with antidepressant drugs. Arch Gen Psychiatry 2006;63:332–9.

[31] Jick H, Kaye J, Jick S. Antidepressants and the risk of suicidal behaviors. JAMA 2004;292: 338–43.
[32] American College of Neuropsychopharmacology, preliminary report of the task force on SSRI's and suicidal behavior in youth. 2004. Available at: www.ancp.org. Accessed December 5, 2011.
[33] U.S. FDA Public Health Advisory: suicidality in children and adolescents being treated with antidepressant medications; 2004.
[34] Olfson M, Shaffer D, Marcus S, et al. Relationship between antidepressant medication treatment and suicide in adolescents. Arch Gen Psychiatry 2003;60:978–82.
[35] Gibbons RD, Brown H, Hur K, et al. Early evidence on the effects of regulators' suicidality warnings on SSRI prescriptions and suicide in children and adolescents. Am J Psychiatry 2007;164:1356–63.
[36] Mamdani MM. Health advisories: when good intentions go bad. CMAJ 2008;178: 1025–6.
[37] Katz Ly, Kozyrskyj AL, Prior HJ, et al. Effects of regulatory warnings on antidepressant prescribing rates, use of health services and outcomes among children, adolescents and young adults. CMAJ 2008;178:1005–11.
[38] Birmaher B, Brent D, Bernet W, et al. Practice parameter for the assessment and treatment of children and adolescents with depressive disorders. J Am Acad Child Adolesc Psychiatry 2007;46:1503–36.
[39] Boyer EW, Shannon M. The serotonin syndrome. N Engl J Med 2005;352:1112–20.
[40] Birmes P, Coppin D, Schmitt L, et al. Serotonin syndrome: a brief review. CMAJ 2003;168: 1439–42.
[41] Coupland NJ, Bell CJ, Potokar JP. Serotonin reuptake inhibitor withdrawal. J Clin Psychopharmacol 1996;16:356–62.
[42] Moses-Kolko EL, Bogen D, Perel J, et al. Neonatal signs after late in utero exposure to serotonin reuptake inhibitors: literature review and implications for clinical applications. JAMA 2005;293:2372–83.
[43] Laine k, Heikkinen T, Ekblad U, et al. Effects of exposure to selective serotonin reuptake inhibitors during pregnancy on serotonergic symptoms in newborns and cord blood monoamine and prolactin concentrations. Arch Gen Psychiatry 2003;60:720–6.
[44] Nordeng H, Lindemann R, Perminov A. Neonatal withdrawal syndrome after in utero exposure to serotonin reuptake inhibitors. Acta Paediatr 2001;90:288–91.
[45] Chambers CD, Hernandez-Diaz S, Van Marter LJ, et al. Selective serotonin reuptake inhibitors and risk of persistent pulmonary hypertension of the newborn. N Engl J Med 2006;354:579–87.
[46] Williams K, Wheeler DM, Silove N, et al. Selective serotonin reuptake inhibitors (SSRI) for autism spectrum disorders (ASD). Cochrane Database Syst Rev 2010;8:CD004677.
[47] King BH, Hollander E, Sikich L, et al. (STAART Psychopharmacology Network): lack of efficacy of citalopram in children with autism spectrum disorders and high levels of repetitive behavior: citalopram ineffective in children with autism. Arch Gen Psychiatry 2009;66(6): 583–90.
[48] Bradley C. The behavior of children receiving benzedrine. Am J Psychiatry 1937;94: 577–85.
[49] Spencer T, Biederman J, Harding M, et al. Growth deficits in ADHD children revisited: evidence for disorder-associated growth delays? J Am Acad Child Adolesc Psychiatry 1996;35:1460–9.
[50] Swanson JM, Elliott GR, Greenhill LL, et al. Effects of stimulant medication on growth rates across 3 years in the MTA follow-up. J Am Acad Child Adolesc Psychiatry 2007;46: 1015–27.
[51] Swanson JM, Hinshaw SP, Arnold LE, et al. Secondary evaluations of MTA 36-month outcomes: propensity score and growth mixture model analyses. J Am Acad Child Adolesc Psychiatry 2007;46:1002–13.

[52] Biederman J, Spencer TJ, Monuteaux MC, et al. A naturalistic 10-year prospective study of height and weight in children with attention-deficit hyperactivity disorder grown up: sex and treatment effects. J Pediatr 2010;157(4):635–40, e1.
[53] Zhang H, Du H, Zhuang H. Impact of long-term treatment of methylphenidate on height and weight of school age children with ADHD. Neuropediatrics 2010;41: 55–9.
[54] Bloch MH, Panza KE, Landeros-Weisenberger A, et al. Meta-analysis: treatment of attention-deficit/hyperactivity disorder in children with comorbid tic disorders. J Am Acad Child Adolesc Psychiatry 2009;48(9):884–93.
[55] Riddle MA, Lynch KA, Scahill L, et al. Effects of methylphenidate discontinuation and reinitiation in children with Tourette's syndrome and ADHD. J Child Adolesc Psychopharmacol 1995;5:205.
[56] Law SF, Schachar RJ. Do typical clinical doses of methylphenidate cause tics in children treated for attention-deficit hyperactivity disorder? J Am Acad Child Adolesc Psychiatry 1999;38(8):944–51.
[57] Gadow KD, Sverd J, Sprafkin J, et al. Efficacy of methylphenidate for attention-deficit hyperactivity disorder in children with tic disorder. Arch Gen Psychiatry 1995;52(6): 444–55.
[58] Gadow KD, Sverd J, Sprafkin J, et al. Long term methylphenidate therapy in children with comorbid attention-deficit hyperactivity disorder and chronic multiple tic disorder. Arch Gen Psychiatry 1999;56:330–6.
[59] Poncin Y, Sukhodolsky DG, McGuire J, et al. Drug and non-drug treatments of children with ADHD and tic disorders. Eur Child Adolesc Psychiatry 2007;16(Suppl 1):78–88.
[60] The Tourette's Syndrome Study Group. Treatment of ADHD in children with tics: a randomized controlled trial. Neurology 2002;58:527–36.
[61] Greenhill LL, Findling RL, Swanson JM, ADHD Study Group. A double-blind, placebo-controlled study of modified-release methylphenidate in children with attention-deficit/hyperactivity disorder. Pediatrics 2002;109:e39.
[62] Wigal SB, Wilens TE, Wolraich M, et al. Hematologic and blood biochemistry monitoring during methylphenidate treatment in children with attention-deficit/hyperactivity disorder: 2-year, open-label study results. Pediatrics 2007;120:e120–8.
[63] U.S. Food and Drug Administration (2005) public health advisory for Adderall and Adderall XR. Available at: http://www.fda.gov/cder/drug/advisory/adderall.htm. Accessed January 24, 2006.
[64] Rosack J. US regulators puzzled by Canada's ruling on safety of ADHD drug. Psychiatr News 2005;40:5–9.
[65] Adderall XR [package insert]. Wayne, PA: Shire US Inc; 2010.
[66] Concerta [package insert]. Titusville, NJ: McNeil Pediatrics; 2008.
[67] Focalin XR [package insert]. East Hanover, NJ: Novartis Pharmaceuticals Corporation; 2008.
[68] Vetter VL, Elia J, Erickson C, et al. A scientific statement from the American Heart Association Council on Cardiovascular Disease in the Young Congenital Cardiac Defects Committee and the Council on Cardiovascular Nursing. Circulation 2008;117(18): 2407–23.
[69] Warren AE, Hamilton RM, Belanger SA, et al. Cardiac risk assessment before the use of stimulant medications in children and youth: a joint position statement by the Canadian Paediatric Society, the Canadian Cardiovascular Society, and the Canadian Academy of Child and Adolescent Psychiatry. Can J Cardiol 2009;25(11):625–30.
[70] Wigal SB, Jun A, Wong A. Does prior exposure to stimulants in children with ADHD impact cardiovascular parameters from lisdexamfetamine dimesylate? Postgrad Med 2010;122(5):27–34.
[71] Perrin JM, Friedman RA, Knilans TK. Cardiovascular monitoring and stimulant drugs for attention deficit hyperactivity disorder. Pediatrics 2008;122:451–3.

[72] Wilens TE, Faraone SV, Biederman J, et al. Does stimulant therapy of attention-deficit/hyperactivity disorder beget later substance abuse? a meta-analytic review of the literature. Pediatrics 2003;111:179–85.
[73] Mannuzza S, Klein RG, Truong NL, et al. Age of methylphenidate treatment initiation in children with ADHD and later substance abuse: prospective follow-up into adulthood. Am J Psychiatry 2008;165(5):604–9.
[74] Biederman J, Monuteaux MC, Spencer T, et al. Stimulant therapy and risk for subsequent substance use disorders in male adults with ADHD: a naturalistic controlled 10-year follow-up study. Am J Psychiatry 2008;165(5):597–603.
[75] Disney ER, Elkins IJ, McGue M, et al. Effects of ADHD, conduct disorder, and gender on substance use and abuse in adolescence. Am J Psychiatry 1999;156:1515–21.
[76] Molina BSG, Flory K, Hinshaw SP, et al. Delinquent behavior and emerging substance use in the MTA at 36 months: prevalence, course, and treatment effects. J Am Acad Child Adolesc Psychiatry 2007;46:1028–40.
[77] Wigal SB, Gupta S, Greenhill L, et al. Pharmacokinetics of methylphenidate in preschoolers with attention-deficit/hyperactivity disorder. J Child Adolesc Psychopharmacol 2007;17(2):153–64.
[78] Wigal T, Wigal S, Shanklin A, et al. ADHD in preschoolers: a diagnosis—or just a "PhAse"? Consultant for Pediatricians 2008;8(Suppl):S2–8.
[79] Faraone SV, Beiderman J, Spencer TJ. Comparing the efficacy of medications for ADHD using meta-analysis. Medscape General Medicine 2006;8(4):4.
[80] Donnelly C, Bangs M, Trzepacz P, et al. Safety and tolerability of atomoxetine over 3 to 4 years in children and adolescents with ADHD. J Am Acad Child Adolesc Psychiatry 2009;48(2):176–85.
[81] Loo S, Barkley R. Clinical utility of EEG in attention deficit hyperactivity disorder. Appl Neuropsychol 2005;12(2):64–76.
[82] Gevensleben H, Holl B, Albrecht B, et al. Neurofeedback training in children with ADHD: 6-month follow-up of a randomized controlled trial. Eur Child Adolesc Psychiatry 2010;19(9):715–24.
[83] Gevensleben H, Holl B, Albrecht B, et al. Is neurofeedback an efficacious treatment for ADHD? A randomized controlled clinical trial. J Child Psychol Psychiatry 2009;50(7):780–9.
[84] Patel NC, Crismon ML, Hoagwood K, et al. Trends in the use of typical and atypical antipsychotics in children and adolescents. J Am Acad Child Adolesc Psychiatry 2005;44:548–56.
[85] Olfson M, Blanco C, Liu L, et al. National trends in the outpatient treatment of children and adolescents with antipsychotic drugs. Arch Gen Psychiatry 2006;63(6):679–85.
[86] Vitiello B, Correll C, van Zwieten-Boot B, et al. Antipsychotics in children and adolescents: increasing use, evidence for efficacy and safety concerns. Eur Neuropsychopharmacol 2009;19(9):629–35.
[87] Weiss M, Panagiotopoulos C, Giles L, et al. A naturalistic study of predictors and risks of atypical antipsychotic use in an attention-deficit/hyperactivity disorder clinic. J Child Adolesc Psychopharmacol 2009;19(5):575–82.
[88] Kumar R, Perminder S. Akathesia and second generation antipsychotic drugs. Curr Opin Psychiatry 2009;22(3):293–9.
[89] Cooper BM, Keck PE, Satlin A, et al. Prevalence and severity of akathisia in patients on clozapine. Biol Psychiatry 1991;29:1215–9.
[90] Shirazadi AA, Ghaemi SN. Side effects of atypical antipsychotics: extrapyramidal symptoms and the metabolic syndrome. Harv Rev Psychiatry 2006;14:152–64.
[91] Findling RL. Paediatric psychopharmacology: closing the gap between science and practice. Expert Opin Pharmacother 2001;2:523–5.
[92] Laita P, Cifuentes A, Doll A, et al. Antipsychotic-related abnormal involuntary movements and metabolic and endocrine side effects in children and adolescents. J Child Adolesc Psychopharmacol 2007;17:487–502.

[93] Correll CU, Carlson HE. Endocrine and metabolic adverse effects of psychotropic medications in children and adolescents. J Am Acad Child Adolesc Psychiatry 2006;45:771–91.
[94] Correll CU. Assessing and maximizing the safety and tolerability of antipsychotics used in the treatment of children and adolescents. J Clin Psychiatry 2008;69(Suppl 4): 26–30.
[95] Correll CU, Manu P, Olshanskiy V, et al. Cardiometabolic risk of second generation antipsychotic medications during first time use in child and adolescents. JAMA 2009;302(16): 1765–73.
[96] Kumra S, Oberstar JV, Sikich L, et al. Efficacy and tolerabilityof second-generation antipsychotics in children and adolescent with schizophrenia. Schizophr Bull 2008;34:60–71.
[97] Shaw P, Sporn A, Gogtay N, et al. Childhood-onset schizophrenia: a double-blind, randomized clozapine-olanzapine comparison. Arch Gen Psychiatry 2006;63:721–30.
[98] Lieberman JA, Stroup TS, McEvoy JP, et al. (Clinical Antipsychotic Trials of Intervention Effectiveness (CATIE) Investigators): effectiveness of antipsychotic drugs in patients with chronic schizophrenia. N Engl J Med 2005;353(12):1209–23.
[99] Sikich L, Frazier JA, McClellan J, et al. Double blind comparison of first- and second-generation antipsychotics in early onset schizophrenia: findings from the treatment of early-onset schizophrenia spectrum disorders (TEOSS) study. Am J Psychiatry 2008;165:1420–31.
[100] McCracken JT, Mcgough J, Shah B. Risperidone in children with autism and serious behavior problems. N Engl J Med 2002;347:314–21.
[101] Haupt DW, Rosenblatt LC, Kim E, et al. Prevalence and predictors of lipid and glucose monitoring in commercially insured patients treated with second-generation antipsychotic agents. Am J Psychiatry 2009;166:345.
[102] Correll CU. Antipsychotic use in children and adolescents: minimizing adverse effects to maximize outcomes. J Am Acad Child Adolesc Psychiatry 2008;47(1):9–20.
[103] Foy JM, Kelleher KJ, Laraque D, et al. American Academy of Pediatrics Task Force on Mental Health. Enhancing pediatric mental health care: strategies for preparing a primary care practice. Pediatrics 2010;125(Suppl 3):S87–108.

Advances in Pediatrics 58 (2011) 181–194

ADVANCES IN PEDIATRICS

Management of Pediatric Intestinal Failure

Jeffrey J. Dehmer, MD[a], Megan K. Fuller, MD[a], Michael A. Helmrath, MD[b,*]

[a]Department of Surgery, University of North Carolina at Chapel Hill, 4032 Burnett-Womack Building, CB# 7050, Chapel Hill, NC 27599-7050, USA

[b]Division of Pediatric Surgery, Cincinnati Children's Hospital Medical Center, 3333 Burnet Avenue, MLC 2023, Cincinnati, OH 45229-3039, USA

Patients and families suffering from intestinal failure are exposed daily to physical, emotional, and fiscal burdens that result in an immeasurable amount of distress [1]. Intestinal failure occurs in these patients because of an inability of their bowel to meet fluid and/or nutritional needs required to sustain normal physiology and growth without parenteral nutritional support. In children, short-bowel syndrome (SBS) is the major cause of intestinal failure and results from both congenital disorders and extensive surgical resection. The common causes of SBS include intestinal atresia, abdominal wall defects (primarily gastroschisis), intestinal volvulus, long-segment Hirschsprung disease, complicated meconium ileus, and necrotizing enterocolitis (30% of cases and the most common cause).

Of all pediatric SBS, 80% occurs during the neonatal period. Data on the incidence and mortality related to SBS are sparse. A recent cohort of very low and extremely low birth weight neonates at 16 tertiary centers in the United States demonstrated incidences of SBS at 0.7% and 1.1%, respectively, although this excluded cases in term infants [2]. Given the increase in the overall number and survival of these at-risk patients, it is logical to assume that the overall number of pediatric SBS will continue to increase as well. Mortality in this population of patients occurs in a bimodal fashion, with the first peak corresponding to infants who undergo massive initial bowel resections and a later peak corresponding to complications of SBS, namely central venous catheter sepsis and intestinal failure–associated liver disease (IFALD). Survival rates for children with SBS have been quoted as 73% to 89%, with lower rates in patients requiring chronic total parenteral nutrition (TPN) [3–6].

Recently, the development of formal multidisciplinary programs has greatly improved the care provided to these patients by reducing both the morbidity and mortality associated with intestinal failure [7]. In general, these programs

*Corresponding author. *E-mail address:* Michael.Helmrath@cchmc.org

0065-3101/11/$ – see front matter
doi:10.1016/j.yapd.2011.03.012

consist of gastroenterologists, pediatric surgeons, advanced care providers dedicated to intestinal rehabilitation, intestinal failure nutritionists, pharmacists with advanced training in parenteral nutrition (PN), and social workers. As intestinal rehabilitation centers care for children within their institutions as well as accepting numerous referrals both nationally and internationally, administrative support that provides these families and referring physicians easy access to the program is invaluable. This includes access to people who can help provide timely information on how to receive a consult and recommendations from the team, coordinate referrals and transport to the center, and provide continuity of care when they return home. After discharge, ongoing communication with the referring physicians and provision of detailed care plans can avoid many of the complications that contribute to the morbidity associated with intestinal failure.

The care of patients at risk for intestinal failure begins at birth for those with congenital problems and in the operating room for patients undergoing massive intestinal resection. Although the time course of intestinal adaptation predicts that many of these patients will eventually be able to obtain enteral autonomy, waiting for the few patients to declare themselves as having chronic intestinal failure misses an opportunity for prevention. Early treatment paradigms designed to minimize morbidity and establish early controlled feedings will likely benefit all patients at risk by reducing the overall need for parental nutritional support. Decisions made at this time should take into account several key points:

1. Rapid intestinal growth occurs during the third trimester and continues into the first year of life, therefore short segments of intestine have the potential for significant increased growth [8,9].
2. The intestine has a remarkable ability to heal after ischemic injury and it is often impossible to predict the fate of the bowel without the benefit of time [10]. This supports the liberal use of second-look operations before committing to resection. When the outcome remains in question after a period of time, we recommend a diverting stoma and leaving the bowel in place with a mucous fistula to provide easy access for evaluation in 4 to 6 weeks. At this point, if the bowel has healed, slow refeeding of stoma output through the mucous fistula can help with fluid and electrolyte imbalance and the timing of reanastomosis can be planned. In conditions such as necrotizing enterocolitis (NEC), procedures such as "clip and drop" have demonstrated that areas of bowel initially deemed nonviable will survive and can function in the future, further emphasizing the point that the bowel has a remarkable ability to recover [11]. We strongly encourage directed operative resections of intestine in patients with NEC to avoid increased loss of bowel length.
3. Enteral nutrition is the most influential driver of intestinal adaptation. The initial operative plan should consider options for early initiation of feeds. The placement of a gastrostomy tube initially helps to decompress the proximal bowel and later enhances early feeds. In addition, careful placement of intestinal stomas and distal mucous fistulas can obviate the need for an extensive laparotomy in the future when reestablishing intestinal continuity. This approach

avoids potential complications and long postoperative periods without enteral nutrition. This also allows early restoration of intestinal continuity, which in turn augments the adaptive response and may minimize complications, including PN-associated liver disease and central venous catheter infections [12]. Preoperative evaluation of the distal intestine with radiographic studies before surgery is essential. Although there is a disadvantage with 2 stomas in close proximity with regard to wound complications and application of the ostomy appliance, this is outweighed by the potential avoidance of additional intestinal injury during extensive operative mobilization.

ASSESSMENT OF THE CHILD WITH INTESTINAL FAILURE

A careful clinical assessment of the child with SBS is invaluable in gauging his or her overall status. Anthropometric data should be obtained frequently and compared with growth curves after adjustment for gestational age. Precise estimates of intake and output are important, as is monitoring of electrolytes, micronutrients, minerals, and trace elements (zinc, calcium, magnesium, copper, manganese, iron, chromium, selenium, and lead), especially in TPN-dependent children. If a surgical resection was performed at a referring institution, the location and type of stomas present is important both for planning reanastomosis and possibly introducing distal mucous fistula feeds. An estimate of the actual length of bowel remaining is helpful and should be recorded as a percentage of expected bowel length. The location and status of any existing central venous access sites should be assessed and a history of any catheter-related infections (CRIs) documented with culture and sensitivity data if available. Studies to evaluate the patency of central veins should be obtained in all patients, as vascular complications from long-term central venous access can limit the ability to provide PN and may be an indication for transplant evaluation.

Aggressive surgical strategies to reestablish intestinal continuity are beneficial in the management of children with intestinal failure. In patients with high stoma output, as commonly seen with proximal jejunostomies, correction of fluid and electrolytes in balance with enteral feeding is not achievable without the benefit of having the distal intestine in continuity. The presence of any defunctionalized loops of bowel should be noted and if possible they should be salvaged at the time of surgery. Before any attempt at reanastomosis, contrast studies should be performed to assess the anatomy of the remnant bowel and to help formulate a surgical plan.

FEEDING STRATEGIES

The ultimate goal in treating children with SBS is a gastrointestinal tract that can meet the nutritional requirements sufficient to continue growth and normal physiology. This often requires continuous feeds to maximize the percentage of enteral feeds over a 24-hour period. Secure enteral access is required to meet this goal. As many of these patients have difficulty with gastric emptying, evaluating the ability of the patient to tolerate nasogastric

(NG) feeds can provide very useful clinical information before placement of a gastric feeding tube (GT). In general, patients who tolerate NG feeds will also tolerate GT feeds. In cases of poor gastric emptying and high residuals, placement of a nasojejunal feeding tube (NJ) provides important additional clinical data regarding the ability of the bowel to tolerate enteral nutrition. If tolerated, placement of gastrojejunal feeding tubes (GJ) will allow distal feeding while simultaneously decompressing the stomach. This also provides a way to start oral feeds in patients with poor gastric motility, as the stomach remains vented. We typically avoid performing antireflux procedures in these patients unless their reflux is a limiting factor in the ability to feed via GJ tube.

In general, all at-risk patients for intestinal failure should be treated using protocols designed to minimize complications and enhance adaptation. Most of these patients will require initial support by PN. At our institution, we have established a lipid reduction protocol that limits the amount of fat to less than 1 g/kg/d in all at-risk patients and we have noted a dramatic decrease in the incidence of elevated direct bilirubin and liver enzymes. In select cases with ongoing elevation of liver enzymes and direct bilirubin, intravenous omega-3 fatty acids (Omegaven; Fresenius Kabi AG, Bad Homburg, Germany) appear to be beneficial [13]. Ongoing prospective studies are evaluating these 2 treatment options and should provide useful data in the near future to help establish data-driven practical guidelines regarding the use of these strategies.

Early initial feeds should be provided continuously using breast milk (mother's or donor's) for all infants when available. There are several studies that support the use of breast milk in this patient population for reducing complications associated with SBS [12]. This benefit is likely because of its high levels of immunoglobulin A, nucleotides, long-chain fats, growth factors, and free amino acids, including glutamine present in breast milk. In cases where protein allergies occur, when breast milk is not available, or in older patients, we initially provide an elemental amino acid–based formula.

Advancement of feeds is based on the lack of emesis and abdominal distention, the consistency and amount of stool output, and the presence of skin break down. When the patient experiences feeding intolerance, the feeds should be reduced rather than stopping and restarting all feeds, unless there is evidence of systemic illness or sepsis. In our opinion, the recurrent practice of starting and stopping feeds limits enteral stimulation of adaptation and makes it difficult to identify the amount of enteral feeds that these patients will tolerate. Fluid losses from stoma output and decompressing gastrostomy tubes in the case of jejunal feeds should be carefully measured and replaced mL:mL with an appropriate electrolyte solution. In cases where the stoma output approaches or exceeds 40 mL/kg/d, we consider adding 3% pectin to the formula and frequently use antidiarrheal and antisecretory medication. We do not decrease the rate of feeds in these patients unless there are issues with persistent fluid and electrolyte issues, usually identified by a decreased

CO_2 below 20 on serum chemistries. We do not check for the presence of reducing substances, as this does not provide useful clinical data in our opinion. One important reason to hold or limit feeds is the presence of skin or perineal breakdown. Local wound care in this population can be very difficult and benefits tremendously from established wound care programs.

Oral feedings in neonates with SBS are typically not begun until the patient is tolerating full continuous feedings. During this time, aggressive occupational and physical therapy are provided to help establish oral motor skills. Holding feeds for 1 hour and offering that omitted volume orally begins the transition from continuous feedings. Initially this is done daily or twice a day and then gradually increased. Parenteral nutrition should be decreased as enteral feeding volumes are increased. In general, we decrease by 1 mL/h for each 1-mL/h increase in enteral feeds. In cases of extremely low birth weight and very low birth weight infants, the inability to provide PN below rates of 2 mL/h and the overall limitation of total amount of fluid volume the patient may receive can make achieving the total amount of calories by enteral nutrition a challenge. In situations where early reestablishment of intestinal continuity is possible, we will opt for improved growth with PN rather than pushing or concentrating feeds until after surgery. It is important to recognize that the short-term goal is not to wean off PN, but rather to establish enteral nutrition with fluid and electrolyte balance that results in normal growth. Many of the complications of PN are greatly minimized when enteral feeding provides greater than 50% of the total needs. Morbidity associated with early weaning of PN such as poor weight gain and intestinal damage or bacteremia owing to high formula concentration or volume is outweighed by the risks of low-volume PN.

PREDICTORS OF OUTCOME IN INTESTINAL FAILURE

Several retrospective studies have tried to identify certain characteristics that may be useful in predicting outcomes in children with SBS and/or intestinal failure. Given the wide array of diagnoses that can lead to intestinal failure, it is difficult to isolate predictors of outcome, but there are some general trends (Table 1). The length of remaining bowel and its location are the most logical

Table 1
Factors associated with prognosis in intestinal failure

Positive Factors	Negative Factors
High plasma citrulline levels	Remnant bowel length <10% of expected
Remnant segments include terminal ileum and colon	Cholestasis (direct bilirubin >2.5 mg/dL)
Enteral feeding at least 50% of total needs	Bacterial overgrowth
Care in a multidisciplinary program	Loss of the ileum
	Recurrent sepsis

factors to use in predicting a patient's course with intestinal failure. Neonates have an amazing capacity for adaptation, and this potential is increased in preterm infants [9]. Previous work has shown that patients with less than 10% of their predicted small-bowel length were less likely to wean from PN and they have a higher relative risk of death [5]. This fact makes accurate assessment of small-bowel length at the time of surgery critical for helping to plan a comprehensive treatment regimen and for anticipating complications. The remnant bowel should be measured and documented in the operative notes with each surgical procedure. Using a silk suture along the antimesenteric border of the bowel is a reasonable approach to obtain an accurate length [8].

In addition to length, the location of the remaining bowel is also important. The jejunum is primarily a secretory segment of the gastrointestinal tract, whereas the ileum possesses more absorptive capacity, as well as participating in vitamin B_{12}, fat-soluble vitamin, bile salt, and fatty acid physiology. For this reason, the ileum has a far greater ability to adapt than the jejunum, and therefore the amount of distal bowel required to become independent of PN is far less then that of the jejunum. In addition, the ileocecal valve prevents migration of colonic bacteria into the small bowel, which can hinder absorption further [14]. The idea that the presence or absence of the ileocecal valve itself is a predictor of potential to wean from PN has been recently challenged. As its loss does not appear to be an independent factor contributing to intestinal failure, a more likely explanation is that it is surgically removed in cases associated with the loss of the ileum. Restoring diverted colon back into the enteral steam provides significant absorptive capacity that is greatly beneficial in the maintenance of fluid and electrolyte balance. Equally important is the potential for the colon to reclaim energy from the production of short-chain fatty acids (predominantly butyrate) by colonic microbiota that serve as an energy source and enhance fluid absorption as well as providing strong adaptive hormonal signals back to the proximal small bowel to augment absorption and to slow down intestinal transit time [5].

Across several studies, IFALD remains the most likely predictor of a negative outcome and some estimate that nearly two-thirds of children with intestinal failure end up with liver disease at some point during their course [15,16]. Multiple studies have also indicated that increasing levels of direct hyperbilirubinemia (particularly >2.5 mg/dL) are strongly predictive of mortality [5,17,18]. In addition to predicting mortality, bilirubin levels have been evaluated as predictors of progression to end-stage liver disease [19]. The progression of IFALD is aggravated by episodes of sepsis that may result from CRIs. Prolonged peripheral nutrition can result in transient elevation of bilirubin, transaminases, and GGT that resolve after discontinuing PN. In children requiring PN for extended periods, it can result in cholestasis, periportal inflammation, and fibrosis. With ongoing hepatic damage, cirrhosis, portal hypertension, and other sequelae of chronic liver disease can result. Extensive ileal resection with loss of normal enterohepatic circulation can further exacerbate this process. Aggressive prevention of IFALD is important, as this is one of the main causes of morbidity and mortality in these children. It also hinders adaptation in the remaining bowel [20]. The importance of preventing this complication has led to the development of PN protocols designed specifically to protect the liver, as discussed previously, with the basic premise of these strategies being lipid reduction.

Along with physical characteristics of the bowel, there are several systemic indicators of a patient's course with intestinal failure. A predictive marker would be useful to stratify children and identify earlier those who might benefit from expeditious evaluation for intestinal transplantation [2,18,21,22]. Plasma citrulline levels have been investigated as a surrogate for functional enterocyte mass and intestinal adaptation and may be predictive of PN dependence. Small intestinal enterocytes are unique in their ability to synthesize and export citrulline to the blood. Fasting plasma citrulline levels correlate with residual small-bowel length in patients with SBS [23]. In addition, higher levels of citrulline (>15 μmol/L) may be predictive of achieving independence from PN [24].

OTHER COMPLICATIONS ASSOCIATED WITH INTESTINAL FAILURE

Gastric hypersecretion is a problem after major small-bowel resection, as decreased gastrin breakdown leads to hypergastrinemia and potentially gastroduodenal ulceration [25,26]. In addition, increased acid present in the remnant small bowel can decrease the activity of pancreatic enzymes, which function in a narrow pH range. Acid-reducing therapy, either via proton pump inhibition or histamine blockade can help reduce enteral output. For this reason, we empirically manage all patients on a proton pump inhibitor for at least the first 6 months following intestinal loss. We will consider stopping therapy at that point, especially in patients with recurrent line infections, as the acid in the stomach provides a natural barrier to limit bacterial overgrowth.

As part of the adaptive process, the small bowel undergoes dilation. Along with less effective aboral peristalsis and changes in anatomy, increased secretion may promote abnormal growth of bacteria. Normally, the terminal ileum acts as a transition zone between the proximal small bowel, which contains mostly aerobic bacteria, and the colon, which contains mostly gram-negative organisms and anaerobes. These latter bacteria may be beneficial in the colon, where they are capable of fermenting unabsorbed carbohydrates to short-chain fatty acids (most important is likely butyrate) that can promote epithelial barrier function, sodium and chloride absorption, and serve as an important energy source. The negative consequences that occur with bacterial overgrowth include the production of toxic metabolites, translocation of bacteria into the bloodstream, and altered use of luminal nutrients [27]. If this occurs, it may result in prolonged dependence on PN, liver injury, increased rates of CRIs, and malabsorption [28]. The very high rate of recurrent bloodstream infections in infants with SBS is at least in some part a result of gut barrier dysfunction and impaired immunity, both in the gut and systemically. Translocation of indigenous intestinal microbes has been shown to occur in animal models of SBS, with the translocation being promoted by generalized host immunosuppression, gut-associated immune dysfunction, bacterial overgrowth, and gut barrier dysfunction [28–30].

Correctly diagnosing this condition is difficult, as an invasive endoscopic procedure is required to obtain luminal samples (gold standard) and breath hydrogen tests may not be reliable in patients with SBS; therefore, the diagnosis is often made empirically [31]. Contrast studies may demonstrate diffuse dilation in the absence of obstruction (Fig. 1). Many of the signs and symptoms of bacterial overgrowth are indistinguishable from symptoms of intestinal failure: feeding intolerance, diarrhea, abdominal pain, bloating, unexplained acidosis, and poor weight gain. As a result, the use of antibiotic regimens to decrease bacterial content and shift the balance to luminal flora less detrimental to the patient is an important adjunct. To hinder the production of resistant species, a rotational antibiotic regimen with on and off weeks is recommended. Probiotics may be useful in both the prevention and treatment of bacterial overgrowth. These are live organisms that may provide a benefit by populating the gut with nonpathogenic bacteria. Unfortunately, there are no strong data supporting their use at this time. The use of probiotics during periods of antibiotic regimens to treat bacterial overgrowth is counterproductive and is not recommended.

With impaired carbohydrate absorption, bacterial fermentation in the bowel lumen may also result in the production of D-lactate. In these patients, malabsorbed carbohydrate is fermented by an abnormal bacterial flora in the colon that produces D-lactate, thus resulting in D-lactic acidosis. This anion gap acidosis can result in neurologic symptoms, including altered mental status, slurred speech, and ataxia. The diagnosis is made by the presence of elevated D-lactate

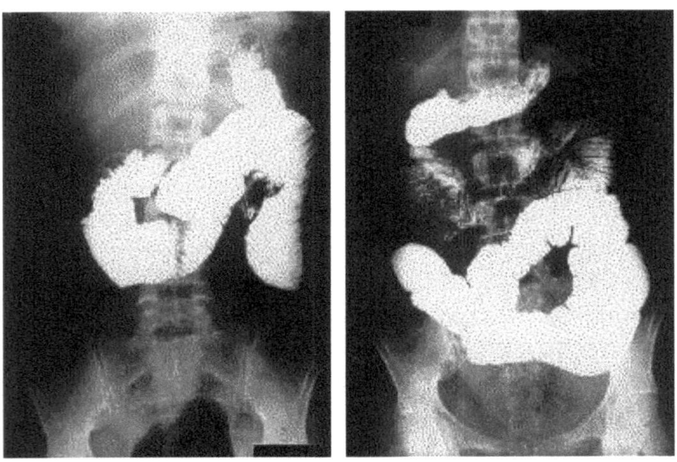

Fig. 1. Upper part of gastrointestinal tract demonstrating small intestinal dilation consistent with intestinal failure. Note the diffuse dilation in the absence of obstruction.

in the blood or urine. D-lactic acidosis is managed by reduction or elimination of carbohydrates and administering sodium bicarbonate along with antibiotics. As there have been no adequate clinical trials of antibiotics or probiotics in children with SBS and bacterial overgrowth, there is currently no approved therapy. However, many antibiotic regimens have proved to be effective in managing this condition when delivered at 1-week to 2-week intervals, with rotation of antibiotic regimens to avoid resistance. Metronidazole (20 mg/kg/d) has achieved the widest popularity; additional options are trimethoprim/sulfamethoxazole (40–50 mg/kg/d), aminoglycosides given orally, or amoxicillin/clavulanic acid. Recently, rifaximin has been shown to be effective in adults and has proven to be useful in some of our resistant pediatric patients [32]. When these conditions fail, surgical management of the dilated intestine has been shown to eliminate recurrent episodes in children with SBS.

In addition to complications intrinsic to the intestinal tract, the frequent requirement for central venous access to provide PN leads to CRIs. The incidence of CRI is also significantly higher in children with SBS than in those without SBS (7.8 vs 1.3 per 1000 catheter days) and enteric organisms are responsible for 62% of catheter sepsis in patients with SBS compared with only 12% in patients without SBS [33]. Successful prevention, diagnosis, and treatment of CRIs are paramount for any child requiring PN. Cuffed, tunneled central venous catheters (CVCs) are preferable to peripherally inserted central catheters (PICC lines), as they are less likely to become infected, dislodged, or migrate from a central location. The Infectious Disease Society of America provides guidelines for obtaining blood cultures to diagnose CRI, as well as strategies for catheter salvage [34]. As peripheral blood cultures are frequently difficult to obtain from children, a criteria-based diagnosis of CRI is often not possible. Maintenance of sterile technique during catheter placement is essential.

Both antibiotic and 70% ethanol locks have been used to prevent and treat CRI in children [35–37]. Both have demonstrated some efficacy, specifically by attacking biofilms that are frequently the proximate cause of CRI, but concerns exist with both modalities. Antibiotic locks can promote proliferation of resistant species and require heparin to maintain patency. Ethanol locks can degrade polyurethane CVCs, although no instances of degradation have been reported with silicone catheters. Additional complications of ethanol intoxication, dizziness, nausea, and dyspnea have been reported, although using a dwell time of 4 hours, 3 times per week with withdrawal of the instilled ethanol before flushing resulted in no reports of adverse events. Ethanol should not be used in patients receiving metronidazole, as it can cause a disulfiramlike reaction. Various reports of ethanol lock use in children demonstrate good reductions in CRI rates and decreased need for catheter removal [34–36].

NEW CONCEPTS IN MEDICAL AND SURGICAL MANAGEMENT

The use of growth hormones and specific nutrients known to stimulate bowel growth have had limited effectiveness clinically. Challenges to their clinical utility include reversal of the adaptive process after termination of hormonal treatment and a lack of overall intestinal muscle growth (effects are limited to the mucosa) [38–43]. Recently, encouraging data from a randomized, placebo-controlled study of teduglutide (glucagon-like peptide-2 analog) administered for 24 weeks to adult patients with chronic intestinal failure demonstrated a decrease in stoma output associated with a decrease in PN requirements [44]. Of note, 3 patients were completely weaned off PN in this study. Based on the observation in the phase 2 trial that the effects of teduglutide are reversible suggests that chronic long-term treatment will be necessary to sustain this observation [45]. Clinical studies evaluating the early administration of GLP-2 and the effect in pediatric patients are needed. Data from murine intestinal resection models suggest that enhanced and sustained expansion of intestinal stem cells may occur with early administration that do not occur at later time points [46].

Glutamine is a nonessential amino acid that is a primary energy source for the enterocyte. It has been shown in animals and adults to prevent mucosal atrophy and deterioration in gut permeability in patients receiving peripheral nutrition. Glutamine administration improves the growth and function of human gut epithelial cells. When supplemented with Glycyl-Gln, PN-dependent individuals demonstrated significantly increased duodenal villus height and decreased intestinal permeability compared with individuals with standard nonsupplemented compositions. In adults, using a combination of enteral glutamine (30 g/d), subcutaneously administered human growth hormone, and a high-fiber (apple pectin), low-fat diet (20% fat, 20% protein, and 60% carbohydrate) led to improvement of intestinal absorptive capacity and weaning or reducing TPN [47]. The data in children are inconclusive at this time regarding the use of enteral glutamine.

Intestinal dilation is associated with intestinal failure [48]. The past 20 years have seen advances in surgical treatment of these patients after maximization of medical therapy. This group of procedures, most appropriately referred to as autologous intestinal reconstruction surgery (AIRS), gives children who have maximized their medical management another option to achieve intestinal autonomy. It is important to note that surgical management of SBS should not be first-line therapy, but rather an adjunct to diligent management of the remaining functional intestinal mucosa. Two major problems intrinsic to the bowel itself are directly affected by AIRS: dysmotility and bacterial stasis and overgrowth secondary to dilation. The most widely used AIRS procedures are the serial transverse enteroplasty (STEP) and longitudinal intestinal lengthening and tailoring (LILT). Despite these advances, up to 45% of patients will have complications and/or no clinical improvement following autologous reconstruction of the bowel [49–51].

Bianchi [52] originally reported the longitudinal intestinal lengthening and tailoring procedure in 1980. This operation bluntly divides the mesentery of the bowel into 2 leaflets, each with its own blood supply sufficient to support one-half of the intestinal diameter with blood flow. Once the mesentery has been partitioned, the intestine is divided and then the ends are anastomosed in an isoperistaltic fashion, in effect doubling the length of the intestine. In 2006, a worldwide review of studies involving LILT was published with mixed results in overall survival and weaning from PN [53]. Reported complications beyond those already associated with SBS include anastomotic strictures and bowel obstruction secondary to adhesions, among others.

The serial transverse enteroplasty was initially described in 2003, and the procedure was performed on a human infant that same year [54,55]. STEP uses serial firings of a stapler perpendicular to the long axis of the bowel, alternating from the mesenteric to the antimesenteric side. This results in a zig-zag appearance to the bowel and a luminal diameter of about 2 cm. In addition to SBS, this procedure has been applied in instances of proximal atresias with significant bowel dilation, as well as recurrent episodes of D-lactic acidosis. Patients frequently experience redilation of the bowel after STEP and may require a second procedure. It is important to note that STEP may be used in asymmetrically dilated bowel, unlike the LILT procedure. A 2007 review found no significant difference in complications between the 2 procedures [56].

The concept of "intestinal lengthening" to improve total absorption and function is likely a simplistic view of these procedures. The term autologous reconstruction highlights that what is being accomplished during this surgical procedure is correction of intestinal dysmotility owing to bowel dilation in a manner that maximizes preservation of mucosal surface area. Careful consideration and timing of these procedures is complex and best performed in a center experienced with the care of patients with intestinal failure. In our opinion, elective autologous reconstruction should be delayed until at least 1 year after the initial insult to allow maximal time for adaptation of the remnant bowel. Earlier surgical procedures that result in unexpected postoperative complications that do not allow feeding, such as anastomotic leak, potentially risk hindering the adaptive process, which cannot be reinitiated once it is disrupted. Consideration to perform autologous reconstruction in addition to other procedures, such as resection of a stricture with associated bowel dilation may be beneficial in the correct circumstances. In general, this would be in a patient with minimal remaining dilated bowel and where clinical advancement of enteral nutrition has plateaued. For patients who exhaust all medical and surgical options, intestinal transplantation has been performed with improved results over the past decade with 75% graft and 80% patient survival at 1 year in 2005 [57].

SUMMARY

In conclusion, the management approach to children with intestinal failure is complex. It requires diligent management of nutrition with maximal effort given to achieving as much as possible via the enteral route, involving enteral tubes if necessary. Optimization of enteral feeding should be in a manner that minimizes starting and stopping feeds frequently. In these challenging patients, timely management and preferably prevention of complications can result in significant clinical benefit. Problems such as gastric hypersecretion, bacterial overgrowth, IFALD, and CRIs are unfortunately common in these challenging patients. Autologous intestinal reconstruction should be considered only after adequate time for physiologic adaptation has occurred. With intestinal failure, even small clinical gains can be profound both financially and emotionally for the patients and their families. Strong consideration should be given to early referral to a specialized center with experience in treating the full spectrum of patients with intestinal failure.

References

[1] Baxter JP, Fayers PM, McKinlay AW. A review of the quality of life of adult patients treated with long-term parenteral nutrition. Clin Nutr 2006;25(4):543–53.
[2] Cole CR, Hansen NI, Higgins RD, et al. Very low birth weight preterm infants with surgical short bowel syndrome: incidence, morbidity and mortality, and growth outcomes at 18 to 22 months. Pediatrics 2008;122(3):e573–82.
[3] Diamond IR, de Silva N, Pencharz PB, et al. Neonatal short bowel syndrome outcomes after the establishment of the first Canadian multidisciplinary intestinal rehabilitation program: preliminary experience. J Pediatr Surg 2007;42(5):806–11.
[4] Modi BP, Langer M, Ching YA, et al. Improved survival in a multidisciplinary short bowel syndrome program. J Pediatr Surg 2008;43(1):20–4.
[5] Spencer AU, Neaga A, West B, et al. Pediatric short bowel syndrome: redefining predictors of success. Ann Surg 2005;242(3):403–9 [discussion: 409–12].
[6] Sudan D, DiBaise J, Torres C, et al. A multidisciplinary approach to the treatment of intestinal failure. J Gastrointest Surg 2005;9(2):165–76 [discussion: 176–7].
[7] Javid PJ, Malone FR, Reyes J, et al. The experience of a regional pediatric intestinal failure program: successful outcomes from intestinal rehabilitation. Am J Surg 2010;199(5): 676–9.
[8] Struijs MC, Diamond IR, de Silva N, et al. Establishing norms for intestinal length in children. J Pediatr Surg 2009;44(5):933–8.
[9] Goday PS. Short bowel syndrome: how short is too short? Clin Perinatol 2009;36(1): 101–10.
[10] Estrada JJ, Petrosyan M, Hunter CJ, et al. Preservation of extracorporeal tissue in closing gastroschisis augments intestinal length. J Pediatr Surg 2008;43(12):2213–5.
[11] Ron O, Davenport M, Patel S, et al. Outcomes of the "clip and drop" technique for multifocal necrotizing enterocolitis. J Pediatr Surg 2009;44(4):749–54.
[12] Andorsky DJ, Lund DP, Lillehei CW, et al. Nutritional and other postoperative management of neonates with short bowel syndrome correlates with clinical outcomes. J Pediatr 2001;139(1):27–33.
[13] Diamond IR, Sterescu A, Pencharz PB, et al. The rationale for the use of parenteral omega-3 lipids in children with short bowel syndrome and liver disease. Pediatr Surg Int 2008;24(7): 773–8.
[14] Goulet O, Ruemmele F, Lacaille F, et al. Irreversible intestinal failure. J Pediatr Gastroenterol Nutr 2004;38(3):250–69.
[15] Carter BA, Shulman RJ. Mechanisms of disease: update on the molecular etiology and fundamentals of parenteral nutrition associated cholestasis. Nat Clin Pract Gastroenterol Hepatol 2007;4(5):277–87.
[16] Cowles RA, Ventura KA, Martinez M, et al. Reversal of intestinal failure-associated liver disease in infants and children on parenteral nutrition: experience with 93 patients at a referral center for intestinal rehabilitation. J Pediatr Surg 2010;45(1):84–7 [discussion: 87–8].

[17] Kelly DA. Intestinal failure-associated liver disease: what do we know today? Gastroenterology 2006;130(2 Suppl 1):S70–7.
[18] Soden JS. Clinical assessment of the child with intestinal failure. Semin Pediatr Surg 2010;19(1):10–9.
[19] Nasr A, Avitzur Y, Ng VL, et al. The use of conjugated hyperbilirubinemia greater than 100 micromol/L as an indicator of irreversible liver disease in infants with short bowel syndrome. J Pediatr Surg 2007;42(2):359–62.
[20] Weber TR, Keller MS. Adverse effects of liver dysfunction and portal hypertension on intestinal adaptation in short bowel syndrome in children. Am J Surg 2002;184(6):582–6 [discussion: 586].
[21] Wales PW, Christison-Lagay ER. Short bowel syndrome: epidemiology and etiology. Semin Pediatr Surg 2010;19(1):3–9.
[22] Bailly-Botuha C, Colomb V, Thioulouse E, et al. Plasma citrulline concentration reflects enterocyte mass in children with short bowel syndrome. Pediatr Res 2009;65(5):559–63.
[23] Crenn P, Coudray-Lucas C, Thuillier F, et al. Postabsorptive plasma citrulline concentration is a marker of absorptive enterocyte mass and intestinal failure in humans. Gastroenterology 2000;119(6):1496–505.
[24] Fitzgibbons S, Ching YA, Valim C, et al. Relationship between serum citrulline levels and progression to parenteral nutrition independence in children with short bowel syndrome. J Pediatr Surg 2009;44(5):928–32.
[25] Hyman PE, Everett SL, Harada T. Gastric acid hypersecretion in short bowel syndrome in infants: association with extent of resection and enteral feeding. J Pediatr Gastroenterol Nutr 1986;5(2):191–7.
[26] Hyman PE, Garvey TQ 3rd, Harada T. Effect of ranitidine on gastric acid hypersecretion in an infant with short bowel syndrome. J Pediatr Gastroenterol Nutr 1985;4(2):316–9.
[27] Cole CR, Ziegler TR. Small bowel bacterial overgrowth: a negative factor in gut adaptation in pediatric SBS. Curr Gastroenterol Rep 2007;9(6):456–62.
[28] Cole CR, Frem JC, Schmotzer B, et al. The rate of bloodstream infection is high in infants with short bowel syndrome: relationship with small bowel bacterial overgrowth, enteral feeding, and inflammatory and immune responses. J Pediatr 2010;156(6):941–7, 947.e941.
[29] Aldazabal P, Eizaguirre I, Barrena MJ, et al. Bacterial translocation and T-lymphocyte populations in experimental short-bowel syndrome. Eur J Pediatr Surg 1998;8(4): 247–50.
[30] Schimpl G, Feierl G, Linni K, et al. Bacterial translocation in short-bowel syndrome in rats. Eur J Pediatr Surg 1999;9(4):224–7.
[31] Corazza GR, Menozzi MG, Strocchi A, et al. The diagnosis of small bowel bacterial overgrowth. Reliability of jejunal culture and inadequacy of breath hydrogen testing. Gastroenterology 1990;98(2):302–9.
[32] Majewski M, Reddymasu SC, Sostarich S, et al. Efficacy of rifaximin, a nonabsorbed oral antibiotic, in the treatment of small intestinal bacterial overgrowth. Am J Med Sci 2007;333(5):266–70.
[33] Kurkchubasche AG, Smith SD, Rowe MI. Catheter sepsis in short-bowel syndrome. Arch Surg 1992;127(1):21–4 [discussion: 24–5].
[34] Mermel LA, Allon M, Bouza E, et al. Clinical practice guidelines for the diagnosis and management of intravascular catheter-related infection: 2009 Update by the Infectious Diseases Society of America. Clin Infect Dis 2009;49(1):1–45.
[35] Jones BA, Hull MA, Richardson DS, et al. Efficacy of ethanol locks in reducing central venous catheter infections in pediatric patients with intestinal failure. J Pediatr Surg 2010;45(6): 1287–93.
[36] Mouw E, Chessman K, Lesher A, et al. Use of an ethanol lock to prevent catheter-related infections in children with short bowel syndrome. J Pediatr Surg 2008;43(6):1025–9.
[37] Toltzis P. Antibiotic lock technique to reduce central venous catheter-related bacteremia. Pediatr Infect Dis J 2006;25(5):449–50.

[38] Brubaker PL, Crivici A, Izzo A, et al. Circulating and tissue forms of the intestinal growth factor, glucagon-like peptide-2. Endocrinology 1997;138(11):4837–43.
[39] Helmrath MA, Shin CE, Erwin CR, et al. The EGF\EGF-receptor axis modulates enterocyte apoptosis during intestinal adaptation. J Surg Res 1998;77(1):17–22.
[40] Jeppesen PB, Szkudlarek J, Hoy CE, et al. Effect of high-dose growth hormone and glutamine on body composition, urine creatinine excretion, fatty acid absorption, and essential fatty acids status in short bowel patients: a randomized, double-blind, crossover, placebo-controlled study. Scand J Gastroenterol 2001;36(1):48–54.
[41] Scolapio JS. Effect of growth hormone and glutamine on the short bowel: five years later. Gut 2000;47(2):164.
[42] Tavakkolizadeh A, Shen R, Jasleen J, et al. Effect of growth hormone on intestinal Na+/glucose cotransporter activity. JPEN J Parenter Enteral Nutr 2001;25(1):18–22.
[43] Yang H, Wildhaber BE, Teitelbaum DH. 2003 Harry M. Vars Research Award. Keratinocyte growth factor improves epithelial function after massive small bowel resection. JPEN J Parenter Enteral Nutr 2003;27(3):198–206 [discussion: 206–7].
[44] Jeppesen PB, Gilroy R, Pertkiewicz M, et al. Randomised placebo-controlled trial of teduglutide in reducing parenteral nutrition and/or intravenous fluid requirements in patients with short bowel syndrome. Gut 2011; [Epub ahead of print]. DOI: 10.1136/gut.2010.218271.
[45] Jeppesen PB, Sanguinetti EL, Buchman A, et al. Teduglutide (ALX-0600), a dipeptidyl peptidase IV resistant glucagon-like peptide 2 analogue, improves intestinal function in short bowel syndrome patients. Gut 2005;54(9):1224–31.
[46] Garrison AP, Dekaney CM, von Allmen DC, et al. Early but not late administration of glucagon-like peptide-2 following ileo-cecal resection augments putative intestinal stem cell expansion. Am J Physiol Gastrointest Liver Physiol 2009;296(3):G643–50.
[47] Byrne TA, Morrissey TB, Nattakom TV, et al. Growth hormone, glutamine, and a modified diet enhance nutrient absorption in patients with severe short bowel syndrome. JPEN J Parenter Enteral Nutr 1995;19(4):296–302.
[48] Wilmore DW, Robinson MK. Short bowel syndrome. World J Surg 2000;24(12):1486–92.
[49] Bianchi A. Longitudinal intestinal lengthening and tailoring: results in 20 children. J R Soc Med 1997;90(8):429–32.
[50] Bueno J, Guiterrez J, Mazariegos GV, et al. Analysis of patients with longitudinal intestinal lengthening procedure referred for intestinal transplantation. J Pediatr Surg 2001;36(1): 178–83.
[51] Miyasaka EA, Brown PI, Teitelbaum DH. Redilation of bowel after intestinal lengthening procedures—an indicator for poor outcome. J Pediatr Surg 2011;46(1):145–9.
[52] Bianchi A. Intestinal loop lengthening—a technique for increasing small intestinal length. J Pediatr Surg 1980;15(2):145–51.
[53] Bianchi A. From the cradle to enteral autonomy: the role of autologous gastrointestinal reconstruction. Gastroenterology 2006;130(2 Suppl 1):S138–46.
[54] Kim HB, Fauza D, Garza J, et al. Serial transverse enteroplasty (STEP): a novel bowel lengthening procedure. J Pediatr Surg 2003;38(3):425–9.
[55] Kim HB, Lee PW, Garza J, et al. Serial transverse enteroplasty for short bowel syndrome: a case report. J Pediatr Surg 2003;38(6):881–5.
[56] Sudan D, Thompson J, Botha J, et al. Comparison of intestinal lengthening procedures for patients with short bowel syndrome. Ann Surg 2007;246(4):593–601 [discussion: 601–4].
[57] Fishbein TM. Intestinal transplantation. N Engl J Med 2009;361(10):998–1008.

Advances in Pediatrics 58 (2011) 195–206

ADVANCES IN PEDIATRICS

Infantile Hypertrophic Pyloric Stenosis: Epidemiology, Genetics, and Clinical Update

Judith D. Ranells, MD[a], Jane D. Carver, PhD, MS, MPH[a], Russell S. Kirby, PhD, MS[a,b,*]

[a]Department of Pediatrics, College of Medicine, University of South Florida, 12901 Bruce B. Downs Boulevard, Tampa, FL 33612, USA

[b]Department of Community and Family Health, College of Public Health, University of South Florida, 13201 Bruce B. Downs Boulevard, MDC56, Tampa, FL 33612, USA

Infantile hypertrophic pyloric stenosis (IHPS), the most common surgical condition producing emesis in infancy, was first described by Hirschsprung [1] in 1888. Ramstedt performed the first successful pyloromyotomy in 1912; however, most cases were lethal at that time. Although advances in medical knowledge and care have resulted in minimal mortality and morbidity today, the cause of IHPS remains unclear [2]. This article provides an update on IHPS, focusing on pathogenesis, diagnosis and treatment, descriptive epidemiology and associated risk factors, and current understanding of the role of genetics.

PATHOGENESIS

In infants with IHPS, the pyloric portion of the stomach becomes abnormally thickened, resulting in narrowing and elongation of the pyloric channel (Fig. 1). A gastric outlet obstruction is produced, with compensatory dilation, hypertrophy, and hyperperistalsis of the stomach. Most infants with IHPS present in the first 2 to 12 weeks of life with forceful or projectile nonbilious vomiting after feeding. The emesis may become blood-tinged because of gastritis. The timing of the presentation is likely related to increasing volumes of enteral feeding acting on abnormal pyloric tissue. Many infants with IHPS are initially believed to have a food allergy or gastroesophageal reflux [2,3]. The narrow window of diagnosis between approximately 2 and 12 weeks may be due to the introduction of enteral feeding, which acts on abnormal pyloric tissue.

As reviewed by Panteli [4], the pyloric sphincter contracts tonically and phasically to effect gastric emptying. Sphincter function is controlled by

*Corresponding author. Department of Community and Family Health, College of Public Health, University of South Florida, 13201 Bruce B. Downs Boulevard, MDC56, Tampa, FL 33612. *E-mail address:* rkirby@health.usf.edu

0065-3101/11/$ – see front matter
doi:10.1016/j.yapd.2011.03.005

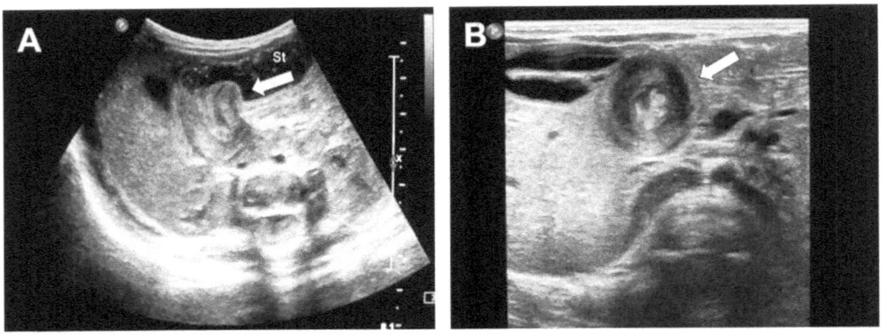

Fig. 1. Congenital hypertrophic pyloric stenosis. Sonogram depicting thick-walled pylorus (*arrow*) in a longitudinal section (*A*) and cross section (*B*). (*Reprinted from* Maheshwari P, Abograra A, Shamam O. Sonographic evaluation of gastrointestinal obstruction in infants: a pictorial essay. J Pediatr Surg 2009;44(10):2038; with permission.)

a complex system involving the enteric nervous system, gastrointestinal hormones, and interstitial cells of Cajal. Abnormalities in hormonal control, extracellular matrix, smooth muscle fibers, growth factors, interstitial cells of Cajal, and pyloric innervations have been implicated in the pathogenesis of IHPS. The muscular layer of the pylorus in IHPS is reportedly characterized by abnormal distribution of nerve terminals [5], reduced intramuscular nerve supporting cells [6], altered peptidergic innervation [7], altered nitric oxide production [8], ultrastructural abnormalities of enteric nerves and the interstitial cells of Cajal [9], and increased insulin-like growth factor production [10]. This constellation of abnormalities leads to failure of the pyloric muscle to relax, increased synthesis of growth factors, and subsequent hypertrophy [11].

EVALUATION

Traditionally, the diagnosis of IHPS was based on a history of projectile vomiting and palpation of the hypertrophied pyloric muscle, which is referred to as an olive because of its size and shape. This method, known as palpating the olive, has a 99% positive predictive value [12]. Positive test feeds can also be used diagnostically; however, this approach has unacceptably high false-positive and false-negative rates and is not used extensively [13,14]. Ultrasound imaging is usually used as a substitute or complement to physical examination or test feeds. Although imaging is more costly, it is highly sensitive, with accuracy and sensitivity approaching 100% [2,12,14]. Measurements of canal length and muscle thickness can support the ultrasonographic diagnosis [14].

The increasing reliance on imaging has resulted in diagnoses being made before alkalosis has developed, and in a shorter clinical course, less morbidity, and a shorter postoperative hospital stay [15]. Fluoroscopic upper gastrointestinal contrast studies can also be used for diagnosis, because the pyloric canal in IHPS is outlined by a string of contrast material. However, fluoroscopy is time consuming, involves radiation exposure, and its sensitivity is dependent on the skill of the examiner. Consequently, real-time ultrasonography has supplanted fluoroscopy as the diagnostic procedure of choice [2,3]. Although ultrasonography is the standard diagnostic procedure, the pylorus is difficult to visualize in patients with gastric overdistension because of displacement of the pyloric muscle dorsally by the gas-filled and fluid-filled stomach. This problem can usually be averted by turning the patient to a right lateral decubitus position, which causes the pylorus to rise to an anterior position, thus allowing it to be imaged [16]. Borderline cases can also be problematic, because the muscle typically does not measure more than 3 mm in thickness [16]. Repeating the ultrasound several days later may confirm the diagnosis [17]. Dehydration resulting from the protracted vomiting can also cause a spuriously low measurement of muscle thickness, which may increase after fluid resuscitation [18]. In borderline cases, it may also be helpful to visualize the relaxation of the pyloric canal following introduction of fluid into the stomach; this finding reliably excludes IHPS [16]. Although radiologists most often make the diagnosis, Copeland and colleagues [16] report that surgeons who have undergone focused training can diagnose the condition without confirmatory testing by a radiologist.

Despite the high specificity and sensitivity of diagnostic methods, the current guidelines may not be sufficient for accurate diagnosis of IHPS in infants younger than 3 weeks because of the thin pyloric muscle thickness [19] and equivocal clinical and biochemical variables [14]. Young infants should be observed and reevaluated in 1 to 2 days when the lesion may be more clinically or radiologically evident [20].

TREATMENT/MANAGEMENT

The vomiting associated with IHPS leads to depletion of sodium, potassium, and hydrochloric acid, resulting in hypokalemic, hypochloremic metabolic acidosis. Because IHPS is not a surgical emergency, fluid and electrolyte losses should be corrected before surgical intervention. This correction typically requires hospitalization and intravenous fluid replacement therapy [2,3].

The practice of evidence-based medicine requires physicians to review evidence to justify medical decisions and treatments. Although general pediatric surgeons perform a great variety of different operations, the number of surgeries performed is small relative to comparable procedures performed in adults. In addition, surgery has lagged behind other disciplines in the conduct of randomized clinical trials. As a result, the evidence base for many pediatric and neonatal surgical procedures is weak [21,22]. There is a paucity of randomized, controlled trials for IHPS treatment, and most are based on collaborations between pediatric surgical units, thus highlighting the importance of creating a network of centers that promote multicenter prospective studies [21].

Extramucosal longitudinal pyloromyotomy, first described in 1908 [23], has been the standard treatment of IHPS for decades. The pyloric muscle is split longitudinally, which allows the submucosal layer to bulge out to the level of the serosa. Most patients have excellent short-term and long-term outcomes, and mortality has been virtually eliminated with the use of appropriate fluid resuscitation, improvements in anesthesia, and a standard surgical approach. Muscle thickness returns to normal within 4 weeks, and is associated with healing of the pyloric muscle and return of function [3].

Laparoscopic pyloromyotomy (LP) was first described in 1990 [24], and it is increasingly the surgical treatment of choice as laparoscopic technology has improved. However, it remains controversial whether LP is superior to open pyloromyotomy. Sola and Neville [25] performed a systematic review and meta-analysis of laparoscopic versus open pyloromyotomy. Six prospective studies with 625 patients (303 laparoscopic, 322 open surgery) met selection criteria. Patients who underwent LP had lower total complication rates (odds ratio [OR] 0.58; 95% CI 0.35, 0.97), mostly because of fewer wound complications, shorter time to full feedings (mean difference −11.52 hours, 95% CI −12.77, −10.27) and shorter postoperative lengths of stay (mean difference −5.71 hours, 95% CI −8.90, −2.52). There were no significant differences in the rates of mucosal perforation, wound infection, postoperative emesis, or operating time. Incomplete pyloromyotomy occurred in 6 patients who underwent LP. As Hall and colleagues [21] point out, major complications such as incomplete pyloromyotomy are rare and individual studies are not powered to detect them. Thus, although rare complications are important, they may not pose a clinically significant risk for individual patients. Because LP is associated with shorter postoperative recovery period and duration of pain, it should be considered a valid technique as long as care and attention are paid to avoiding incomplete pyloromyotomy [21].

Although pyloromyotomy remains the first choice of treatment in Western countries, several investigators, mostly from Asian countries, have reported that some infants respond to intravenous or oral atropine without requiring surgery. The rationale for atropine therapy is that the pathophysiology of IHPS may be due, in part, to impaired function of acetylcholine and muscarinic receptors. Because atropine is an anticholinergic agent with strong antimuscarinic activity, it may decrease intestinal peristalsis by relaxing smooth muscles [26]. In studies conducted in Japan [27–30], Taiwan [31], and India [32], infants with IHPS were treated with intravenous or oral atropine sulfate daily until vomiting ceased, with higher doses given thereafter for varying periods of time. The investigators concluded that medical treatment is a safe and effective treatment option for IHPS, although approximately 10% of patients required pyloromyotomy and prolonged medical treatment was often needed. Meissner and colleagues [33] reported that atropine sulfate was successful in only 25 of 33 IHPS cases treated in Germany, and that clinical improvement was often not observed before the sixth or seventh day of treatment. Because of the persistent vomiting, nearly a quarter of families requested that their child be treated surgically before completing the 7 days of treatment. The investigators conclude that the 75% success rate does not favor atropine in view of the 95% success rate with surgical repair, and that the higher cure rates reported by other investigators were likely caused by prolonged medical therapy. Surgically treated patients are typically discharged within 24 hours of surgery, whereas medical treatment may require 7 days or more of skilled nursing and careful follow-up. Although the investigators conclude that atropine sulfate therapy should not be recommended where standard surgical procedure is available [33], Aspelund and Langer [2] believe it should be considered as an alternative in infants with contraindications to anesthesia or surgery.

EPIDEMIOLOGY

The reported prevalence of IHPS has varied considerably by region and time. Although early case reports date from the eighteenth and nineteenth centuries, from the time of Hirschsprung's initial report (1888) through the mid-twentieth century very few cases were examined in case series reports [34]. More recent reports have been varied both in prevalence estimates and trends over time. The most recent national report on prevalence of birth defects for 2003 to 2007 shows state-level prevalence of IHPS ranging by almost an order of magnitude, from 0.5 to 4.21 per 1000 live births (excluding states with clearly incomplete case ascertainment) [35].

Although the literature on descriptive epidemiology of IHPS seems enigmatic at first glance, a closer look at the data suggests that surveillance and ascertainment issues may account for much of the reported variability. Many reports based on the population-based data focus on small underlying birth populations, increasing the inherent variability in prevalence from year to year. Surveillance methods also vary, ranging from surgery/treatment reports to active case-finding methods, with many studies based primarily on hospital discharge data. Many birth defects surveillance programs include only those diagnoses identifiable from hospital discharge records or made in the first month after birth, whereas others use comprehensive multisource ascertainment throughout the first, and occasionally the second, year of life. Some programs use procedure codes as well as diagnostic codes, and some epidemiologic reports are based on incidence of pyloromyotomy among patients in infancy.

Although numerous studies have examined trends in prevalence of IHPS with time, the cumulative weight of the evidence suggests that the prevalence has been stable over time. Although contemporary prevalence estimates are in the range of 1 to 2 per 1000 infants, many reports examine trends during periods dating to the mid-twentieth century. Although some reports suggest an increasing trend, most of these observations come from regions with a lower initial prevalence estimate. National estimates for the prevalence of IHPS in the United States are not available; IHPS was not selected for inclusion in the most recent report because it generally has onset after the first day of life [36].

IHPS prevalence varies by maternal race/ethnicity. Studies in the United States generally report higher prevalence of IHPS among white non-Hispanic mothers, with significantly lower prevalence among non-Hispanic black mothers. In a recent Texas study, babies born to Hispanic mothers born in the United States had prevalence of IHPS similar to those born to white mothers, whereas the prevalence was significantly lower among those born outside the United States [37]. We reported a similar association between maternal nativity and risk of another complex disorder: gastroschisis [38]. This finding further supports a cause that involves a genetic/environmental interaction. Crude prevalence rates for births to Asian mothers tend to be lower than among white non-Hispanic mothers; in the most recent national surveillance report, IHPS prevalence was lowest among births to Asian mothers in all but 3 states [35].

MacMahon [34] provided a comprehensive review of the descriptive epidemiology of IHPS; this article compares his findings with more recent reports. Studies have shown no consistent association between maternal age and IHPS. However, the prevalence of IHPS seems to decline with increasing birth order, and most reports find the highest prevalence among first-born infants. IHPS is considerably more common among boys, with 4 to 5 times greater prevalence than in girls in most Western European and North American studies. Evidence for an association of IHPS with birth weight remains enigmatic. A recent study from Texas [37] found reduced prevalence among infants born at greater than 4500 g birth weight, whereas the prevalence among infants born at 3500 to 4499 g did not differ from the reference group. Although Wang [37] found no association with low birth weight, Applegate and Druschel [39] found a decreased risk for IHPS among infants born at less than 1500 g. Patterns of IHPS variation with gestational age mirror those for birth weight to some extent. As MacMahon noted [34], although preterm birth does not seem to be a risk factor, symptom onset in relation to maturity dated from conception rather than birth may explain the observed patterns. However, most birth defects registries in the United States do not record infant age at onset for IHPS. Wang [37] used 37 to 39 weeks of gestational age at birth as the reference group, and found higher adjusted prevalence ratios for IHPS among infants born at 28 to 31, 32 to 34, and 35 to 36 weeks' gestation, but lower prevalence among infants born after less than 28 or more than 40 weeks of gestation. Data suggest that maternal smoking may be associated with an increased risk for IHPS but studies have been inconclusive [40]. Studies failed to show increased risk for IHPS associated with *Helicobacter pylori* infection [4,41,42].

Numerous reports have considered the role of socioeconomic status in IHPS. Most studies in the United States have no direct measures of family income or occupation and use maternal education as a proxy measure. In 2 of these studies [37,39], IHPS was inversely associated with maternal education; however, neither study reported a test for trend. A recent report from Scotland suggests an increasing prevalence of IHPS with higher levels of social deprivation [43].

Several researchers have examined the time trends in sudden infant death syndrome (SIDS) and IHPS. Persson and colleagues [44] found a correlation of +0.57 between the 2 conditions in Stockholm, Sweden in the period 1970 to 1997, and Sommerfield and colleagues [43] reported an even stronger correlation ($r = +0.89$) in Scotland in the period 1981 to 2004. Although these observations raise the possibility that public health interventions to promote safe sleeping practices may be associated with reductions in incidence of both conditions, the hypothesis that IHPS may be associated with infant sleep position requires more detailed study.

Several recent meta-analyses have examined associations between maternal health status and prenatal behaviors and birth defects. Among those that included IHPS as an outcome, Browne [45] found no association with maternal caffeine consumption in pregnancy, Goh and colleagues [46] found no association with use of prenatal vitamins with supplements, and a meta-analysis by Stothard and colleagues [47] found insufficient evidence to support an association between in the literature to support meta-analysis of the association with maternal overweight or obesity.

GENETICS

IHPS is a complex condition, resulting from interaction of genetic and environmental factors. Genetic predisposition to IHPS was established by Carter and Powell [48] and Carter [49], who described the multifactorial sex-modified threshold model of inheritance of IHPS, with a male preponderance of 4 to 1. There is significant variation in incidence between populations, with IHPS being most common in white and Hispanic people, and less common in those of African and Asian heritage. The existence of a major dominant gene of low penetrance with a multifactorial background was considered likely in several families described in the literature [50,51]. Large, multigenerational families consistent with autosomal dominant transmission of IHPS have been reported [52–54]. The male sex bias tends to be less pronounced in familial cases [54]. Re-analysis of several previously published family studies led to the conclusion that the familial recurrence pattern of IHPS is compatible with multifactorial threshold inheritance or the effects of multiple interacting loci [55].

An analysis of cases of IHPS in Denmark occurring in a 31-year period confirmed strong familial aggregation of IHPS, with a nearly 200-fold increase among monozygotic twins and 20-fold increase among dizygotic twins and siblings [56]. The lack of increased risk among dizygotic twins compared with siblings suggests that intrauterine environmental factors are not significant in IHPS. High heritability of IHPS was further supported by strong aggregation of cases, even in third-degree and fourth-degree relatives. They observed similar rates of IHPS regardless of sex of the index case, sex of the affected relative, or presence of the affected relative in maternal or paternal side of the family. These findings are also at odds with the multifactorial threshold model, which predicts that male offspring of affected females would be at higher risk because of higher genetic and environmental liability for this trait. The investigators concluded that familial aggregation of IHPS is caused by shared genes that may affect responses to postnatal factors.

Five genetic loci associated with IHPS have been identified [57]. The gene for nitric oxide synthetase, *NOS1* (IHPS1; chromosomal locus 12q24.2-q24.31) was identified as a candidate gene for IHPS because lack of neuronal nitric oxide in pyloric tissue seems to be responsible for pylorospasm and hypertrophy in IHPS [58,59]. Two loci, IHPS2 (16p13-p12) and IHPS5 (16q24.3), are associated with autosomal dominant forms of the disease. This finding is not surprising, because identification of monogenic subtypes of complex traits has become common. This genetic heterogeneity is consistent with the multiple variables and complex molecular pathways underlying the development of IHPS. IHPS3 (11q14-q22) and IHPS4 (Xq23-q24) were identified via genome-wide linkage analysis of families with 2 or more affected individuals [60]. It is notable that the X chromosome locus could provide a basis for the increased frequency of IHPS in boys. The IHPS3 and IHPS4 regions each include a candidate gene from the family of canonical transient receptor potential (TRPC) cation channels. Further analysis led to identification of an additional locus on chromosome 3q12-q25, a region including the candidate gene TRPC1. These genes, TRPC6 (IHPS3), TRPC5 (IHPS4), and TRPC1, are expressed in smooth muscle and have been implicated in smooth muscle hypertrophy. TRPC1 and TRPC6 are also believed to be mechanosensitive, responding to stimuli from food present in the stomach [61]. In this way, they may interact with environmental factors such as prone position for sleep.

IHPS has been described in a variety of syndromes including Cornelia de Lange, Apert, Opitz FG, Marden-Walker, Smith-Lemli-Opitz, Zellweger, trisomy 21, trisomy 18, duplication 1q, duplication 9q, deletion 11q, ring 12 [62], Denys-Drash [63], and paramyotonia congenita [64].

ENVIRONMENTAL FACTORS

A variety of environmental and mechanical factors have been implicated in the occurrence of IHPS. A study of isolated IHPS in Sicily by Bianca and colleagues [65] established the association of IHPS with primiparity and low parity status. There was a suggestion that the increased ratio of affected boys to affected girls may be associated with greater parity. There was no association with birth weight or maternal age. Increased incidence of IHPS has been reported in infants exposed prenatally to thalidomide, hydantoins, and trimethadione [62] and those exposed postnatally to erythromycin [66–69]. Possible postnatal environmental factors include feeding practices, maternal smoking, and infant sleeping position [56].

Prone sleeping may be an environmental risk factor for IHPS, which could account for lower occurrence of IHPS in Asian people, who routinely place infants in a supine position for sleep [57]. It has been speculated that pooling of a feed in the antrum, with prone sleep position, may lead to dysmotility of the stomach or pylorus caused by the effects on function of the stomach and/or pylorus via proteins sensitive to change in volume, pressure, or solute concentration.

The gene for motilin (*MLN*), a hormone that induces gastric contractions, was investigated as a candidate gene for IHPS because treatment with erythromycin, a motilin agonist, is associated with increased risk for IHPS. No association was found between *MLN* sequence variants and IHPS, although this does not exclude a role for motilin in the pathogenesis of this disorder [70]. Larger milk curds produced by artificial milk formulas may be more likely to cause obstruction in association with pylorospasm. A 30-year retrospective study in Nigeria suggests that exclusive breastfeeding was associated with reduced risk for IHPS [71]; however, this observation requires confirmation with a larger study that includes a control group.

Rogers [72] proposed that inheritance of high parietal cell mass results in hyperacidity, which causes repeated pyloric contraction, leading to pyloric hypertrophy and stenosis. Neonates normally have higher levels of gastrin, with higher acidity level, which can explain the development of IHPS within the first few weeks of life. Godwin and colleagues [73] found increased incidence of pyloric stenosis in Canada after grain products were fortified with folic acid for prevention of neural tube defects. However, no causal relationship was established and there was evidence that the rate of IHPS was increasing independently of folic acid supplementation.

SUMMARY

This review summarizes the current knowledge concerning the pathogenesis, cause, genetics, epidemiology, and treatment of idiopathic hypertrophic pyloric stenosis of infancy. Pyloromyotomy remains the treatment of choice in Western countries, with the laparoscopic approach favored because of shorter recovery time and lower rate of wound complications. Treatment with IV or oral atropine has been successful predominantly in Asian countries, although this may require a week or more and surgery is ultimately necessary in approximately 10%–25% of cases.

Variability in reported prevalence of IHPS may reflect variations in surveillance and ascertainment. The true prevalence of the condition does not seem to be changing. IHPS is more prevalent in children of white, non-Hispanic mothers, and considerably less prevalent among offspring of non-Hispanic black and Asian mothers. Prevalence is highest in first-born infants and is 4 to 5 times more common in boys than in girls. IHPS may be less prevalent in infants born at less than 28 weeks and more than 40 weeks of gestation.

Our review of the available literature suggests that IHPS is a complex disorder resulting from the interaction of genetic and environmental factors. Five genetic loci linked to IHPS have been identified, and 2 of these are associated with autosomal dominant inheritance of the trait. The gene for nitric acid synthetase and others implicated in smooth muscle hypertrophy are among the few candidate genes under investigation. Gastric hyperacidity seems to be a contributing factor. Putative environmental risk factors include prone sleeping, treatment with erythromycin, and use of artificial milk formula; however, confirmatory evidence remains elusive. We anticipate that research into the genetic, molecular, and environmental basis for IHPS will provide insights into prevention and treatment of this complex disorder.

References

[1] Hirschsprung H. Falle von angeborener Pylorusstenose, beobachtet bei Sauglingen. Jahrb Kinderheilk 1888;27:61 [in German].
[2] Aspelund G, Langer JC. Current management of hypertrophic pyloric stenosis. Semin Pediatr Surg 2007;16(1):27–33.
[3] Magnuson DK, Schwartz MZ. Stomach and duodenum. In: Oldham KT, Colombani PM, Foglia RP, et al, editors. Principles and practice of pediatric surgery. Philadelphia: Lippincott Williams & Wilkins; 2005. p. 1149–79.
[4] Panteli C. New insights into the pathogenesis of infantile pyloric stenosis. Pediatr Surg Int 2009;25(12):1043–52.
[5] Okazaki T, Yamataka A, Fujiwara T, et al. Abnormal distribution of nerve terminals in infantile hypertrophic pyloric stenosis. J Pediatr Surg 1994;29(5):655–8.
[6] Kobayashi H, O'Briain DS, Puri P. Selective reduction in intramuscular nerve supporting cells in infantile hypertrophic pyloric stenosis. J Pediatr Surg 1994;29(5):651–4.
[7] Malmfors G, Sundler F. Peptidergic innervation in infantile hypertrophic pyloric stenosis. J Pediatr Surg 1986;21(4):303–6.
[8] Kusafuka T, Puri P. Altered messenger RNA expression of the neuronal nitric oxide synthase gene in infantile hypertrophic pyloric stenosis. Pediatr Surg Int 1997;12(8):576–9.
[9] Langer JC, Berezin I, Daniel EE. Hypertrophic pyloric stenosis: ultrastructural abnormalities of enteric nerves and the interstitial cells of Cajal. J Pediatr Surg 1995;30(11):1535–43.
[10] Ohshiro K, Puri P. Increased insulin-like growth factor-I mRNA expression in pyloric muscle in infantile hypertrophic pyloric stenosis. Pediatr Surg Int 1998;13(4):253–5.
[11] Oue T, Puri P. Smooth muscle cell hypertrophy versus hyperplasia in infantile hypertrophic pyloric stenosis. Pediatr Res 1999;45(6):853–7.
[12] White MC, Langer JC, Don S, et al. Sensitivity and cost minimization analysis of radiology versus olive palpation for the diagnosis of hypertrophic pyloric stenosis. J Pediatr Surg 1998;33(6):913–7.
[13] Huddy SP. Investigation and diagnosis of hypertrophic pyloric stenosis. J R Coll Surg Edinb 1991;36(2):91–3.
[14] Mullassery D, Mallappa S, Shariff R, et al. Negative exploration of pyloric stenosis - is it preventable? BMC Pediatr 2008;8:37.
[15] Hulka F, Campbell TJ, Campbell JR, et al. Evolution in the recognition of infantile hypertrophic pyloric stenosis. Pediatrics 1997;100(2):E9.
[16] Copeland DR, Cosper GH, McMahon LE, et al. Return of the surgeon in the diagnosis of pyloric stenosis. J Pediatr Surg 2009;44(6):1189–92 [discussion: 1192].
[17] Shaoul R, Toubi A. The evolution of infantile pyloric stenosis. Isr Med Assoc J 2006;8(1):71–2.
[18] Starinsky R, Klin B, Siman-Tov Y, et al. Does dehydration affect thickness of the pyloric muscle? An experimental study. Ultrasound Med Biol 2002;28(4):421–3.
[19] Leaphart CL, Borland K, Kane TD, et al. Hypertrophic pyloric stenosis in newborns younger than 21 days: remodeling the path of surgical intervention. J Pediatr Surg 2008;43(6): 998–1001.
[20] Misra D, Akhter A, Potts SR, et al. Pyloric stenosis: is over-reliance on ultrasound scans leading to negative explorations? Eur J Pediatr Surg 1997;7(6):328–30.
[21] Hall NJ, Eaton S, Pierro A. The evidence base for neonatal surgery. Early Hum Dev 2009;85(11):713–8.
[22] Ostlie DJ, St Peter SD. The current state of evidence-based pediatric surgery. J Pediatr Surg 2010;45(10):1940–6.
[23] Dufur H, Fredet P. Le sténose hypertrophique du pylore chez le nourrisson et son traitement chir surgical. Rev Chir 1908;37:208 [in French].
[24] Alain JL, Grousseau D, Longis B, et al. Extramucosal pyloromyotomy by laparoscopy. Eur J Pediatr Surg 1996;6(1):10–2.
[25] Sola JE, Neville HL. Laparoscopic vs open pyloromyotomy: a systematic review and meta-analysis. J Pediatr Surg 2009;44(8):1631–7.

[26] Brown JH. Atropine, scopolamine and related antimuscarinic drugs. In: Gilman AG, Rall TW, Nies AS, et al, editors. Goodman and Gilman's pharmacological basis of therapeutics. Tokyo: Pergamon Press; 1990. p. 150–65.
[27] Nagita A, Yamaguchi J, Amemoto K, et al. Management and ultrasonographic appearance of infantile hypertrophic pyloric stenosis with intravenous atropine sulfate. J Pediatr Gastroenterol Nutr 1996;23(2):172–7.
[28] Yamataka A, Tsukada K, Yokoyama-Laws Y, et al. Pyloromyotomy versus atropine sulfate for infantile hypertrophic pyloric stenosis. J Pediatr Surg 2000;35(2):338–41 [discussion: 342].
[29] Kawahara H, Imura K, Nishikawa M, et al. Intravenous atropine treatment in infantile hypertrophic pyloric stenosis. Arch Dis Child 2002;87(1):71–4.
[30] Kawahara H, Takama Y, Yoshida H, et al. Medical treatment of infantile hypertrophic pyloric stenosis: should we always slice the "olive"? J Pediatr Surg 2005;40(12):1848–51.
[31] Huang YC, Su BH. Medical treatment with atropine sulfate for hypertrophic pyloric stenosis. Acta Paediatr Taiwan 2004;45(3):136–40.
[32] Singh UK, Kumar R, Prasad R. Oral atropine sulfate for infantile hypertrophic pyloric stenosis. Indian Pediatr 2005;42(5):473–6.
[33] Meissner PE, Engelmann G, Troeger J, et al. Conservative treatment of infantile hypertrophic pyloric stenosis with intravenous atropine sulfate does not replace pyloromyotomy. Pediatr Surg Int 2006;22(12):1021–4.
[34] MacMahon B. The continuing enigma of pyloric stenosis of infancy: a review. Epidemiology 2006;17(2):195–201.
[35] National Birth Defects Prevention Network. Selected birth defects data from population-based birth defects surveillance programs in the United States, 2003–2007. Birth Defects Res A Clin Mol Teratol 2010;88(12):1062–174.
[36] Parker SE, Mai CT, Canfield MA, et al. Updated National Birth Prevalence estimates for selected birth defects in the United States, 2004–2006. Birth Defects Res A Clin Mol Teratol 2010;88(12):1008–16.
[37] Wang J, Waller DK, Hwang LY, et al. Prevalence of infantile hypertrophic pyloric stenosis in Texas, 1999–2002. Birth Defects Res A Clin Mol Teratol 2008;82(11):763–7.
[38] Salemi JL, Pierre M, Tanner JP, et al. Maternal nativity as a risk factor for gastroschisis: a population-based study. Birth Defects Res A Clin Mol Teratol 2009;85(11):890–6.
[39] Applegate MS, Druschel CM. The epidemiology of infantile hypertrophic pyloric stenosis in New York State, 1983 to 1990. Arch Pediatr Adolesc Med 1995;149(10):1123–9.
[40] Sorensen HT, Norgard B, Pedersen L, et al. Maternal smoking and risk of hypertrophic infantile pyloric stenosis: 10 year population based cohort study. BMJ 2002;325(7371):1011–2.
[41] Sherwood W, Choudhry M, Lakhoo K. Infantile hypertrophic pyloric stenosis: an infectious cause? Pediatr Surg Int 2007;23(1):61–3.
[42] Dahshan A, Donovan KG, Halabi IM, et al. Helicobacter pylori and infantile hypertrophic pyloric stenosis: is there a possible relationship? J Pediatr Gastroenterol Nutr 2006;42(3):262–4.
[43] Sommerfield T, Chalmers J, Youngson G, et al. The changing epidemiology of infantile hypertrophic pyloric stenosis in Scotland. Arch Dis Child 2008;93(12):1007–11.
[44] Persson S, Ekbom A, Granath F, et al. Parallel incidences of sudden infant death syndrome and infantile hypertrophic pyloric stenosis: a common cause? Pediatrics 2001;108(4):E70.
[45] Browne ML. Maternal exposure to caffeine and risk of congenital anomalies: a systematic review. Epidemiology 2006;17(3):324–31.
[46] Goh YI, Bollano E, Einarson TR, et al. Prenatal multivitamin supplementation and rates of congenital anomalies: a meta-analysis. J Obstet Gynaecol Can 2006;28(8):680–9.
[47] Stothard KJ, Tennant PW, Bell R, et al. Maternal overweight and obesity and the risk of congenital anomalies: a systematic review and meta-analysis. JAMA 2009;301(6):636–50.
[48] Carter CO, Powell BW. Two-generation pyloric stenosis. Lancet 1954;263(6815):746–8.
[49] Carter CO. The inheritance of congenital pyloric stenosis. Br Med Bull 1961;17:251–4.

[50] Carter CO, Evans KA. Inheritance of congenital pyloric stenosis. J Med Genet 1969;6:233–54.
[51] Lalouel JM, Morton NE, MacLean CJ, et al. Recurrence risks in complex inheritance with special regard to pyloric stenosis. J Med Genet 1977;14:408–14.
[52] Finsen VR. Infantile hypertrophic pyloric stenosis–unusual familial incidence. Arch Dis Child 1979;54(9):720–1.
[53] Fried K, Aviv S, Nisenbaum C. Probable autosomal dominant infantile pyloric stenosis in a large kindred. Clin Genet 1981;20(5):328–30.
[54] Capon F, Reece A, Ravindrarajah R, et al. Linkage of monogenic infantile hypertrophic pyloric stenosis to chromosome 16p12-p13 and evidence for genetic heterogeneity. Am J Hum Genet 2006;79(2):378–82.
[55] Mitchell LE, Risch N. The genetics of infantile hypertrophic pyloric stenosis. A reanalysis. Am J Dis Child 1993;147(11):1203–11.
[56] Krogh C, Fischer TK, Skotte L, et al. Familial aggregation and heritability of pyloric stenosis. JAMA 2010;303(23):2393–9.
[57] Chung E. Infantile hypertrophic pyloric stenosis: genes and environment. Arch Dis Child 2008;93(12):1003–4.
[58] Vanderwinden JM, Mailleux P, Schiffmann SN, et al. Nitric oxide synthase activity in infantile hypertrophic pyloric stenosis. N Engl J Med 1992;327(8):511–5.
[59] Huang PL, Dawson TM, Bredt DS, et al. Targeted disruption of the neuronal nitric oxide synthase gene. Cell 1993;75(7):1273–86.
[60] Everett KV, Chioza BA, Georgoula C, et al. Genome-wide high-density SNP-based linkage analysis of infantile hypertrophic pyloric stenosis identifies loci on chromosomes 11q14-q22 and Xq23. Am J Hum Genet 2008;82(3):756–62.
[61] Everett KV, Chioza BA, Georgoula C, et al. Infantile hypertrophic pyloric stenosis: evaluation of three positional candidate genes, TRPC1, TRPC5 and TRPC6, by association analysis and re-sequencing. Hum Genet 2009;126(6):819–31.
[62] Stevenson RE, Hall JG, editors. Human malformations and related anomalies. 2nd edition. New York: Oxford University Press; 2006.
[63] Hu M, Craig J, Howard N, et al. A novel mutation of WT1 exon 9 in a patient with Denys-Drash syndrome and pyloric stenosis. Pediatr Nephrol 2004;19(10):1160–3.
[64] Ay B, Gercek A, Dogan VI, et al. Pylorotomy in a patient with paramyotonia congenita. Anesth Analg 2004;98(1):68–9.
[65] Bianca S, Barbagallo MA, Ingegnosi C, et al. Isolated hypertrophic pyloric stenosis and perinatal factors. Genet Couns 2003;14(1):101–3.
[66] Cooper WO, Griffin MR, Arbogast P, et al. Very early exposure to erythromycin and infantile hypertrophic pyloric stenosis. Arch Pediatr Adolesc Med 2002;156(7):647–50.
[67] SanFilippo A. Infantile hypertrophic pyloric stenosis related to ingestion of erythromycine estolate: a report of five cases. J Pediatr Surg 1976;11(2):177–80.
[68] Honein MA, Paulozzi LJ, Himelright IM, et al. Infantile hypertrophic pyloric stenosis after pertussis prophylaxis with erythromycin: a case review and cohort study. Lancet 1999;354(9196):2101–5.
[69] Mahon BE, Rosenman MB, Kleiman MB. Maternal and infant use of erythromycin and other macrolide antibiotics as risk factors for infantile hypertrophic pyloric stenosis. J Pediatr 2001;139(3):380–4.
[70] Svenningsson A, Lagerstedt K, Omrani MD, et al. Absence of motilin gene mutations in infantile hypertrophic pyloric stenosis. J Pediatr Surg 2008;43(3):443–6.
[71] Osifo DO, Evbuomwan I. Does exclusive breastfeeding confer protection against infantile hypertrophic pyloric stenosis? A 30-year experience in Benin City, Nigeria. J Trop Pediatr 2009;55(2):132–4.
[72] Rogers IM. The true cause of pyloric stenosis is hyperacidity. Acta Paediatr 2006;95(2):132–6.
[73] Godwin KA, Sibbald B, Bedard T, et al. Changes in frequencies of select congenital anomalies since the onset of folic acid fortification in a Canadian birth defect registry. Can J Public Health 2008;99(4):271–5.

Advances in Pediatrics 58 (2011) 207–241

ADVANCES IN PEDIATRICS

rhGH Safety and Efficacy Update

Bradley S. Miller, MD, PhD

Division of Endocrinology, Department of Pediatrics, University of Minnesota Amplatz Children's Hospital, MMC 8952D, East Building Room MB671, 2450 Riverside Avenue, Minneapolis, MN 55455, USA

Growth hormone (GH) has been used to treat patients with GH deficiency (GHD) since 1960 when it was originally extracted from cadaveric pituitary glands [1]. In 1985, several cases of Creutzfeldt-Jakob disease were identified and attributed to pituitary-derived GH. Later that year, recombinant human GH (rhGH) was approved by the US Food and Drug Administration (FDA). The availability of an unlimited supply of rhGH improved access to therapy for children with GHD and the frequency of dosing increased from 3 times each week to 6 or 7 days each week [2]. The increased supply of rhGH allowed investigation into treatment of multiple conditions associated with short stature not associated with GHD leading to FDA approval for treatment of children with growth failure associated with chronic renal insufficiency (1993), Turner syndrome (TS; 1996), Prader-Willi Syndrome (PWS; 2000), small for gestational age (SGA) without adequate catch-up growth (2001), idiopathic short stature (ISS; 2003), short stature homeobox (SHOX) deficiency (2006), and Noonan syndrome (NS, 2007). In addition, rhGH therapy was FDA approved for acquired immune deficiency syndrome (AIDS) wasting (1996), adult GHD (1996), and short bowel syndrome (2003) (Table 1). Guidelines for the use of GH therapy have been reported previously by the American Association of Clinical Endocrinologists (AACE), Growth Hormone Research Society (GRS), and The Lawson Wilkins Pediatric Endocrinology Society (LWPES) [2–4].

GH registries have been an invaluable resource for determining the safety and efficacy of GH. These registries were originally mandated by the FDA in 1985 because rhGH was the first product approved in the United States derived from recombinant DNA technology. The FDA required Genentech to conduct a 5-year phase IV postmarketing safety study. However, the National Cooperative Growth Study (NCGS) was extended as a phase IV postmarketing safety and efficacy study until 2010 [5]. Other GH registries include GHMonitor^{SM} (Serono) and the ongoing international registries American Norditropin Studies: Web Enabled Research (ANSWER; Novo Nordisk), Genetics and

E-mail address: mille685@umn.edu

0065-3101/11/$ – see front matter
doi:10.1016/j.yapd.2011.05.001

Table 1
FDA-approved indications for GH therapy by manufacturer

Indication	Genentech	Lilly	Novo nordisk	Pfizer	Sandoz	Serono	Teva
Pediatric GHD	**Protropin 10/85-12/02** Nutropin 3/94 Nutropin AQ 1/96 Nutropin Depot 12/99-6/04	Humatrope 3/87	Norditropin 3/97	Genotropin 8/95	Omnitrope 5/06	Saizen 10/96	Tev-Tropin 5/95
Chronic renal insufficiency	**Nutropin 11/93** Nutropin AQ 1/96						
Adult GHD	Nutropin 12/97 Nutropin AQ 12/97	**Humatrope 8/96**	Norditropin 3/97	Genotropin 10/97	Omnitrope 5/06	Saizen 11/04	
Turner syndrome	**Nutropin 12/96** Nutropin AQ 4/97	Humatrope 3/97	Norditropin 9/07	Genotropin 4/06			
Prader-Willi syndrome				**Genotropin 6/00**	Omnitrope 4/10		
SGA		Humatrope 3/09	Norditropin 10/08	**Genotropin 7/01**	Omnitrope 4/10		
ISS	Nutropin AQ 6/05	**Humatrope 7/03**		Genotropin 6/08	Omnitrope 8/10		
SHOX deficiency		**Humatrope 11/06**					
NS			**Norditropin 6/07**				
AIDS wasting						**Serostim 8/96**	
Short bowel syndrome						**Zorbtive 12/03**	

Bold indicates that the product was the first to be approved for a given indication.
Bio-Tropin (Ferring, 5/95), Valtropin (LG Life, 4/07), and Accretropin (Cangene Corporation, 1/08) are rhGH products that have also been approved by the FDA, but are not yet commercially available in the United States.

Neuroendocrinology of Short Stature International Study (GeNeSIS, Eli Lilly), and Pfizer International Growth Study (formerly Kabi International Growth Study [KIGS]) as well as national and pharmaceutical registries in many individual countries. Some countries continue to mandate safety and efficacy registries for children receiving GH therapy. The cumulative safety and efficacy data from these multiple studies involves more than 120,000 children treated for nearly half a million patient years. Numerous publications from these studies have educated the pediatric and adult endocrinology community about the safety and efficacy of GH therapy in children and adults.

GH registries have been, and continue to be, primarily conducted through entry of data relating to patient care without requiring adherence to specific practice guidelines. Thus, the data collected reflect the variation in clinical practice among the investigators who participate in the trial. Attempts have been made to use the registries to provide evidence to guide clinical practice [6] and to compare practice patterns with reported knowledge, attitudes, and beliefs [7]. However, one major weakness of these registries is the vast amount of data that are not entered by the participating sites. Although the study sites are compensated for the time required for data entry, because of the volume of data and work involved the number of fields required for payment were limited to high-priority items. Therefore, items not required for payment are less likely to be recorded. However, the sheer volume of these registries overcomes these limitations to some degree.

This article focuses on efficacy data for FDA-approved indications for promoting linear growth in children and available safety data related to rhGH treatment of all conditions in children. Effects that can occur after rhGH therapy is completed, or in individuals who continue rhGH therapy into adulthood, are also addressed.

EFFICACY

Since rhGH became available, numerous clinical trials have been performed to show its efficacy in improving linear growth, quality of life, body composition, and bone mineral density [8–11]. Prospective, phase III clinical trials showing efficacy and safety have formed the basis of FDA approval for the numerous indications described earlier. Although small clinical trials have also shown efficacy in numerous other conditions associated with growth failure, including inflammatory bowel disease, chronic steroid use, cystic fibrosis, skeletal dysplasias, hypophosphatemic rickets, and juvenile rheumatoid arthritis, rhGH has not been FDA approved for these conditions. Phase IV postmarketing surveillance and efficacy studies (ie, registries) have also provided significant efficacy and safety information regarding FDA-approved indications and numerous other conditions treated with rhGH.

Pediatric GHD

rhGH was first approved for the treatment of childhood-onset GHD on October 18, 1985. The efficacy of GHD depends on several variables including cause, rhGH dose, and dosing schedule. Children with organic causes of GHD, including congenital panhypopituitarism, multiple pituitary hormone deficiency, and suprasellar tumors, tend to be more sensitive to rhGH and grow well in response to lower doses. However, the growth response in children with idiopathic GHD (IGHD) is more variable and may be predicted by the results of the GH stimulation tests [9]. GHD is diagnosed in children using auxologic features (short stature and/or poor growth velocity), radiologic investigations (bone age, magnetic resonance imaging of brain with focus on pituitary), and biochemical testing (insulin-like growth factor [IGF]-1, IGFBP-3, and GH stimulation testing). Peak GH responses of less than 10 ng/mL to two separate secretory stimuli have been considered the cutoff for abnormally low GH secretion and support a diagnosis of GHD. Because of the variability and lack of reproducibility of GH stimulation tests (GHSTs), a trial of GH therapy has been suggested as part of the diagnostic evaluation of a child who otherwise fits the criteria for GHD but has normal response to GHST. The recommended rhGH dose for children with GHD in the United States is 0.175 to 0.35 mg/kg/wk with 0.3 mg/kg/wk being used most commonly [2–4,6]. Because of the GH sensitivity of children with GHD, at some point in the dose curve, increasing the dosage does not translate into improvement in growth response (Fig. 1) [12]. Adjustment of rhGH dosing (0.4–0.7 mg/kg/wk) during puberty in an attempt to match the normal increase in GH secretion during puberty has also been shown to improve growth velocity during puberty [13]. A stepwise increase in rhGH dose with pubertal stages has been shown to improve near-adult height by 3.6 cm (or +0.49 mean height standard deviation score [SDS]) compared with age-matched historical controls [14].

The use of serum IGF-1 values to adjust rhGH dosing has been debated since the reliable assays for IGF-1 (formerly Somatomedin C) became available [15]. The impact of this treatment paradigm was shown in a clinical trial in which weight-based dosing of rhGH was compared with dosing of rhGH to

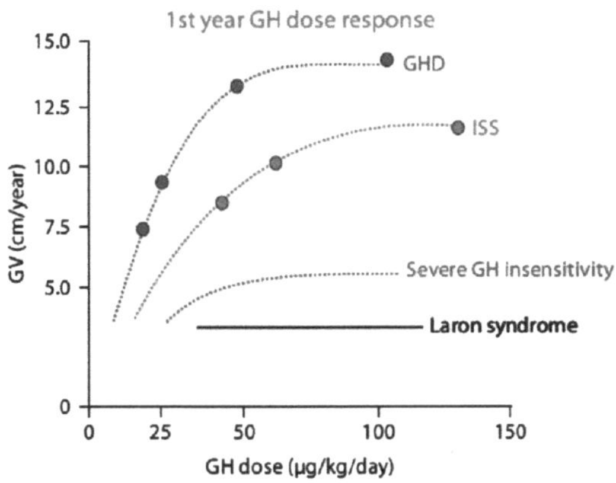

Fig. 1. First-year response to rhGH therapy. (*From* Keni J, Cohen P, Keni J, et al. Optimizing growth hormone dosing in children with idiopathic short stature. Horm Res 2009;71 Suppl 1: 71; with permission.)

target an IGF-1 value at the mean (0 SDS) or top of the normal range for age (+2 SDS) [16]. Children in the weight-based dosing arm of the study grew similarly to those titrated to an IGF-1 at 0 SDS. However, children whose rhGH doses were titrated to IGF-1 levels at +2 SDS grew significantly better than either other group. An important finding in this study was that the spectrum of rhGH doses that children required to achieve a particular target was highly variable. The weight-based arm was treated with 0.28 mg/kg/wk, whereas the 0 SDS target arm received an average of 0.23 mg/kg/wk and the GHD subjects in the +2 SDS target arm received an average of 0.46 mg/kg/wk. Children with GHD also showed better growth response to treatment in all 3 arms. In a 2006 survey of pediatric endocrinologists, 72% reported that they routinely monitor IGF-1 values in children receiving rhGH [7]. Demonstration of the use of IGF-based dosing in clinical practice was done by reviewing NCGS that which showed that 41% of children with GHD had IGF-1 values entered into the registry between 2000 and 2005 [7]. However, the long-term efficacy of IGF-based dosing has not been tested. In addition, the safety of the higher doses of rhGH required in some children to achieve a serum IGF-1 target of +2 SDS is unclear [17].

Short-term growth responses to rhGH in GHD have been reported in multiple articles [8–11]. The growth velocity (GV) seen in the first 12 months is characteristically the highest GV seen during therapy, with subsequent years remaining at more than the pretreatment values. In mathematical growth prediction models, growth in children with the first-year growth response has been shown to be inversely correlated with age and height deficit, but positively correlated with body weight, birth weight, and GH dose [18]. A recent analysis of data from the NCGS provides expected growth responses to rhGH in prepubertal children for the first year of therapy (Fig. 2A–D). This analysis also shows that responsiveness to rhGH decreases with age [6].

Efficacy may also be termed lack of failure. However, growth parameters for failure to respond to rhGH therapy have not been well established. Criteria that have been used include a doubling of the pretreatment growth velocity, 2 cm/y faster than pretreatment GV, and 50% faster than pretreatment GV. It has been proposed that the children whose GV is greater than −1 SDS on the Bakker charts are showing an adequate response to therapy. The relationship of the early growth response to rhGH therapy has been shown to correlate with final adult height [19].

Determination of long-term growth response to rhGH using near-adult height has been done for 2 large GH registries [19,20]. In the NCGS, height improved in children with IGHD from −2.7 (± 0.7) SDS to −1.4 (± 1.0) SDS [20]. Enrollment height and GHST response were significant predictors for Δ height SDS in this cohort. In KIGS, median height SDS at the start of treatment were −2.4 (IGHD) and −2.9 (MPHD) for white boys and −2.6 (IGHD) and −3.4 (MPHD) for girls, respectively. With rhGH treatment, height improved to −0.8 (IGHD) and −0.7 (MPHD) for white boys and −1.0 (IGHD) and −1.1 (MPHD) for girls, respectively [19] The first-year increase in height SDS and prepubertal height gain was highly correlated with total height gain.

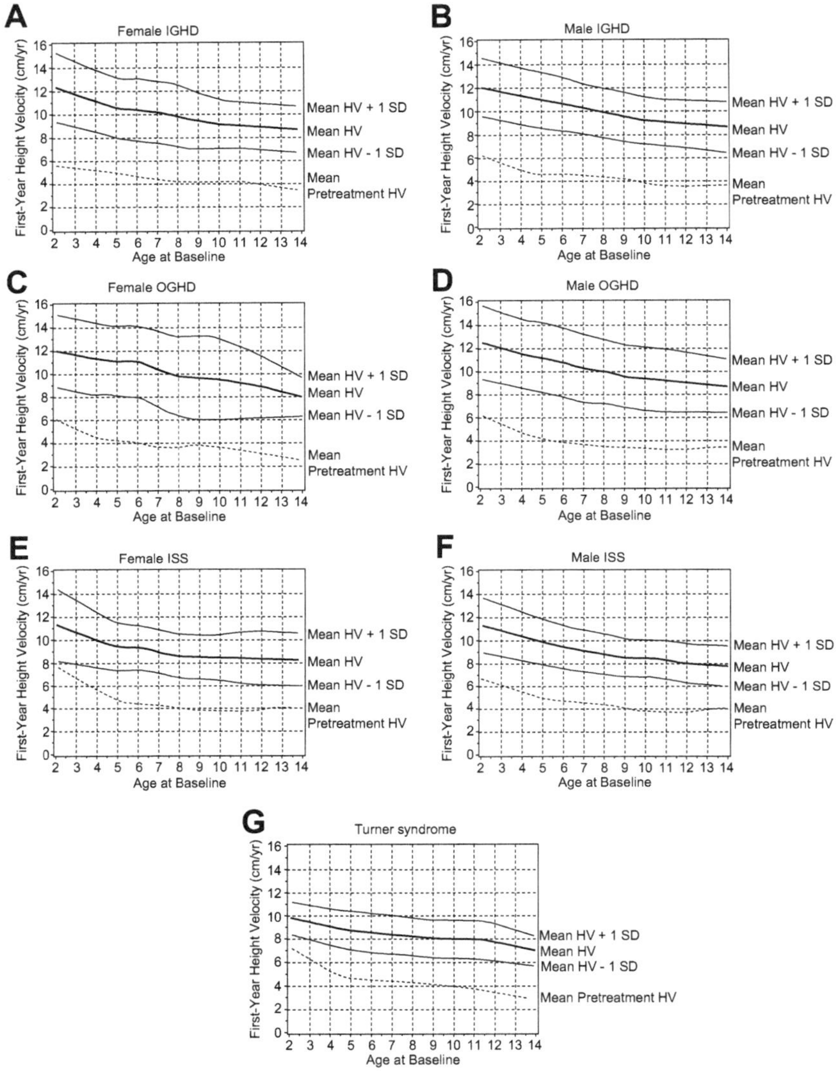

Fig. 2. First-year growth responses to daily rhGH. First-year growth responses to daily GH expressed as height velocity (HV) at age of treatment onset (x-axis) in naive, prepubertal girls and boys with IGHD (*A, B*), organic GHD (OGHD) (*C, D*), and ISS (*E, F*), and girls with TS (*G*). Data given for mean and mean ± 1 SD. (*From* Bakker B, Frane J, Anhalt H, et al. Height velocity targets from the National Cooperative Growth Study for first-year growth hormone responses in short children. J Clin Endocrinol Metab 2008;93(2):355; with permission.)

Chronic renal insufficiency before transplantation

Children with chronic renal insufficiency (CRI) frequently have growth failure that, if untreated, leads to adult short stature. Growth failure in CRI is multifactorial, with GH resistance playing a major role [21]. Before consideration of rhGH therapy, management of modifiable factors that may impair growth in CRI (eg, malnutrition, acidosis, metabolic bone disease, and/or the iatrogenic impact of therapies for CRI) needs to be optimized. rhGH therapy for children with growth failure (height <−1.88 SDS) in the setting of CRI before renal transplant was approved in 1993. GH treatment is recommended at a dosage of 0.35 mg/kg/wk, divided into 6 or 7 doses [2,22]. Treatment with rhGH is effective and has been shown to improve final adult height [22–24]. A recent analysis of data from the NCGS provides expected growth responses to rhGH in prepubertal children with CRI for the first year of therapy (Fig. 3) [25]. To maximize response to rhGH therapy in CRI, it is important that continued attention is paid to the management of modifiable factors that may impair growth. Long-term rhGH treatment of children with CRI showed improvement of height from −2.6 to −0.7 SDS after 5 years [26]. Final adult height was analyzed in a study of 38 children with CRI, showing that rhGH therapy led to improvement from a height of −3.1 ± 1.2 to −1.6 ± 1.2 SDS [23]. A group of 50 age-matched controls with CRI without growth failure at baseline did not receive rhGH therapy and had worsening of their height in the same time period, with a loss of 0.5 SDS [23]. Analysis of adult height in 49 patients with baseline height SDS between −2 and −3 revealed that 65% had an adult height of more than −2 SDS [27].

RhGH therapy following renal transplantation has been controversial and is not FDA approved despite multiple studies showing efficacy [28]. Despite a lack of FDA approval, analysis of the North American Pediatric Renal Transplant

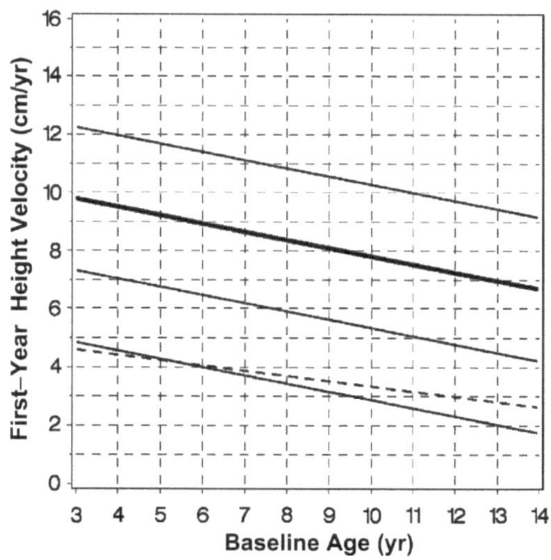

Fig. 3. First-year growth responses to daily rhGH in CRI. First-year growth response (fitted curves) expressed in HV for prepubertal children with chronic kidney disease during rhGH treatment compared with pretreatment HV for the same children. (*From* Mahan JD, Warady BA, Frane J, et al. First-year response to rhGH therapy in children with CKD: a National Cooperative Growth Study report. Pediatr Nephrol 2010;25(6):1128; with permission.)

Cooperative Study (NAPRTCS) database has shown that the number of children receiving rhGH more than 5 years after transplantation is 9% of all patients and 14% of those whose height was less than −1.88 SDS 6 months after transplant [28]. In this population, there was a modest improvement in height of approximately +0.5 SDS following 5 years of rhGH use [28]. Analysis of NAPRTCS data shows that the final adult height in renal transplant recipients who received rhGH therapy (n = 71) compared with renal transplant recipients who did not receive rhGH therapy (n = 669) showed a height gain of +0.77 SDS (−1.83 ± 0.14 rhGH vs −2.60 ± 0.05, $P<.001$) [29].

Turner syndrome

Short stature is the most common clinical characteristic of TS. A significant proportion of the height deficit in girls with TS is caused by the presence of only a single copy of the SHOX gene (haploinsufficiency). The SHOX gene is a homeobox gene that regulates the growth of long bones. The SHOX gene is located in the pseudoautosomal region of both sex chromosomes and its actions are gene dose related [30]. Growth in children with TS is characterized by a slight intrauterine growth retardation (−1 SD), slow growth during infancy and childhood, and lack of pubertal growth spurt. More than half of girls with TS are at less than the fifth percentile by 2 years of age [31]. The average height of an adult woman with TS who has not received rhGH therapy is 143 cm, approximately 20 cm (8 inches) less than the average adult woman [32].

rhGH therapy was FDA approved in 1996 for treatment of short stature in TS, has been shown to significantly improve adult height in girls with TS, and may allow achievement of height in the normal adult female range [33–36]. Earlier diagnosis and initiation of GH treatment in children with TS should help patients to attain heights near the normal range at a younger age. Early initiation of rhGH therapy enables the children to start estrogen supplementation in a more age-appropriate manner [37]. According to the 2006 Turner Syndrome Consensus Study Group, puberty should not be delayed to promote statural growth because this approach undervalues the psychosocial importance of age-appropriate pubertal maturation [38]. Treatment with rhGH should commence when the child has experienced growth deceleration or is less than or equal to −2SD less than the target adult height based on midparental height. Earlier rhGH treatment of young patients with TS can abrogate the height loss compared with their peers [39]. If the rhGH is initiated later than 10 years, or in cases of extreme short stature, adjunct therapy with nonaromatizable androgens should be considered [40]. Therapy should be continued until final adult height is reached or the height achieved is acceptable [41]. Final height gains may be as high as 8 to 10 cm with or without delaying estrogen-replacement therapy [42–45]. A typical rhGH dose for treatment in children with TS is 0.35 mg/kg/wk [2,6] and is FDA approved up to 0.469 mg/kg/wk. Higher doses of rhGH may be associated with increased height gain [46], although the potential for adverse late effects has not been evaluated adequately. rhGH dose seems to be the most important predictor of height velocity in the first year of rhGH therapy, whereas, for height gain in years 2 to 4 of therapy, the velocity during the previous year is the most important predictor [46]. A recent analysis of data from the NCGS provides expected growth responses to rhGH in prepubertal children with TS for the first year of therapy (see Fig. 2G) [6].

The usefulness of monitoring IGF-1 levels during rhGH therapy in TS has not been well studied. In one study of 24 prepubertal children with TS, IGF-1 values were low at baseline, improved at 3 and 6 months after starting rhGH therapy, but returned to baseline at 12 months [47]. Although the IGF-1 response does not seem to have a clear relationship with rhGH dose [47] in girls with TS, rhGH-induced IGF-1 levels have been shown to correlate with the growth response [48]. In the largest randomized study of rhGH therapy for TS treated to near-final height, in which 232 children with TS received either 0.27 or 0.36 mg/kg/wk, baseline IGF-I concentrations were low normal and remained within 2 SDS of the mean during GH therapy in all but 2 subjects [34].

Short stature from prader-willi syndrome

RhGH treatment was FDA approved in 2000 for the treatment of growth failure in children with PWS. The FDA-approved dose is 0.24 mg/kg/wk with recommended rhGH dosing between 0.24 and 0.35 mg/kg/wk [4]. rhGH treatment in PWS has been proved to improve linear growth and increase muscle mass/body fat ratios [49–51]. Improved muscle tone and strength have also been clinically observed in children with PWS treated with rhGH [49–51]. GH therapy has also been shown to provide neurodevelopmental benefits in young children with PWS [51]. This finding suggests additional benefits of rhGH treatment of younger PWS children with growth failure and hypotonia. Near-adult height in PWS is also shown to be improved with rhGH therapy. In a study of 22 children with genetically-confirmed PWS treated with rhGH (0.30 mg/kg/wk) from age 6.9 to 18.1 years, the near-adult height for all children was within midparental height median −0.5 SDS (−1.4 to 0.7) and 0.9 SDS (0.1–1.9) for girls and boys, respectively [52]. Analysis of growth data in the Pfizer International Growth Study (KIGS) shows that two-thirds of children with PWS achieved a height within the normal range [52,53].

The impact of rhGH treatment on obesity in children with PWS is controversial, and stringent weight management techniques are necessary for all children with PWS regardless of rhGH treatment status. However, multiple studies with rhGH have shown overall improvement in body composition. KIGS data indicate that there is a decrease in body mass index (BMI) in the first year of GH therapy. BMI then tends to stabilize as a result of an increase in muscle mass and a decrease in fat mass associated with rhGH therapy [53]. Furthermore, at final adult height, body composition has been shown to be improved, but not normalized [52].

Small for gestational age

SGA (<−2 SD for birth weight and/or birth length) is defined at different gestational ages based on data from Usher and McLean [54]. The incidence of children born SGA in the United States has been estimated at 8.6% [55]. Eighty-five percent of children born SGA catch up to the normal curve by the age of 2 years, with most of them catching up by the age of 6 months [56,57]. Children who have not shown adequate catch-up growth by 2 years of age are unlikely to attain a normal adult height without rhGH therapy [56,58]. Children who are SGA have relative GH resistance, but rhGH therapy has been shown to improve final adult height and was FDA approved in 2001 [59,60]. Approved rhGH doses for treatment of SGA are up to 0.49 mg/kg/wk. Mathematic prediction models of the growth response of SGA children to rhGH show that rhGH dose is the most important predictor of the first-year growth response [61]. Age at start of therapy is negatively correlated with the first-year growth response [61]. Subsequent growth is dependent on the first-year response to rhGH therapy. Investigations comparing continuous and intermittent rhGH therapy in SGA children showed similar growth responses over time [59]. However, because of the degree of catch-down growth seen between therapy courses with intermittent therapy, continuous therapy has been adopted [62]. In a final height study of continuous rhGH therapy, 54 children started treatment with rhGH at 8.1 ($\pm$1.9) years at a dose of 0.23 or 0.46 mg/kg/wk. Final adult height was -1.1 ($\pm$ 0.7) SDS in those who received 0.23 mg/kg/wk and -0.9 ($\pm$0.8) SDS in those who received 0.46 mg/kg/wk. rhGH treatment resulted in an adult height more than -2 SDS in 85% of the children after a mean rhGH treatment period of 7.8 ($\pm$ 1.7) years [57].

Idiopathic short stature

Short stature is commonly defined as a height less than the third percentile (2 SD <the mean) compared with children of the same age and gender. Using this statistical definition, 1.8 million children (aged 5–14 years) in the United States have short stature at any given time [63]. The prevalence of short stature (<third percentile) and poor growth (GV<5 cm/y) has been predicted as 0.7% of children (420,000; 1:143) in a school-based study [64]. The rate of referral of children with short stature and poor growth has a major impact on the number of children prescribed GH. Estimates of the referral rate vary from 2.5% by records review (Adda Grimberg, personal communications, 2006) to 34% by hypothetical survey [65]. Assuming a 20% referral rate, 84,000 children could be expected to be evaluated at some point between the ages of 4 and 15 years. If 35% of children referred to a pediatric endocrinologist for short stature have a known pathologic condition that would respond to GH therapy [5,66], 65% of referrals (54,600 children) for short stature and poor growth to have no known cause for their growth failure. This value correlates well with data from the NCGS showing that 60.2% of children receiving GH therapy are in a combined category of IGHD and ISS [67].

By definition, ISS excludes known causes of short stature [68]. However, ISS most certainly includes a subset of children with GHD that have a normal response to GHST. The basis of the diagnosis can affect the interpretation of efficacy. For example, the cutoff for the GH peak is moved following GHST to diagnose GHD from less than 10 down to less than 7, less than 5, or less than 3, the spectrum of ISS and its response to rhGH therapy expands. Therefore, the ability to describe the cause of short stature in children with ISS is limited by the current diagnostic tools [69]. Many children with undiagnosed conditions that result in severe short stature respond to rhGH therapy [70–72].

The use of rhGH in ISS has been the focus of both ethical and financial controversies. Multiple natural history studies report that children with ISS have short stature as adults. Hintz and colleagues [70] showed that GH treatment in children with ISS resulted in an increase in final height of 5 cm compared with predicted height. A larger increase (9 cm) was seen when the final height of treated patients was compared with historical controls. In the only randomized, placebo-controlled trial of rhGH therapy for 68 children with ISS to final height, adult height was greater in the rhGH-treated group (-1.81 ± 0.11 SDS) than in the placebo-treated group (-2.32 ± 0.17 SDS) by 0.51 SDS (3.7 cm) [71]. In a meta-analysis of 40 studies of GH therapy in ISS, the investigators concluded that adult height was increased by 4 to 6 cm in those treated with GH [73]. However, they estimated the cost of treatment at $35,000 per inch. In May, 2003, the FDA approved the use of rhGH at a dose of up to 0.37 mg/kg/wk in children with ISS who are less than −2.25 height SDS and who are unlikely to catch up in height. A subsequent final height trial with higher dose and more frequent administration showed improved height outcome. This study compared the adult height of 50 patients with ISS given daily injections of GH at dosages of 0.24 mg/kg/wk, 0.24 mg/kg/wk for the first year and 0.37 mg/kg/wk thereafter, or 0.37 mg/kg/wk [72]. Mean height SDS increased by 1.55, 1.52, and 1.85, respectively. Final heights were 7.2 cm and 5.4 cm more than pretreatment predicted final heights for the 0.37 mg/kg/wk and 0.24 mg/kg/wk dose groups, respectively [72]. In addition, in those children who received 0.24 mg/kg/wk, 71% of final height SDS values were within the normal range and in those who received 0.37 mg/kg/wk, 94% of final height SDS values (all but 1) were within the normal range.

Determination of long-term growth response to rhGH for children with ISS using near-adult height has been done for 2 large GH registries [20,74]. In the NCGS, height improved in children with ISS from −2.8 (±0.6) SDS to −1.6 (±1.0) SDS [20]. The Δ height SDS for ISS was similar to that seen for IGHD. However, enrollment height and GHST response were not significant predictors of growth response in ISS. In the Pfizer International Growth Study (formerly KIGS), height improved in children with ISS from −2.5 to −1.4 SDS [74]. Age at onset of rhGH therapy and first-year responsiveness are the strongest predictors of long-term growth response in ISS.

The use of serum IGF-1 values to adjust rhGH dosing in ISS is also controversial. The impact of this treatment paradigm in ISS was shown in a clinical trial in which weight-based dosing of rhGH was compared with dosing of rhGH to target an IGF-1 value at the mean (0 SDS) or top of the normal range for age (+2 SDS) [16]. Children in the weight-based dosing arm of the study grew similarly to those titrated to an IGF-1 at 0 SDS. However, children whose rhGH doses were titrated to IGF-1 levels at +2 SDS grew significantly better than either other group. An important finding in this study was that the spectrum of rhGH doses that children required to achieve a particular target was highly variable. The weight-based arm was treated with 0.28 mg/kg/wk, whereas the 0 SDS target arm received an average of 0.23 mg/kg/wk and the ISS subjects in the +2 SDS target arm received a much higher average of 0.83 mg/kg/wk. This finding indicates that ISS represents partial GH insensitivity. Children with ISS also showed a poorer growth response to treatment in all 3 arms compared with children with GHD: Δ height SDS was 2.04 (±0.17) for GHD and 1.33 (±0.09) for ISS groups in those with IGF-1 values targeted at +2 SDS and 1.41 (±0.13) for children with GHD, and 0.84 (±0.07) for those with ISS with IGF-1 values targeted at 0 SDS [75]. This result indicates that ISS also represents a state of partial IGF-1-insensitivity. Demonstration of the use of IGF-based dosing in clinical practice was done by evaluation of IGF-1 data entered into NCGS, which showed that, when children with ISS were growing poorly, the dose was more likely to be changed if an IGF-1 value was obtained [7]. However, the long-term efficacy of IGF-based dosing in ISS has not been tested. In addition, the safety of the higher doses of rhGH required in some children to achieve a serum IGF-1 target of +2 SDS is unclear [17].

SHOX deficiency

SHOX is produced by the short stature homeobox gene in the pseudoautosomal regions on the distal ends of the X and Y chromosomes. Absence of 1 copy (haploinsufficiency) of the *shox* gene, caused by absence of X chromosome material, is a significant component of short stature in TS. The *shox* gene encodes a transcription factor that is important in regulating the growth of long bones. SHOX deficiency (SHOX-D), through mutation or deletion of the *shox* gene, is present in most individuals (~70%) with Leri-Weill dyschondrosteosis (LWD) and in a small, but significant, number (2%–15%) of children with ISS [76–78].

There is a single published, randomized trial of rhGH in short prepubertal children with a molecularly proved SHOX gene defect [30]. In this multinational study, children with SHOX-D with both ISS and LWD phenotypes were randomized to treatment with rhGH. A comparison group of prepubertal girls with TS also received rhGH therapy. After 1 year, children with SHOX-D receiving rhGH therapy (n = 27, 12 boys; 0.35 mg/kg/wk; 8.7 ± 0.3 cm/y) showed a significant improvement in growth compared with untreated controls (n = 25, 12 boys; 5.2 ± 0.2 cm/y, *P*<.0001). The 1-year growth response was also comparable with a group of rhGH-treated children with TS (n = 26; 0.35 μg/kg/wk; 8.9 ± 0.4 cm/y, *P*= .592). After 2 years, rhGH-treated SHOX-deficient children had grown 5.9 cm more and gained +0.9 height SDS more than untreated controls (*P*<.001) [30]. rhGH therapy for SHOX-D was FDA approved in 2006 at a dose of 0.35 mg/kg/wk. A retrospective analysis of rhGH therapy showed similar height gain at final height in individuals with SHOX-D (n = 14, + 1.1± 0.2 SDS) to those with TS (n = 157, + 1.2 ± 0.1

SDS, $P = .708$) [79]. However, individuals with SHOX-D showed a trend toward shorter final heights than those with TS (149.0 ± 6.7 vs 151.4 ± 5.1 cm, $P = .109$) and had a lower final adult height SDS (-2.2 ± 0.8 vs -1.7 ± 0.8, $P = .016$) [79]. Further studies are needed to provide additional near-adult height efficacy data in this condition.

Noonan syndrome

NS, characterized by hypertelorism, down-slanting palpebral fissures, low-set posteriorly rotated ears, small chin, short neck, short stature, chest deformities, and heart defects (especially valvular pulmonic stenosis), was first described in 1963 and has an estimated incidence of 1 in 1000 to 1 in 2500 live births [80]. Mutations in multiple different genes involved in intracellular signaling (PTPN11, K-Ras, SOS1, Raf1, B-Raf, SHOC2, and N-Ras) have been found to cause NS in 61% of cases [80]. Short stature during childhood, caused by postnatal growth failure, is seen in more than 50% of individuals with NS. In untreated individuals with NS, mean adult height at age 19 years has been reported as 162.5 (±5.4) cm in men and 152.7 (±5.7) cm in girls [81]. However, because of the delayed puberty common to NS, untreated final adult height of boys with NS in another cohort was 167.4 cm [82]. The adult height of untreated North American individuals with NS is less than the third percentile in 54.5% of women (<151 cm) and 38% of men (<163.2 cm) [80]. There is a genotype-phenotype correlation, with individuals with NS caused by SOS1 mutations more likely to have normal stature and individuals with PTPN11 mutations more likely to have short stature [83,84]. Reports of GH secretion vary in the incidence of GHD in NS [85]. However, IGF-1 deficiency is a frequent finding in individuals with NS [80,85,86].

rhGH was FDA approved for the treatment of short stature in NS in 2007 at a dose of up to 0.462 mg/kg/wk. Early studies of rhGH therapy in NS showed only mildly improved height SDS and GV with therapy [87] or variable improvement with definite responders and nonresponders [88]. Short-term treatment studies showed poorer linear growth and IGF-1 generation to rhGH therapy in those with PTPN11 mutations [86,89]. However, long-term rhGH treatment studies have shown no difference in growth response between PTPN11-positive and PTPN11-negative individuals [90]. Long-term efficacy is shown in Table 2, with improved outcomes occurring with earlier initiation and longer duration of rhGH therapy [80]. Long-term height gains range from +1.3 to 1.7 SDS or 9.5 to 13 cm in boys and 9.0 to 9.8 cm in girls [80].

SAFETY

When considering a therapy for a medical condition, one of the guiding principles for physicians is Primum non nocere (First, do no harm). Therefore, when considering GH therapy for treatment of GHD and short stature, the medical, physical, psychological, and psychosocial impacts of the disease or condition need to be considered. The potential therapeutic benefit of rhGH therapy then needs to be balanced with the known and potential short-term

Table 2
Baseline and treatment growth data from studies that reported adult height outcomes in individuals with NS treated with GH

References	Patients, n (n female)	Baseline age (y)	Baseline SDS[a]	GH Dose, (mg/kg/wk)	Duration therapy (y)	Δ Height SDS	Height gain (cm)
[91]	4(4)	13.5	(−0.6)	0.19 for 1 y, then 0.31	3.5	−0.48	NA
[88]	10(4)	12	−3.1 (−0.7)	0.3	5.3		3.1
[92]	18(11)	8.6 (boys), 7.7 (girls)	−2.9 (−0.3)	0.23 (n = 10), 0.46 (n = 15) for 2 y, then dose titration[b]	7.5	1.7	13 (boys), 9.8 (girls)
[93]	24(NA)	10.2 (median)	−3.24 (median)	0.24 (median (range:0.17–0.77))	7.59 (median)	0.61 (0.97)	NA
[90]	29(8)	11	−2.8 (0.0)	0.35	6.4 (median)	1.3 (1.3)	9.5 (boys), 9.0 (girls)
[94]	65(30)	11.6	−3.5	0.33	5.6	1.4	10.9 (boys), 9.2 (girls)

Results are mean values unless specified otherwise. SDS, SD score; NA, not applicable.
[a]Height SDS is reported according to population standards and/or NS standards.
[b]Estimated mean: 0.35 mg/kg/wk.
Data from Romano AA, Allanson JE, Dahlgren J, et al. Noonan syndrome: clinical features, diagnosis, and management guidelines. Pediatrics 2010;126(4):753.

and long-term side effects. This article defines the short-term side effects as those that can occur while receiving rhGH therapy during childhood, and the long-term side effects as those that occur after rhGH therapy has been discontinued or in those individuals who continue rhGH therapy into adulthood.

Short-term safety

GH registries have been an invaluable resource for determining the safety and efficacy of GH. Such postmarketing surveillance is necessary to accurately assess the safety profile of a drug because of the inability of clinical trials to identify rare side effects. In addition, spontaneous postmarketing adverse event reporting may be incomplete and does not allow for the determination of incidence rates for side effects. The cumulative safety data from the 2 largest studies (KIGS and NCGS) represent more than 120,000 children treated for nearly half a million patient years. Based on the most recent NCGS safety publication, the cumulative enrollment in the NCGS from December 1985 to January 1 2006 was 54,996 patients comprising 195,419 patient years of treatment with Genentech's rhGH products [95]. Additional safety data were collected with continued enrollment in NCGS until December 2010 and data collection until June 2011 when the study was discontinued. Based on the most recent KIGS safety publication, the cumulative enrollment in the KIGS from January 1987 to August, 2008 was 58,603 patients comprising 197,173 patient years of treatment with Kabi, Pharmacia, and Pfizer's rhGH products [96]. Additional safety and efficacy data continue to be collected with ongoing US and international enrollment in KIGS. GHMonitor^{SM} enrolled 1335 subjects from January 2003 to August 2006 and is no longer collecting US data [97]. Safety and efficacy data also continue to be collected in the ongoing international registries ANSWER (5797 subjects enrolled from January 2002 to November 2009) [98] and GeNeSIS (estimated enrollment 23,500 from April 1999 to March 2010) [99].

The major safety questions that have been raised regarding rhGH therapy have been the risks of mortality and malignancy. The risk of mortality has focused particularly on sudden death in children with PWS, aortic dissection in children with TS, and cancer survivors. The risk of malignancy has focused particularly on children at increased risk for malignancy, including cancer survivors and those with genetic conditions predisposed to tumor formation.

Short-term risk of mortality

From the 54,996 patients enrolled in NCGS, there were 174 reported deaths, 19 (11%) of which were assessed as related to rhGH by the investigator, 4 were designated as not assessable, and no causality was provided for 21. Most of the 19 deaths assessed as related to rhGH (12 of 19) were caused by neoplasms (Table 3) [95]. The other 7 deaths assessed as related to rhGH were isolated cases as follows: cerebral edema in a patient with a glioma resection, and cerebral edema in a patient with a mitochondrial myopathy and hypertrophic cardiomyopathy; arrhythmia in a patient with 2 renal transplants with hypertrophic cardiomyopathy and coronary atherosclerosis at autopsy;

Table 3
Incidence of targeted events by indication

	All NCGS	IGHD	OGHD	TS	CRI	ISS	Other
n	54,996	23,393	8351	5127	1778	9778	6569
AE	6.2	4.4	12.0	7.6	10.9	3.6	7.3
SAE	2.4	1.2	6.8	1.9	6.5	0.7	3.1
Deaths	0.3	0.1	1.0	0.1	1.2	0.0	0.5
Malignancy[a]	0.1	0.0	0.1	0.1	0.0	0.0	0.0
IC tumor recurrence	0.3	0.0	1.8	0.0	0.1	0.0	0.0
Leukemia[a,b]	0.0	0.0	0.0	0.0	0.0	0.0	0.0
Second neoplasm	0.1	0.0	0.5	0.0	0.1	0.0	0.0
AI[b]	0.0	0.0	0.1	0.0	0.0	0.0	0.0
DM	0.1	0.0	0.1	0.2	0.2	0.1	0.2
IH	0.1	0.1	0.2	0.2	0.3	0.0	0.1
SCFE	0.1	0.1	0.4	0.2	0.3	0.0	0.1
Scoliosis	0.4	0.2	0.5	0.7	0.1	0.2	0.6
Pancreatitis	0.0	0.0	0.0	0.1	0.0	0.0	0.0

Data are expressed as percentages.

Abbreviations: AE, adverse event; AI, adrenal insufficiency; DM, diabetes mellitus; IC, intracranial; IGHD, idiopathic GHD; IH, intracranial hypertension; OGHD, organic GHD; SAE, serious adverse event; SCFE, slipped capital femoral epiphysis.

[a]New onset, no risk factors.

[b]Based on fewer than 15 reports.

Data from Bell J, Parker KL, Swinford RD, et al. Long-term safety of recombinant human growth hormone in children. J Clin Endocrinol Metab 2010;95(1):169.

diabetic hyperosmolar coma in a patient with craniopharyngioma who was receiving rhGH at the time the hyperosmolar coma developed; depression after stopping rhGH in a 21-year-old man with thalassemia major, with subsequent death from an overdose of street drugs; complications of neurofibromatosis in a patient with an optic glioma, an odontoma, ataxia, and facial swelling; and sudden death in a 4-year-old boy with PWS [95].

Mortality in prader-willi syndrome

The annual mortality in PWS has been described as 3% across all age groups and is increased particularly in relation to complications of obesity [100]. A review of all reported deaths in PWS conducted in 2007 identified 64 deaths in children up to age 19 years with PWS (42 boys) [101]. Twenty-eight (44%) of these children received rhGH treatment. Respiratory disorders were the most common cause of death (61%; 68% of rhGH treated, 56% of untreated). Seventy-five percent of deaths occurred in the first 9 months after the initiation of rhGH therapy. No significant differences were found between the groups in gender, prevalence of obesity, or sleep apnea. More deaths in the untreated group occurred in children less than 3 years of age (25 deaths, 22 untreated). However, deaths in those receiving rhGH were more evenly distributed by age.

It has been hypothesized that the causal connection between rhGH therapy and sudden death in PWS is the induction of tonsillar and adenoid hypertrophy. However, sleep studies have shown an improvement of sleep apnea, particularly central apnea, and 1 death has been reported in a child with a normal polysomnograph before and after initiation of rhGH therapy [102,103].

Increases in IGF-1 are associated with tonsillar hypertrophy. This finding suggests that it may be safer to start at low doses of rhGH and titrate the rhGH dose using IGF-1 values. However, there are no studies to support this practice. Tonsillectomy and adenoidectomy have also been proposed as a treatment of sleep apnea. However, this treatment may be dangerous in children with PWS and may not improve the sleep apnea [102].

Therefore, although polysomnography has been recommended before starting rhGH treatment, particularly in the presence of snoring or obesity, there is limited evidence that polysomnography is beneficial, because a normal result cannot guarantee 100% safety. It should be emphasized that PWS is a condition with an inherently high mortality risk. Children with PWS, particularly with obesity, sleep apnea, and respiratory illness, require careful clinical management whether or not they are receiving rhGH therapy. In those children with PWS receiving rhGH therapy, awareness of the risk for sudden death should always be present, but particularly during the first 9 months of treatment. Although a causal link between rhGH therapy, respiratory illness, and sudden death has not been established, discontinuation of rhGH therapy is recommended during respiratory illnesses. In addition, despite the potential metabolic and body composition benefits, rhGH therapy in severely obese children with PWS is contraindicated.

Mortality in turner syndrome

Aortic dissection, an often fatal event, occurs in 1% to 2% of the TS population and is usually preceded by dilatation of the aortic root and/or ascending aorta. Dissection occurs early in life, at a median age of 35 years (range 18–61 years) [104]. Longitudinal imaging every 5 to 10 years to assess aortic diameters is recommended, even in those with a normal initial cardiac study [105]. In the NCGS, 5 deaths from aortic dissection/rupture were reported among 5127 patients with TS [95].

Short-term risk of malignancy

Since the inception of GH therapy, there has been ongoing concern about the potential for GH therapy to promote tumorigenesis either during therapy or in the period following therapy. Increased levels of IGF-I are associated with an increased risk of developing breast, prostate, and colon cancer in adults [106–108]. In addition, GH and IGF-1 signaling have become adjunctive targets in the treatment of certain forms of cancer [109]. Lessons from animal models have suggested that GH and IGF-1 play permissive rather than causative roles in tumorigenesis [110,111]. However, since the first report of leukemia in a child receiving rhGH in 1988 [112], the possibility of an increased risk of cancer in patients receiving rhGH therapy has been investigated. Because of evidence of a link between increased IGF-1 levels and certain forms of cancer [106–108], the concern about the potential of rhGH therapy as a child affecting the long-term risk of cancer after GH therapy resulted in long-term follow-up studies of GH-treated individuals. In one such study of childhood pituitary-derived GH-treated individuals, 2 cases of colorectal cancer were identified in a population in which 1 or less was expected [113]. In the Childhood Cancer Survivor Study, long-term follow-up of childhood cancer survivors has shown that there is an increased risk of second neoplasm developing in GH-treated children years after treatment (Fig. 4) [114]. In this study, the rate ratio of GH-treated survivors developing a second neoplasm was 2.15 (95% confidence interval [CI], 1.3–3.5; $P<.002$) compared with non–GH-treated survivors (Table 4) [114].

This study included data from children who received pituitary-derived GH, rhGH, or both. Meningiomas were the most common second neoplasm (9/20). All individuals who developed meningiomas as second neoplasms had previously received radiation to the head or brain [114]. After adjusting for covariates, the relative risk of death for GH-treated patients compared with those not treated with GH was not statistically increased (1.20; 95% CI, 0.81–1.79; $P = .36$).

In the KIGS database, a total of 32 new malignant neoplasms were reported in 58,603 patients, versus the 25.3 expected (incidence, 16.4 per 100,000 patient years; standardized incidence ratio [SIR] 1.26; 95% CI, 0.86–1.78; Table 5) [96]. These 32 new malignant neoplasms were diagnosed at a mean age of 11.9 years (range, 5.0–17.6 years). The mean duration of rhGH therapy in KIGS before the diagnosis of cancer was 3.6 years (range, 0.08–9.70 years). Eight of 32 patients with a new cancer were treated with rhGH before enrollment in KIGS for a median of 0.7 years (range, 0.06–4.5 years). In 6 of 7626 patients observed in KIGS after rhGH was discontinued, a malignant neoplasm

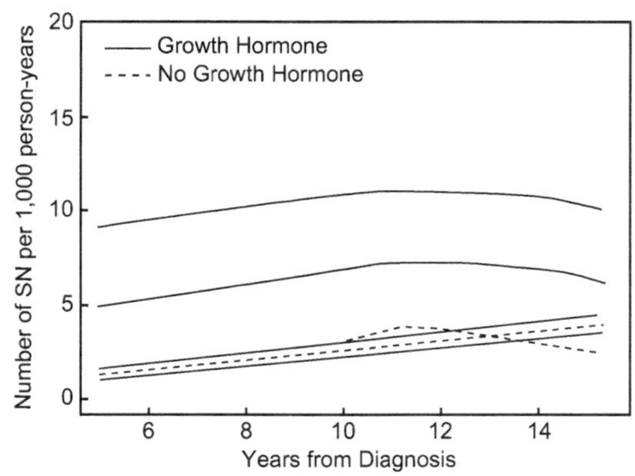

Fig. 4. Incidence of second neoplasms. Comparison of the number of second neoplasms estimated per 1000 person years for survivors who did and did not receive treatment with rhGH, plotted against time from diagnosis. The plot includes 95% confidence intervals. (*From* Ergun-Longmire B, Mertens AC, Mitby P, et al. Growth hormone treatment and risk of second neoplasms in the childhood cancer survivor. J Clin Endocrinol Metab 2006;91(9):3496; with permission.)

Table 4
Risk factors for occurrence of second neoplasms

Covariate	Risk ratio (95% CI)	*P*
Univariate model		
Sex	—	<0.0001
Female	1.00	—
Male	0.53 (0.44–0.62)	—
Age at primary diagnosis (risk/y)	1.08 (1.06–1.09)	<0.0001
Alkylating agent	—	0.0002
No	1.00	—
Yes	1.41 (1.18–1.69)	—
Radiation	—	<0.0001
No	1.00	—
Yes	3.00 (2.32–3.87)	—
Chemotherapy	—	0.67
No	1.00	—
Yes	0.96 (0.78–1.17)	—
GH	—	0.004
No	1.00	—
Yes	1.92 (1.22–2.99)	—
Multivariate model	—	—
Sex	—	<0.0001
Female	1.00	—
Male	0.52 (0.43–0.63)	—
Age at diagnosis (risk/y)	1.07 (1.06–1.09)	<0.0001
Alkylating agent	—	0.004
No	1.00	—
Yes	1.30 (1.09–1.56)	—
Radiation	—	<0.0001
No	1.00	—
Yes	2.88 (2.20–3.78)	—
GH	—	0.002
No	1.00	—
Yes	2.15 (1.33–3.47)	—

Data from Ergun-Longmire B, Mertens AC, Mitby P, et al. Growth hormone treatment and risk of second neoplasms in the childhood cancer survivor. J Clin Endocrinol Metab 2006;91(9):3496.

was reported for as long as 3.1 years after stopping GH. The mean dose of GH in patients in whom a neoplasm developed was 0.26 (±0.08) mg/kg/wk (range, 0.12–0.48). Serum IGF-I levels measured 1 to 12 months before the onset of a neoplasm were only available for 7 patients. Three patients had IGF-I SDS greater than 0 (range, 0.6–1.7), 4 patients had IGF SDS between −0.6 and −1.9, and none were greater than the normal range.

In the NCGS database, intracranial malignancies were reported in 243 patients, 44 of which were new-onset malignancies. Of the 44 new-onset intracranial malignancies, 15 had no predisposing factors. Extracranial malignancies, including leukemia, were reported in 87 patients, with 63 new-onset

Table 5
Observed and expected number of tumor cases

Site or malignant neoplasm (ICD-10 classification)	Number of observed cases	Number of expected cases	SIR (95% CI)
Any primary cancer (C00–C97, except C44[a])	32	25.3	1.26 (0.86–1.78)
Brain/CNS (C70–C72)	9	4.0	224 (1.02–4.25)
Testis (C62)	3	1.2	2.55 (0.51–7.46)
Non-Hodgkin lymphoma (C82–C85, C96)	3	2.1	1.41 (0.28–4.11)
Leukemia (C91–C94)	3	6.2	0.48 (0.10–1.41)
Adrenal gland (C74)	2	0.25	7.93 (0.89–28.6)
Malignant melanoma (C43)	2	0.8	2.57 (0.29–9.27)
Kidney (C64)	2	0.7	2.98 (0.33–10.8)
Trachea and long (C33 + C34)	1	0.1	9.98 (0.13–55.5)
Bone (C40–C41)	1	2.05	0.49 (0.01–2.71)
Mesothelioma (C45E)	1	0.05	22.0 (0.29–123)
Peripheral nerves, connective and soft tissue (C47, C49)	1	1.2	0.85 (0.01–4.72)
Ovary (C56)	1	0.7	1.36 (0.02–7.57)
Thyroid (C73)	1	0.75	1.33 (0.02–7.40)
Hodgkin lymphoma (C81)	1	2.5	0.40 (0.01–2.24)
Other and unspecified (026, 039, 048, 076, 080)	1	0.3	3.43 (0.04–19.1)
All other cancer sites excluding nonmelanoma skin tumors	0	2.4	Not applicable

Observed and expected number of tumor cases, estimated standardized incidence ratio with 95% CI by site of malignant neoplasm in 58,603 patients treated with rhGH in KIGS with no known factors conveying an a priori increased risk of cancer.

Abbreviation: ICD-10, International Statistical Classification of Diseases, 10th Revision.

[a]Other malignant neoplasm of skin (eg, basal cell carcinoma).

Data from Wilton P, Mattsson AF, Darendeliler F, et al. Growth hormone treatment in children is not associated with an increase in the incidence of cancer: experience from KIGS (Pfizer International Growth Database). J Pediatr 2010;157(2):268.

malignancies. Of the 63 new-onset tumors, 21 had no predisposing factors (Tables 6 and 7) [95]. Using the 29 children with new-onset tumors with confirmed NCGS enrollment, a comparison with the risk of new-onset tumor in the general pediatric population yielded an SIR that was not significantly increased (1.12; 95% CI 0.75–1.61; see Table 4 and Bell and colleagues [95]).

Based on these results, the large volume of data from the KIGS and NCGS databases provide no evidence that rhGH therapy in childhood growth disorders results in an increased risk of developing cancer relative to that expected in the normal population. However, surveillance for an extended time should continue to allow further assessment [96].

Table 6
New-onset malignancies in patients without risk factors: tumor types in 2 or more patients

Malignancy	No. of patients (%)
Unspecified brain neoplasm	5 (13.8)
Glioma	4 (11.1)
Lymphoma	4 (11.1)
Leukemia	3 (8.3)
Thyroid carcinoma	3 (8.3)
Astrocytoma	2 (5.5)
Germ cell tumor	2 (5.5)
Osteogenic sarcoma	2 (5.5)
Soft tissue sarcoma	2 (5.5)
Other	9 (25.0)
Total	36 (100)

Data from Bell J, Parker KL, Swinford RD, et al. Long-term safety of recombinant human growth hormone in children. J Clin Endocrinol Metab 2010;95(1):171.

Other targeted safety events

Based on data collected during preclinical trials and postmarketing surveillance registries, the product insert for the various rhGH products includes several safety concerns. Many of these, including headaches and otitis media, are common in the general pediatric population and are minor concerns. Injection site lipoatrophy is a cosmetic concern that can be eliminated by using appropriate rotation of injection sites. Injection site rashes and allergic reactions are concerns with any injectable material and may be related to the diluent rather than the rhGH. Borderline hypothyroidism (primary or secondary) may be uncovered with rhGH therapy. Therefore, thyroid functions should be monitored during rhGH treatment. Fluid retention and edema are common

Table 7
New-onset malignancies in patients without risk factors

Age (y)	Years of GH exposure	Expected rate per 100,000 y of exposure	Observed cases	Expected cases
0–4	11,348	20.4	1	2.32
5–9	44,585	11.4	6	5.08
10–14	85,909	12.9	12	11.08
15–19	36,082	20.0	9	7.22
20–24	540	34.9	1	0.19
Total	178,464	14.5[a]	29	25.88

SIR, 1.12; 95% CI, 0.75, 1.61.

[a] Age-standardized expected rate.

Data from Bell J, Parker KL, Swinford RD, et al. Long-term safety of recombinant human growth hormone in children. J Clin Endocrinol Metab 2010;95(1):171.

side effects of rhGH therapy in adults, but are seen less in children and adolescents. Other targeted safety events including diabetes mellitus, intracranial hypertension, scoliosis, pancreatitis, adrenal insufficiency, and slipped capital femoral epiphysis are described later. In addition, concerns about rhGH therapy for short stature caused by CRI before or following renal transplantation are discussed.

Diabetes mellitus

Diabetes mellitus (DM) has been reported in 65 patients; 37 type 1 DM (T1DM), 20 type 2 DM (T2DM), and 8 unclassifiable [95]. The 33 T1DM cases, compared with that expected and adapted to an age-matched population, yielded an SIR of 0.90 (observed 33; expected 36.8). Based on the mechanism of action of rhGH, it would be unexpected that the incidence of T1DM would be increased. However, because of the relative insulin resistance caused by increased GH secretion or rhGH administration, it would be more likely for a child to develop T2DM while receiving rhGH therapy. If the 8 unclassifiable cases are considered T2DM, the incidence would be 14 per 100,000 patient years. However, it is difficult to compare this incidence with the general pediatric population because of the changing incidence of T2DM during the years of the NCGS database. It is also difficult to determine whether rhGH therapy causes a long-term increase in the risk of T2DM because the insulin resistance would be reduced once rhGH therapy was discontinued.

Intracranial hypertension

Although intracranial hypertension (IH), also known as pseudotumor cerebri, has been identified in children receiving rhGH therapy, no known mechanism has been identified. The annual incidence of IH in the general pediatric population is 0.9 per 100,000 [115]. IH was reported in 61 confirmed patients in the NCGS, with most events occurring within 6 months of starting rhGH [95]. Thus, the incidence of IH in children receiving rhGH therapy reported in the NCGS is 31 per 100,000 patient years [95]. IH was reported in 41 children with confirmed KIGS receiving rhGH therapy, with an incidence of 28 per 100,000 patient years [116].The highest incidence is seen in children with TS, organic GHD, PWS, and CRI [95,116]. Even though only 2 cases of IH have been seen in ISS, this is still higher than the general population [95]. It is unclear whether this is an ascertainment bias. However, IH in children receiving rhGH is generally resolved with discontinuation of rhGH therapy for a brief period followed by resumption of rhGH at a lower dose.

Scoliosis

rhGH therapy does not cause scoliosis. However, it can make it worse so that previously unrecognized scoliosis becomes evident or known scoliosis progresses. Scoliosis was reported in 238 patients in the NCGS of which 76 were preexisting. Scoliosis was more common in TS and PWS. Among the 64 patients with serious scoliosis, 37 reported surgical treatment. It is recommended that clinicians monitor regularly for the development or worsening of scoliosis. If scoliosis is present and/or worsening, involvement of a pediatric orthopedist is recommended. rhGH therapy in children with severe or worsening scoliosis should be monitored closely and should involve ongoing communication between the pediatric orthopedist and pediatric endocrinologist.

Pancreatitis

Pancreatitis has been reported in 10 children receiving rhGH therapy in the NCGS database and 1 individual 5 months after discontinuation of rhGH therapy. These data provide an incidence of 5.2 per 100,000 in rhGH-treated individuals, and yield an SIR of 1.44 and 95% CI of 0.70 to 2.67 [95]. The annual background incidence of pancreatitis is 3.6 per 100,000 in the pediatric age group [117]. These data fail to show a clearly significant relationship between rhGH therapy and pancreatitis.

Adrenal insufficiency

Concern about adrenal insufficiency (AI) in children with multiple pituitary hormone deficiencies has arisen because of the impact of GH on cortisol metabolism. The microsomal enzyme 11β-hydroxysteroid dehydrogenase type 1 (11βHSD-1) is required for conversion of cortisone to its active metabolite, cortisol. GH inhibits 11βHSD-1 activity [118]. Therefore, children with unrecognized central AI may develop an adrenal crisis caused by rhGH therapy. Alternatively, individuals with known central AI may require higher maintenance and stress doses of steroids when rhGH therapy is initiated [119]. Close dose monitoring and possible increase would be particularly needed in individuals receiving prednisone or cortisone acetate who require 11βHSD-1 activity for conversion to cortisol. In patients with organic GHD (OGHD) and idiopathic panhypopituitarism in the NCGS, 11 events consistent with acute AI, including 4 deaths, were recorded [95]. The time from onset of rhGH therapy to the event of AI ranged from within 24 hours of initiation to 7.4 years, with a mean of 2.5 years. Five nonfatal cases were assessed as serious by the investigator. Although rhGH may facilitate the occurrence of AI, patients with hypopituitarism are at lifelong risk for AI and sudden death whether or not they are receiving rhGH [120,121].

Slipped capital femoral epiphysis

The annual incidence of slipped capital femoral epiphysis (SCFE) in the general pediatric population is 2 to 13 per 100,000 [122,123]. The risk of SCFE is increased in obesity, hypogonadism, multiple pituitary hormone deficiency, and rapid growth during puberty. SCFE was reported in 93 confirmed patients in the NCGS receiving rhGH [95]. Thus the incidence of SCFE in children receiving rhGH therapy reported in the NCGS is 48 per 100,000 patient years [95]. SCFE was reported in 52 confirmed children in the KIGS receiving rhGH therapy, with an incidence of 73 per 100,000 patient years [116].The highest incidence is seen in children with TS, organic GHD, and CRI [95,116]. Wider growth plates and relative osteopenia seen in GHD, SHOX deficiency in TS, and metabolic bone disease in CRI may predispose the growth plates to slip during rapid growth [95,116].

Chronic renal insufficiency after transplantation

Primarily, there has been concern that rhGH therapy would increase the frequency of solid organ rejection. Data from the NAPRTCS showed no increase in rejection episodes in children receiving rhGH therapy after renal transplant compared with children not receiving rhGH. A potential increased risk of rejection was seen in patients receiving rhGH with a history of frequent previous rejection episodes [124,125]. However, the risk of rejection is also increased in children with a history of frequent previous rejection episodes who have not received rhGH. The use of rhGH before transplantation was associated with a borderline higher risk for posttransplant lymphoproliferative disorder (PTLD; odds ratio 1.88, 95% CI 1.00–3.55, $P = .05$). In contrast, use of rhGH during dialysis or after transplantation only was not associated with a higher risk for PTLD [126]. Because of these concerns, rhGH therapy in children following renal transplantation should be carefully considered by a multispecialty team including pediatric nephrologists, pediatric endocrinologists, and transplant surgeons.

Long-term safety

For the purposes of this article, long-term side effects are defined as those that occur after rhGH therapy has been discontinued or in those individuals who continue rhGH therapy into adulthood. In children with organic GHD and severe isolated GHD, rhGH therapy should be considered replacement therapy and, if replacement doses are not excessive, is not expected to have long-term negative side effects. However, subcutaneous doses given once daily are unlikely to match the natural profile of pulsatile GH secretion. If larger doses are given for OGHD or IGHD, or when treating conditions without GHD, then there may be more risk of long-term negative effects. The relative safety of rhGH during therapy, as documented in numerous publications and described earlier in this article ,makes long-term side effects less likely.

Measurement of IGF-1 and IGFBP-3 levels during therapy started as a measure of efficacy and compliance [15]. With the identification of a correlation between high IGF-1 levels and an increased risk of cancer in adults, monitoring IGF-1 and IGFBP-3 has become a safety practice [15]. However, it is unclear whether increased levels of IGF-1 or IGFBP-3 during childhood correlate with any adverse effects in adults. Studies showing an increased risk of cancer with high IGF-1 levels in adults show that the highest risk occurs in those with increased IGF-1 and low IGFBP-3 (Fig. 5) [15]. This finding may be caused by increased levels of free IGF-1, reduced IGF-independent actions of IGFBP-3, or both. Low levels of IGF-1 with high IGFBP-3 in adulthood are associated with an increased risk of cardiovascular disease [15].

Children treated with rhGH typically have low or low normal levels of IGF-1 before therapy. During rhGH therapy, IGF-1 and IGFBP-3 levels increase in

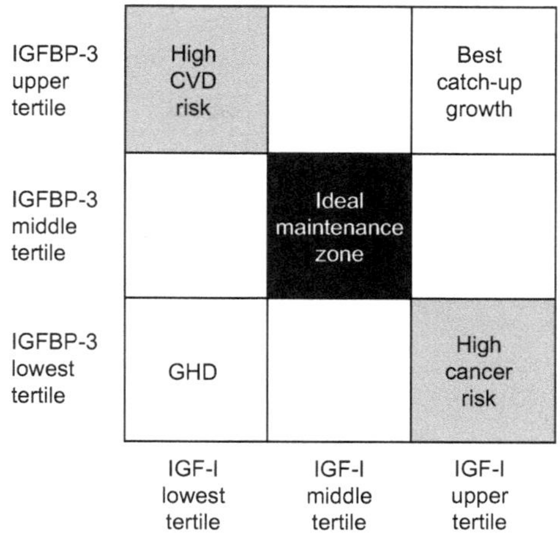

Fig. 5. The relationships between IGF-1, IGFBP-3, and rhGH treatment for GHD, catch-up growth, malignancy risk, and cardiovascular disease (CVD) risk shown in a two-dimensional grid. (*Data from* Park P, Cohen P. The role of insulin-like growth factor I monitoring in growth hormone-treated children. Horm Res 2004;62 Suppl 1:61.)

tandem, a combination with a low cancer risk profile. The degree of increase of IGF-1 and IGFBP-3 during rhGH therapy is dependent on the rhGH dose, compliance, and GH-responsiveness. Following completion of rhGH therapy, IGF-1 and IGFBP-3 levels are likely to revert to pretreatment ranges with low IGF-1 and BP-3 that have a low cancer risk profile. It is unclear whether the temporary, although prolonged, increase of IGF-1 and IGFBP-3 levels during rhGH therapy has any long-term impact on the cancer risk or any other health risk factors. Although it has been proposed as a safety measure, it also remains unclear whether monitoring IGF-1 and IGFBP-3 levels, targeting IGF-1 and/or IGFBP-3 values to a certain range, or reducing rhGH doses if IGF-1 levels are high, has any impact on the long-term safety of rhGH therapy [16,17].

Although GH registries have been invaluable in the determination of safety and efficacy during rhGH therapy, once children discontinue therapy, they are not typically entered into the registries and frequently no longer see the pediatric endocrinologist. Therefore, long-term safety data in this population are sparse. There have been several studies that have attempted to investigate long-term effects of rhGH therapy in childhood. In one study, the risk of cancer was investigated in adults who received pituitary-derived GH between 1959 and 1985 [113]. There was no overall increase in the incidence of cancer in this study. However, this study raised concerns about an increased risk of colorectal cancer (SIR 7.9; 1.0–28.7, $P = .05$) and Hodgkin lymphoma (SIR 2.3; 0.3–8.5, $P = .42$) occurring in individuals with IGHD. Two cases of each type of these cancers were identified in this population. One of the cases of colorectal cancer occurred in an individual with an unclear history of possible polyposis coli. If that case is excluded, neither tumor had a significantly increased incidence compared with the normal population.

Because of the unanswered questions regarding long-term safety of rhGH therapy, further long-term follow-up studies are necessary. These studies could be prospective cohort studies or cross-sectional studies. One such effort is the ongoing retrospective observational study entitled Safety and Appropriateness of Growth Hormone Treatments in Europe (SAGhE). On December 10 2010, the French drug agency Agence Francaise de Securite Sanitaire des Produits de Santé and the European Medicines Agency (EMA) issued press releases based on preliminary mortality data from the French portion of this study, Santé Adulte GH Enfant (FrSAGhE) regarding potential increased mortality in adults previously treated with rhGH [127,128]. According to the reports, the FrSAGhE study evaluated data from about 7000 patients who had received rhGH during childhood, initiated between 1985 and 1996, for treatment of IGHD (~75% of the cohort) or ISS/SGA. They reported an increased risk of all-cause mortality (93 deaths) compared with the general French population (70 deaths estimated), with an abnormally high death rate caused by cerebrovascular complications and bone tumors. The risk was also reported to be associated with higher doses of rhGH.

The Committee for Medicinal Products (CHMP) for Human Use of the EMA reviewed the available data and determined "that there is no need for regulatory action based on the presented data." On December 16 2010, the CHMP of the EMA issued the following statement reporting their plans for further review of the safety of rhGH: "While this review is ongoing, the CHMP confirms that there is no immediate concern. However, prescribers are reminded to strictly follow the indications and the approved doses. The maximum recommended dose of 50 μg/kg weight/day for somatropin-containing medicines should not be exceeded." [129] The FDA issued a similar report on December 22 2010 [130]. The EMA and FDA reported that they would review all available information on the potential risk of rhGH therapy and communicate any new recommendations once the review was complete. The FDA issued the following statement: "At this time, FDA believes the benefits of recombinant GH continue to outweigh its potential risks" [130].

These preliminary results regarding potential mortality related to rhGH therapy emphasize the need for ongoing long-term studies of adults previously treated with rhGH. It is also necessary to ensure that appropriate reference or control populations are evaluated to determine whether the risk is related to rhGH therapy or a predisposition related to the underlying condition (IGHD, ISS, or SGA). It is unclear whether there is a selection bias for individuals participating in such a study that may influence the risk of reporting adverse events. Studies of cancer survivors have shown that the increased risk of second neoplasms compared with the reference population was reduced simply by extension of the follow-up period [114]. This argues that long-term studies are necessary to determine the risk of long-term side effects related to rhGH therapy. The CHMP of the EMA has emphasized the need for the

European SAGhE study to continue. Similar studies should be considered in the United States where the prescribed rhGH doses are typically higher than in Europe. However, tracking individuals previously treated with rhGH over time may be difficult.

Overall, the rhGH short-term safety profile is reassuring, with the fewest adverse events occurring in children with ISS. It is unclear whether rhGH treatment during childhood has any long-term impact on morbidity and mortality. However, because short stature has low morbidity and mortality, it would not be acceptable to expose children to even a small increase in the long-term risk of a serious adverse event related to rhGH treatment for the relative improvement in growth. Therefore, the pediatric endocrinology community, rhGH manufacturers, and research funding and regulatory agencies need to work together to design studies that will identify the long-term risk of rhGH therapy.

FUTURE DIRECTIONS

This article focuses on currently available data regarding safety and efficacy of rhGH therapy. The use of rhIGF-1, approved in 2005 for severe primary IGF-1 deficiency, for treatment of children with less severe growth issues as a single agent or in combination with rhGH therapy has been the subject of clinical trials [131,132]. The safety data for rhIGF-1 alone, or in combination with rhGH, for this population is limited to small clinical trials. The short-term and long-term safety of rhIGF-1 is currently being studied in a postmarketing surveillance registry [133]. Long-term safety after rhIGF-1 therapy also needs to be monitored in the future.

Long-acting rhGH was previously available as Nutropin Depot. The safety profile of this medication was similar to that of daily rhGH [134]. However, the medication was only commercially available for 4.5 years and no long-term studies have been reported. Efficacy of Nutropin Depot was diminished compared with daily rhGH [134]. Several forms of long-acting rhGH are currently in development and may soon be commercially available [135]. If these long-acting rhGH preparations are approved, it will be important to establish their short-term and long-term safety and efficacy.

References

[1] Sizonenko PC, Clayton PE, Cohen P, et al. Diagnosis and management of growth hormone deficiency in childhood and adolescence. Part 1: diagnosis of growth hormone deficiency. Growth Horm IGF Res 2001;11(3):137–65.

[2] Gharib H, Cook DM, Saenger PH, et al. American Association of Clinical Endocrinologists medical guidelines for clinical practice for growth hormone use in adults and children–2003 update. Endocr Pract 2003;9(1):64–76.

[3] Growth Hormone Research Society. Consensus guidelines for the diagnosis and treatment of growth hormone (GH) deficiency in childhood and adolescence: summary statement of the GH Research Society. GH Research Society [see comment]. J Clin Endocrinol Metab 2000;85(11):3990–3.

[4] Wilson TA, Rose SR, Cohen P, et al. Update of guidelines for the use of growth hormone in children: the Lawson Wilkins Pediatric Endocrinology Society Drug and Therapeutics Committee. J Pediatr 2003;143(4):415–21.
[5] August GP, Lippe BM, Blethen SL, et al. Growth hormone treatment in the United States: demographic and diagnostic features of 2331 children. J Pediatr 1990;116(6): 899–903.
[6] Bakker B, Frane J, Anhalt H, et al. Height velocity targets from the National Cooperative Growth Study for first-year growth hormone responses in short children. J Clin Endocrinol Metab 2008;93(2):352–7.
[7] Miller BS, Shulman DI, Shillington A, et al. Consensus and discordance in the management of growth hormone-treated patients: results of a knowledge, attitudes, beliefs, and practices survey. Int J Pediatr Endocrinol 2010;2010:891571.
[8] Ranke MB, Lindberg A, Board KI, et al. Observed and predicted growth responses in prepubertal children with growth disorders: guidance of growth hormone treatment by empirical variables. J Clin Endocrinol Metab 2010;95(3):1229–37.
[9] Ranke MB, Lindberg A, Chatelain P, et al. Derivation and validation of a mathematical model for predicting the response to exogenous recombinant human growth hormone (GH) in prepubertal children with idiopathic GH deficiency. KIGS International Board. Kabi Pharmacia International Growth Study. J Clin Endocrinol Metab 1999;84(4): 1174–83.
[10] Ranke MB, Lindberg A, Ranke MB, et al. Predicting growth in response to growth hormone treatment. Growth Horm IGF Res 2009;19(1):1–11.
[11] Tanaka T, Cohen P, Clayton PE, et al. Diagnosis and management of growth hormone deficiency in childhood and adolescence–part 2: growth hormone treatment in growth hormone deficient children. Growth Horm IGF Res 2002;12(5):323–41.
[12] Keni J, Cohen P, Keni J, et al. Optimizing growth hormone dosing in children with idiopathic short stature. Horm Res 2009;71(Suppl 1):70–4.
[13] Mauras N, Attie KM, Reiter EO, et al. High dose recombinant human growth hormone (GH) treatment of GH-deficient patients in puberty increases near-final height: a randomized, multicenter trial. Genentech, Inc, Cooperative Study Group. J Clin Endocrinol Metab 2000;85(10):3653–60.
[14] Riddick L, Alter C, Davis DA, et al. A stepwise increase in recombinant human growth hormone dosing during puberty achieves improved pubertal growth: a National Cooperative Growth Study report. J Pediatr Endocrinol 2009;22(7):623–8.
[15] Park P, Cohen P. The role of insulin-like growth factor I monitoring in growth hormone-treated children. Horm Res 2004;62(Suppl 1):59–65.
[16] Cohen P, Rogol AD, Howard CP, et al. Insulin growth factor-based dosing of growth hormone therapy in children: a randomized, controlled study. J Clin Endocrinol Metab 2007;92(7):2480–6.
[17] Baron J. Editorial: growth hormone therapy in childhood: titration versus weight-based dosing? J Clin Endocrinol Metab 2007;92(7):2436–8.
[18] Ranke MB, Lindberg A, Martin DD, et al. The mathematical model for total pubertal growth in idiopathic growth hormone (GH) deficiency suggests a moderate role of GH dose. J Clin Endocrinol Metab 2003;88(10):4748–53.
[19] Reiter EO, Price DA, Wilton P, et al. Effect of growth hormone (GH) treatment on the near-final height of 1258 patients with idiopathic GH deficiency: analysis of a large international database. J Clin Endocrinol Metab 2006;91(6):2047–54.
[20] Frindik JP, Kemp SF, Hunold JJ, et al. Near adult heights after growth hormone treatment in patients with idiopathic short stature or idiopathic growth hormone deficiency. J Pediatr Endocrinol 2003;16(Suppl 3):607–12.
[21] Tonshoff B, Kiepe D, Ciarmatori S. Growth hormone/insulin-like growth factor system in children with chronic renal failure. Pediatr Nephrol 2005;20(3):279–89.

[22] Fine RN, Kohaut EC, Brown D, et al. Growth after recombinant human growth hormone treatment in children with chronic renal failure: report of a multicenter randomized double-blind placebo-controlled study. Genentech Cooperative Study Group. J Pediatr 1994;124(3):374–82.
[23] Haffner D, Schaefer F, Nissel R, et al. Effect of growth hormone treatment on the adult height of children with chronic renal failure. German Study Group for Growth Hormone Treatment in Chronic Renal Failure. N Engl J Med 2000;343(13):923–30.
[24] Koch VH, Lippe BM, Nelson PA, et al. Accelerated growth after recombinant human growth hormone treatment of children with chronic renal failure. J Pediatr 1989;115(3):365–71.
[25] Mahan JD, Warady BA, Frane J, et al. First-year response to rhGH therapy in children with CKD: a National Cooperative Growth Study report. Pediatr Nephrol 2010;25(6):1125–30.
[26] Fine RN, Kohaut E, Brown D, et al. Long-term treatment of growth retarded children with chronic renal insufficiency, with recombinant human growth hormone. Kidney Int 1996;49(3):781–5.
[27] Berard E, Andre JL, Guest G, et al. Long-term results of rhGH treatment in children with renal failure: experience of the French Society of Pediatric Nephrology. Pediatr Nephrol 2008;23(11):2031–8.
[28] Fine RN, Martz K, Stablein D, et al. What have 20 years of data from the North American Pediatric Renal Transplant Cooperative Study taught us about growth following renal transplantation in infants, children, and adolescents with end-stage renal disease? Pediatr Nephrol 2010;25(4):739–46.
[29] Fine RN, Stablein D, Fine RN, et al. Long-term use of recombinant human growth hormone in pediatric allograft recipients: a report of the NAPRTCS Transplant Registry. Pediatr Nephrol 2005;20(3):404–8.
[30] Blum WF, Crowe BJ, Quigley CA, et al. Growth hormone is effective in treatment of short stature associated with short stature homeobox-containing gene deficiency: two-year results of a randomized, controlled, multicenter trial. J Clin Endocrinol Metab 2007;92(1):219–28.
[31] Davenport ML, Punyasavatsut N, Stewart PW, et al. Growth failure in early life: an important manifestation of Turner syndrome. Horm Res 2002;57(5–6):157–64.
[32] Lippe B. Turner syndrome. Endocrinol Metab Clin North Am 1991;20(1):121–52.
[33] Carel JC, Mathivon L, Gendrel C, et al. Near normalization of final height with adapted doses of growth hormone in Turner's syndrome. J Clin Endocrinol Metab 1998;83(5):1462–6.
[34] Quigley CA, Crowe BJ, Anglin DG, et al. Growth hormone and low dose estrogen in Turner syndrome: results of a United States multi-center trial to near-final height. J Clin Endocrinol Metab 2002;87(5):2033–41.
[35] Rosenfeld RG, Attie KM, Frane J, et al. Growth hormone therapy of Turner's syndrome: beneficial effect on adult height. J Pediatr 1998;132(2):319–24.
[36] Stephure DK, Canadian Growth Hormone Advisory Committee. Impact of growth hormone supplementation on adult height in Turner syndrome: results of the Canadian randomized controlled trial. J Clin Endocrinol Metab 2005;90(6):3360–6.
[37] Reiter EO, Blethen SL, Baptista J, et al. Early initiation of growth hormone treatment allows age-appropriate estrogen use in Turner's syndrome. J Clin Endocrinol Metab 2001;86(5):1936–41.
[38] Bondy CA, Turner Syndrome Study Group. Care of girls and women with Turner syndrome: a guideline of the Turner Syndrome Study Group. J Clin Endocrinol Metab 2007;92(1):10–25.
[39] Davenport ML, Crowe BJ, Travers SH, et al. Growth hormone treatment of early growth failure in toddlers with Turner syndrome: a randomized, controlled, multicenter trial. J Clin Endocrinol Metab 2007;92(9):3406–16.

[40] Rosenfeld RG, Hintz RL, Johanson AJ, et al. Methionyl human growth hormone and oxandrolone in Turner syndrome: preliminary results of a prospective randomized trial. J Pediatr 1986;109(6):936–43.
[41] Frias JL, Davenport ML, Committee on Genetics and Section on Endocrinology. Health supervision for children with Turner syndrome. Pediatrics 2003;111(3):692–702.
[42] Chernausek SD, Attie KM, Cara JF, et al. Growth hormone therapy of Turner syndrome: the impact of age of estrogen replacement on final height. Genentech, Inc, Collaborative Study Group. J Clin Endocrinol Metab 2000;85(7):2439–45.
[43] Plotnick L, Attie KM, Blethen SL, et al. Growth hormone treatment of girls with Turner syndrome: the National Cooperative Growth Study experience. Pediatrics 1998;102(2 Pt 3): 479–81.
[44] Saenger P. Growth-promoting strategies in Turner's syndrome. J Clin Endocrinol Metab 1999;84(12):4345–8.
[45] van Pareren YK, de Muinck Keizer-Schrama SM, Stijnen T, et al. Final height in girls with Turner syndrome after long-term growth hormone treatment in three dosages and low dose estrogens. J Clin Endocrinol Metab 2003;88(3):1119–25.
[46] Ranke MB, Lindberg A, Chatelain P, et al. Prediction of long-term response to recombinant human growth hormone in Turner syndrome: development and validation of mathematical models. KIGS International Board. Kabi International Growth Study. J Clin Endocrinol Metab 2000;85(11):4212–8.
[47] Darendeliler F, Aycan Z, Cetinkaya E, et al. Effects of growth hormone on growth, insulin resistance and related hormones (ghrelin, leptin and adiponectin) in Turner syndrome. Horm Res 2007;68(1):1–7.
[48] Collett-Solberg PF, Pessoa de Queiroz AN, Cardoso ME, et al. The correlation of the IGF-I, IGFBP-3, and ALS generation test to height velocity after 6 months of recombinant growth hormone therapy in girls with Turner syndrome. Growth Horm IGF Res 2006;16(4): 240–6.
[49] Carrel AL, Myers SE, Whitman BY, et al. Long-term growth hormone therapy changes the natural history of body composition and motor function in children with Prader-Willi syndrome. J Clin Endocrinol Metab 2010;95(3):1131–6.
[50] Carrel AL, Moerchen V, Myers SE, et al. Growth hormone improves mobility and body composition in infants and toddlers with Prader-Willi syndrome. J Pediatr 2004;145(6): 744–9.
[51] Myers SE, Whitman BY, Carrel AL, et al. Two years of growth hormone therapy in young children with Prader-Willi syndrome: physical and neurodevelopmental benefits. Am J Med Genet A 2007;143(5):443–8.
[52] Lindgren AC, Lindberg A. Growth hormone treatment completely normalizes adult height and improves body composition in Prader-Willi syndrome: experience from KIGS (Pfizer International Growth Database). Horm Res 2008;70(3):182–7.
[53] Tauber M, Cutfield W, Tauber M, et al. KIGS highlights: growth hormone treatment in Prader-Willi syndrome. Horm Res 2007;68(Suppl 5):48–50.
[54] Usher R, McLean F. Intrauterine growth of live-born Caucasian infants at sea level: standards obtained from measurements in 7 dimensions of infants born between 25 and 44 weeks of gestation. J Pediatr 1969;74(6):901–10.
[55] Hediger ML, Overpeck MD, Maurer KR, et al. Growth of infants and young children born small or large for gestational age: findings from the Third National Health and Nutrition Examination Survey. Arch Pediatr Adolesc Med 1998;152(12):1225–31.
[56] Karlberg JP, Albertsson-Wikland K, Kwan EY, et al. The timing of early postnatal catch-up growth in normal, full-term infants born short for gestational age. Horm Res 1997;1:17–24.
[57] Van Pareren Y, Mulder P, Houdijk M, et al. Adult height after long-term, continuous growth hormone (GH) treatment in short children born small for gestational age: results of a randomized, double-blind, dose-response GH trial. J Clin Endocrinol Metab 2003;88(8): 3584–90.

[58] Albertsson-Wikland K, Karlberg J. Postnatal growth of children born small for gestational age. Acta Paediatr Suppl 1997;423:193–5.
[59] de Zegher F, Albertsson-Wikland K, Wollmann HA, et al. Growth hormone treatment of short children born small for gestational age: growth responses with continuous and discontinuous regimens over 6 years. J Clin Endocrinol Metab 2000;85(8):2816–21.
[60] Ranke M, Wilton P, editors. Growth hormone therapy in KIGS: 10 years' experience. Heidelberg (Germany): Barth Verlag; 1999.
[61] Ranke MB, Lindberg A, Cowell CT, et al. Prediction of response to growth hormone treatment in short children born small for gestational age: analysis of data from KIGS (Pharmacia International Growth Database). J Clin Endocrinol Metab 2003;88(1):125–31.
[62] Fjellestad-Paulsen A, Simon D, Czernichow P, et al. Short children born small for gestational age and treated with growth hormone for three years have an important catch-down five years after discontinuation of treatment. J Clin Endocrinol Metab 2004;89(3):1234–9.
[63] US Census Bureau. Profile of general demographic characteristics. Geographic area: United States. US Census 2000. Table DP-1.
[64] Lindsay R, Feldkamp M, Harris D, et al. Utah growth study: growth standards and the prevalence of growth hormone deficiency. J Pediatr 1994;125(1):29–35.
[65] Finkelstein BS, Silvers JB, Marrero U, et al. Insurance coverage, physician recommendations, and access to emerging treatments: growth hormone therapy for childhood short stature [see comment]. JAMA 1998;279(9):663–8.
[66] Lifshitz F, Cervantes C. Short stature. In: Lifschitz F, editor. Pediatric endocrinology. 3rd edition. New York: Marcel Dekker; 1996. p. 1–18.
[67] Wilson DM, Frane J. A brief review of the use and utility of growth hormone stimulation testing in the NCGS: do we need to do provocative GH testing? Growth Horm IGF Res 2005;15(Suppl A):S21–5.
[68] Cohen P, Rogol AD, Deal CL, et al. Consensus statement on the diagnosis and treatment of children with idiopathic short stature: a summary of the Growth Hormone Research Society, the Lawson Wilkins Pediatric Endocrine Society, and the European Society for Paediatric Endocrinology Workshop. J Clin Endocrinol Metab 2008;93(11):4210–7.
[69] Miller BS, Zimmerman D. Idiopathic short stature in children. Pediatr Ann 2004;33(3): 177–81.
[70] Hintz RL, Attie KM, Baptista J, et al. Effect of growth hormone treatment on adult height of children with idiopathic short stature. Genentech Collaborative Group [see comment]. N Engl J Med 1999;340(7):502–7.
[71] Leschek EW, Rose SR, Yanovski JA, et al. Effect of growth hormone treatment on adult height in peripubertal children with idiopathic short stature: a randomized, double-blind, placebo-controlled trial [see comment]. J Clin Endocrinol Metab 2004;89(7):3140–8.
[72] Wit JM, Rekers-Mombarg LT, Cutler GB, et al. Growth hormone (GH) treatment to final height in children with idiopathic short stature: evidence for a dose effect [see comment]. J Pediatr 2005;146(1):45–53.
[73] Finkelstein BS, Imperiale TF, Speroff T, et al. Effect of growth hormone therapy on height in children with idiopathic short stature: a meta-analysis. Arch Pediatr Adolesc Med 2002;156(3):230–40.
[74] Ranke MB, Lindberg A, Price DA, et al. Age at growth hormone therapy start and first-year responsiveness to growth hormone are major determinants of height outcome in idiopathic short stature. Horm Res 2007;68(2):53–62.
[75] Cohen P, Germak J, Rogol AD, et al. Variable degree of growth hormone (GH) and insulin-like growth factor (IGF) sensitivity in children with idiopathic short stature compared with GH-deficient patients: evidence from an IGF-based dosing study of short children. J Clin Endocrinol Metab 2010;95(5):2089–98.
[76] Binder G, Ranke MB, Martin DD, et al. Auxology is a valuable instrument for the clinical diagnosis of SHOX haploinsufficiency in school-age children with unexplained short stature. J Clin Endocrinol Metab 2003;88(10):4891–6.

[77] Huber C, Rosilio M, Munnich A, et al. High incidence of SHOX anomalies in individuals with short stature. J Med Genet 2006;43(9):735–9.
[78] Rappold GA, Fukami M, Niesler B, et al. Deletions of the homeobox gene SHOX (short stature homeobox) are an important cause of growth failure in children with short stature. J Clin Endocrinol Metab 2002;87(3):1402–6.
[79] Blum WF, Cao D, Hesse V, et al. Height gains in response to growth hormone treatment to final height are similar in patients with SHOX deficiency and Turner syndrome. Horm Res 2009;71(3):167–72.
[80] Romano AA, Allanson JE, Dahlgren J, et al. Noonan syndrome: clinical features, diagnosis, and management guidelines. Pediatrics 2010;126(4):746–59.
[81] Ranke MB, Heidemann P, Knupfer C, et al. Noonan syndrome: growth and clinical manifestations in 144 cases. Eur J Pediatr 1988;148(3):220–7.
[82] Shaw AC, Kalidas K, Crosby AH, et al. The natural history of Noonan syndrome: a long-term follow-up study. Arch Dis Child 2007;92(2):128–32.
[83] Zenker M, Buheitel G, Rauch R, et al. Genotype-phenotype correlations in Noonan syndrome. J Pediatr 2004;144(3):368–74.
[84] Ko JM, Kim JM, Kim GH, et al. PTPN11, SOS1, KRAS, and RAF1 gene analysis, and genotype-phenotype correlation in Korean patients with Noonan syndrome. J Hum Genet 2008;53(11–12):999–1006.
[85] Noordam C, van der Burgt I, Sweep CG, et al. Growth hormone (GH) secretion in children with Noonan syndrome: frequently abnormal without consequences for growth or response to GH treatment. Clin Endocrinol 2001;54(1):53–9.
[86] Limal JM, Parfait B, Cabrol S, et al. Noonan syndrome: relationships between genotype, growth, and growth factors. J Clin Endocrinol Metab 2006;91(1):300–6.
[87] MacFarlane CE, Brown DC, Johnston LB, et al. Growth hormone therapy and growth in children with Noonan's syndrome: results of 3 years' follow-up. J Clin Endocrinol Metab 2001;86(5):1953–6.
[88] Kirk JM, Betts PR, Butler GE, et al. Short stature in Noonan syndrome: response to growth hormone therapy. Arch Dis Child 2001;84(5):440–3.
[89] Ferreira LV, Souza SA, Arnhold IJ, et al. PTPN11 (protein tyrosine phosphatase, nonreceptor type 11) mutations and response to growth hormone therapy in children with Noonan syndrome. J Clin Endocrinol Metab 2005;90(9):5156–60.
[90] Noordam C, Peer PG, Francois I, et al. Long-term GH treatment improves adult height in children with Noonan syndrome with and without mutations in protein tyrosine phosphatase, non-receptor-type 11. Eur J Endocrinol 2008;159(3):203–8.
[91] Municchi G, Pasquino AM, Pucarelli I, et al. Growth hormone treatment in Noonan syndrome: report of four cases who reached final height. Horm Res 1995;44(4): 164–7.
[92] Osio D, Dahlgren J, Wikland KA, et al. Improved final height with long-term growth hormone treatment in Noonan syndrome. Acta Paediatr 2005;94(9):1232–7.
[93] Raaijmakers R, Noordam C, Karagiannis G, et al. Response to growth hormone treatment and final height in Noonan syndrome in a large cohort of patients in the KIGS database. J Pediatr Endocrinol 2008;21(3):267–73.
[94] Romano AA, Dana K, Bakker B, et al. Growth response, near-adult height, and patterns of growth and puberty in patients with Noonan syndrome treated with growth hormone. J Clin Endocrinol Metab 2009;94(7):2338–44.
[95] Bell J, Parker KL, Swinford RD, et al. Long-term safety of recombinant human growth hormone in children. J Clin Endocrinol Metab 2010;95(1):167–77.
[96] Wilton P, Mattsson AF, Darendeliler F, et al. Growth hormone treatment in children is not associated with an increase in the incidence of cancer: experience from KIGS (Pfizer International Growth Database). J Pediatr 2010;157(2):265–70.

[97] Pitukcheewanont P, Desrosiers P, Steelman J, et al. Issues and trends in pediatric growth hormone therapy–an update from the GHMonitor observational registry. Pediatr Endocrinol Rev 2008;5(Suppl 2):702–7.
[98] Ross J, Lee PA, Gut R, et al. Factors influencing the one- and two-year growth response in children treated with growth hormone: analysis from an observational study. Int J Pediatr Endocrinol 2010;2010:494656.
[99] ClinicalTrials.gov. Observational study of somatropin treatment in children (GeNeSIS). 2011. Available at: http://clinicaltrials.gov/ct2/show/NCT01088412. Published 2010. Updated 3/16/10. Accessed May 3, 2011.
[100] Whittington JE, Holland AJ, Webb T, et al. Population prevalence and estimated birth incidence and mortality rate for people with Prader-Willi syndrome in one UK Health Region. J Med Genet 2001;38(11):792–8.
[101] Tauber M, Diene G, Molinas C, et al. Review of 64 cases of death in children with Prader-Willi syndrome (PWS). Am J Med Genet A 2008;146(7):881–7.
[102] Festen DA, de Weerd AW, van den Bossche RA, et al. Sleep-related breathing disorders in prepubertal children with Prader-Willi syndrome and effects of growth hormone treatment. J Clin Endocrinol Metab 2006;91(12):4911–5.
[103] Miller J, Silverstein J, Shuster J, et al. Short-term effects of growth hormone on sleep abnormalities in Prader-Willi syndrome. J Clin Endocrinol Metab 2006;91(2):413–7.
[104] Gravholt CH, Landin-Wilhelmsen K, Stochholm K, et al. Clinical and epidemiological description of aortic dissection in Turner's syndrome. Cardiol Young 2006;16(5):430–6.
[105] Davenport ML, Davenport ML. Approach to the patient with Turner syndrome. J Clin Endocrinol Metab 2010;95(4):1487–95.
[106] Chan JM, Stampfer MJ, Giovannucci E, et al. Plasma insulin-like growth factor-I and prostate cancer risk: a prospective study. Science 1998;279(5350):563–6.
[107] Giovannucci E, Pollak M, Platz EA, et al. Insulin-like growth factor I (IGF-I), IGF-binding protein-3 and the risk of colorectal adenoma and cancer in the Nurses' Health Study. Growth Horm IGF Res 2000;10(Suppl A):S30–1.
[108] Hankinson SE, Willett WC, Colditz GA, et al. Circulating concentrations of insulin-like growth factor-I and risk of breast cancer. Lancet 1998;351(9113):1393–6.
[109] Sachdev D, Yee D, Sachdev D, et al. Disrupting insulin-like growth factor signaling as a potential cancer therapy. Mol Cancer Ther 2007;6(1):1–12.
[110] Perry JK, Emerald BS, Mertani HC, et al. The oncogenic potential of growth hormone. Growth Horm IGF Res 2006;16(5–6):277–89.
[111] Yakar S, Leroith D, Brodt P, et al. The role of the growth hormone/insulin-like growth factor axis in tumor growth and progression: lessons from animal models. Cytokine Growth Factor Rev 2005;16(4–5):407–20.
[112] Watanabe S, Tsunematsu Y, Fujimoto J, et al. Leukaemia in patients treated with growth hormone. Lancet 1988;1(8595):1159–60.
[113] Swerdlow AJ, Higgins CD, Adlard P, et al. Risk of cancer in patients treated with human pituitary growth hormone in the UK, 1959–85: a cohort study. Lancet 2002;360(9329):273–7.
[114] Ergun-Longmire B, Mertens AC, Mitby P, et al. Growth hormone treatment and risk of second neoplasms in the childhood cancer survivor. J Clin Endocrinol Metab 2006;91(9):3494–8.
[115] Gordon K. Pediatric pseudotumor cerebri: descriptive epidemiology. Can J Neurol Sci 1997;24(3):219–21.
[116] Darendeliler F, Karagiannis G, Wilton P, et al. Headache, idiopathic intracranial hypertension and slipped capital femoral epiphysis during growth hormone treatment: a safety update from the KIGS database. Horm Res 2007;68(Suppl 5):41–7.

[117] Nydegger A, Heine RG, Ranuh R, et al. Changing incidence of acute pancreatitis: 10-year experience at the Royal Children's Hospital, Melbourne. J Gastroenterol Hepatol 2007;22(8):1313–6.
[118] Gelding SV, Taylor NF, Wood PJ, et al. The effect of growth hormone replacement therapy on cortisol-cortisone interconversion in hypopituitary adults: evidence for growth hormone modulation of extrarenal 11 beta-hydroxysteroid dehydrogenase activity. Clin Endocrinol 1998;48(2):153–62.
[119] Giavoli C, Libe R, Corbetta S, et al. Effect of recombinant human growth hormone (GH) replacement on the hypothalamic-pituitary-adrenal axis in adult GH-deficient patients. J Clin Endocrinol Metab 2004;89(11):5397–401.
[120] Mills JL, Schonberger LB, Wysowski DK, et al. Long-term mortality in the United States cohort of pituitary-derived growth hormone recipients. J Pediatr 2004;144(4):430–6.
[121] Shulman DI, Palmert MR, Kemp SF, et al. Adrenal insufficiency: still a cause of morbidity and death in childhood. Pediatrics 2007;119(2):e484–94.
[122] Henrikson B. The incidence of slipped capital femoral epiphysis. Acta Orthop Scand 1969;40(3):365–72.
[123] Kelsey JL, Keggi KJ, Southwick WO. The incidence and distribution of slipped capital femoral epiphysis in Connecticut and Southwestern United States. J Bone Joint Surg Am 1970;52(6):1203–16.
[124] Fine RN, Stablein D, Cohen AH, et al. Recombinant human growth hormone post-renal transplantation in children: a randomized controlled study of the NAPRTCS. Kidney Int 2002;62(2):688–96.
[125] Tonshoff B, Haffner D, Mehls O, et al. Efficacy and safety of growth hormone treatment in short children with renal allografts: three year experience. Members of the German Study Group for Growth Hormone Treatment in Children with Renal Allografts. Kidney Int 1993;44(1):199–207.
[126] Dharnidharka VR, Talley LI, Martz KL, et al. Recombinant growth hormone use pretransplant and risk for post-transplant lymphoproliferative disease–a report of the NAPRTCS. Pediatr Transplant 2008;12(6):689–95.
[127] European Medicines Agency. European Medicines Agency to review the safety of somatropin-containing medicines. Available at: http://www.ema.europa.eu/docs/en_GB/document_library/Press_release/2010/12/WC500099699.pdf. Published 2010. Updated 12/10/2010. Accessed May 3, 2011.
[128] AFSSAPS. Hormone de Croissance synthétique (somatropine recombinante): premiers résultats de l'étude épidémiologique sur la tolérance à long terme - communiqué. Available at: http://www.afssaps.fr/Infos-de-securite/Communiques-Points-presse/Hormone-de-Croissance-synthetique-somatropine-recombinante-Premiers-resultats-de-l-etude-epidemiologique-sur-la-tolerance-a-long-terme-Communique. Published 2010. Updated 12/10/2010. Accessed May 3, 2011.
[129] European Medicines Agency. Update on somatropin-containing medicines Available at: http://www.ema.europa.eu/docs/en_GB/document_library/Press_release/2010/12/WC500099936.pdf. Published 2010. Updated 12/16/2010. Accessed May 3, 2011.
[130] U.S. Food & Drug Administration. Recombinant human growth hormone (somatropin): ongoing safety review - possible increased risk of death. Available at: http://www.fda.gov/Safety/MedWatch/SafetyInformation/SafetyAlertsforHumanMedicalProducts/ucm237969.htm. Published 2010. Updated 12/22/2010. Accessed May 3, 2011.
[131] ClinicalTrials.gov. rhGH and rhIGF-1 combination therapy in children with short stature associated with IGF-1 deficiency. Available at: http://clinicaltrials.gov/ct2/show/NCT00572156. Published 2007. Updated 9/14/10. Accessed May 3, 2011.
[132] Midyett LK, Rogol AD, Van Meter QL, et al. Recombinant insulin-like growth factor (IGF)-I treatment in short children with low IGF-I levels: first-year results from a randomized clinical trial. J Clin Endocrinol Metab 2010;95(2):611–9.

[133] ClinicalTrials.gov. IGFD Registry: a patient registry for monitoring long-term safety and efficacy of increlex. Available at: http://clinicaltrialsgov/ct2/show/NCT00747604. Published 2008. Updated 1/26/2011. Accessed May 3, 2011.
[134] Silverman BL, Blethen SL, Reiter EO, et al. A long-acting human growth hormone (Nutropin Depot): efficacy and safety following two years of treatment in children with growth hormone deficiency. J Pediatr Endocrinol 2002;15(Suppl 2):715–22.
[135] Fuhr U, Tuculanu D, Berghout A, et al. Bioequivalence between novel ready-to-use liquid formulations of the recombinant human GH Omnitrope and the original lyophilized formulations for reconstitution of Omnitrope and Genotropin. Eur J Endocrinol 2010;162(6): 1051–8.

Advances in Pediatrics 58 (2011) 243–258

ADVANCES IN PEDIATRICS

Update on Precocious Puberty: Girls are Showing Signs of Puberty Earlier, but Most Do Not Require Treatment

Paul Kaplowitz, MD, PhD

Division of Endocrinology, Children's National Medical Center, George Washington University School of Medicine and the Health Sciences, 111 Michigan Avenue, North West, Washington, DC 20010, USA

Precocious puberty is one of the most common endocrine disorders seen by primary care physicians and continues to be a major source of concern for both parents and providers. Since the author's previous review on this subject in *Advances In Pediatrics* in 2004 [1], there have been several reports that have added to the knowledge base and confirmed that signs of puberty in girls are appearing earlier than in the past in the United States as well as in other countries. In this article, the author reviews what pediatricians should know about the physical findings seen during normal puberty and their hormonal basis. The evidence that signs of puberty are appearing earlier than 30 to 40 years ago, at least in girls, and the major theories about why this might be occurring are also discussed. However, the key point to be made is that pediatricians should be able to recognize the benign causes of early breast and pubic hair development, which are, at least in the United States, far more common than the cases that might benefit from treatment. The current state of knowledge concerning the diagnosis and treatment of central (true) precocious puberty (CPP) and the red flags that might point toward one of the rare causes of gonadotropin-independent precocious puberty (GIPP) are then reviewed.

REVIEW OF NORMAL PUBERTY

In girls, the first sign of true puberty is breast development, caused by estrogens produced by the ovaries, under the influence of increased pituitary secretion of the gonadotropin, luteinizing hormone (LH). There is also an increase in follicle-stimulating hormone (FSH), which is more critical for maturation of the immature oocytes. Traditionally, it has been thought that the normal age range for this event, also called thelarche, is between 8 and 13 years; however, as discussed later, there is ample evidence that in many healthy girls, this event can occur before the age of 8 years. Shortly after breasts appear, the pubertal growth spurt starts, and menarche occurs 2 to 3 years later because

E-mail address: pkaplowi@cnmc.org

0065-3101/11/$ – see front matter
doi:10.1016/j.yapd.2011.03.004

gonadotropin secretion increases so that there is a midcycle surge of LH, which triggers ovulation.

According to a recent longitudinal study, the appearance of pubic and/or axillary hair follows the appearance of breast tissue in 66% of girls [2]. This occurrence is often confused with the onset of puberty, but has a different hormonal basis, due to an increase in the production of weak adrenal androgens, primarily dehydroepiandrosterone (DHEA), an event known as adrenarche. In the average girl, adrenarche starts between the ages of 9 and 11 years but is not uncommon in girls aged 6 to 8 years, a situation called premature pubarche or premature adrenarche (PA), which is discussed below.

In boys, the earliest reliable sign of puberty is enlargement of the testes (>3 cm^3 in volume or >2.5 cm in diameter) under the influence of increased FSH secretion, which occurs at an average age of 11 to 12 years but can occur as early as age 9 years. It typically takes 12 to 18 months after testicular enlargement for testosterone production, under the influence of increasing LH secretion, to increase and cause penile growth and the growth spurt, which in the average boy peaks at 13 to 14 years of age. A recent longitudinal study found that testicular enlargement preceded pubic hair development in 91% of boys [2], but pubic hair may occur several years earlier than genital development because of increased adrenal androgen secretion.

ARE GIRLS MATURING EARLIER? IF SO, HOW SHOULD WE DEFINE WHEN PUBERTAL DEVELOPMENT IS PRECOCIOUS?

For many years, going back to the classic study of Marshall and Tanner [3] in the 1960s, which was based on a nonrandom sample of 192 white British girls living in a group home, the age at which puberty was considered precocious in girls was by consensus thought to be 8 years. A landmark study in 1997, based on 17,000 girls aged 3 to 12 years examined in 65 pediatric offices participating in the Pediatric Research in Office Settings (PROS) network, confirmed what many had already suspected: that appearance of breasts and pubic hair in girls before age 8 years was common [4]. In 8-year-old girls (defined as from the eighth birthday to the day before the ninth birthday), 37.8% of black and 10.5% of white girls had at least Tanner stage 2 breast development, and a similar percentage had pubic hair. Even for 7-year-old girls, the numbers were high, 15.4% of black and 5% of white girls had breast development. An article written by the author suggested revising the definition of precocious puberty in girls downward to age 7 years in white girls and age 6 years in black girls to take into account this new data [5]. However, many objected to this recommendation on the basis that the PROS study was flawed because of the participants not being a randomized sample. In addition, because the Tanner staging was done mainly by inspection and not palpation, the results may have been biased because of the problems distinguishing breast tissue from fat tissue in chubby girls. However, similar results were found in the National Health and Nutrition Examination Survey (NHANES-III), which from 1988 to 1994 examined pubertal status in 1623 girls between the ages of 8 and 16 years who were scientifically selected to represent the general population [6]. Recently, new data were reported by Biro and coworkers [7] who examined a cohort of 1239 girls aged 7 and 8 years recruited from 3 centers in East Harlem (NY), greater Cincinnati (OH), and the San Francisco Bay area (CA). The investigators found that the proportion of girls in this group with breast development confirmed by palpation may be even higher than in the 2 earlier studies. The results of these 3 studies are summarized in Table 1. Although there are differences in the numbers reported, the key point is that all studies show a high incidence of early breast development and pubic hair in girls aged 7 to 8 years from all regions of the United States, with the highest percentages seen in black girls.

Another way of looking at pubertal trends in girls is to calculate the mean age of 2 pubertal milestones: thelarche and menarche. The PROS and NHANES-III studies found that the mean age of thelarche, 10.0 to 10.3 years in white girls and 8.8 to 9.5 years in black girls, was earlier than that in previous studies done in the United States and the United Kingdom, which had indicated that the mean age was closer to 11 years. Until recently, most studies from Europe and other industrialized countries had not found any decrease in the mean age of breast development from the 1960s to the 1990s. However, the Copenhagen Puberty Study done from 2006 to 2008 found that girls attained stage 2 breast development at a mean age of 9.86 years, a full year earlier than the previous study done in 1991 to 1993 by the same research group, using the same methodology [8]. Even when adjustments were made for body mass index (BMI), which changed little between the 2 cohorts, the difference remained significant. Furthermore, a recent study on more than 20,000 healthy girls living in China found that the median age for Tanner stage 2 breast development was only 9.2 years, with the median age for Tanner 2 pubic hair significantly later at 11.16

Table 1
Proportion of 7- and 8-year-old girls[a] with breast development and pubic hair from 3 recent US studies

	Percentage with breast development			Percentage with pubic hair		
	PROS (%)	NHANES III (%)	Biro et al (%) [7]	PROS (%)	NHANES III (%)	Biro et al (%) [7]
White (7 y)	5.0	—	10.4	2.8	—	6.4
Black (7 y)	15.4	—	23.4	17.6	—	20.0
Hispanic (7 y)	—	—	14.9	—	—	6.7
White (8 y)	10.5	11.4	18.3	7.7	6.5	10.1
Black (8 y)	37.8	27.8	42.9	34.3	30.4	31.6
Hispanic (8 y)	—	25.4	30.9	—	6.7	18.9

[a]In all the studies mentioned in this table, the definition of 7-year-old girls is any age from the seventh birthday to the day before their eighth birthday, and similarly for 8-year-old girls. Only the NHANES III study is a nationally representative sample.

Data from Refs. [4,6,7].

years and the median age at menarche 12.27 years [9]. Despite the rather dramatic declines reported for the mean age of thelarche, changes in the mean age at menarche have been more modest. In the United States, the PROS study found no decrease in age at menarche when compared with an earlier study in 1966 to 1970 (both 12.7–12.8 years), whereas in the NHANES III study, age at menarche decreased slightly to 12.5 years [6]. A more recent NHANES survey done from 1999 to 2004 found the mean age at menarche for women born from 1980 to 1984 to be 12.4 years [10]. In the Copenhagen study, the mean age at menarche declined from 13.42 years in 1991 to 13.13 years in 2006, again less than the magnitude of the decline in the mean age at thelarche [8]. It is also noteworthy that the mean interval from thelarche to menarche was (13.13–9.82) 3.3 years, much longer than the mean interval of 2.3 ± 1.1 years reported by Marshall and Tanner [3]. This finding suggests either 1) that it now takes long for most girls to progress from thelarche to menarche than in the past or 2) that a significant number of contemporary girls have a nonprogressive or slowly progressive variant of puberty and may not progress at all for a year or two after the first sign of breast development [11].

The key question pediatricians struggle with remains this: given that many studies show a trend toward earlier breast (as well as pubic hair) development, at what age should signs of puberty in girls be considered abnormal and thus trigger a referral to an endocrinologist. As noted earlier, a 1999 review suggested that the age limits for when puberty is considered precocious should be decreased to 7 years in white and 6 years in black girls [5]. Although the proportion of 7-year-old girls with signs of puberty is quite high, most specialists and pediatricians still feel more comfortable with the traditional cutoff of 8 years, even though this cutoff labels many girls as abnormal who are undoubtedly at the lower end of the current normal range for pubertal maturation. The author believes that rather than focusing on one age as separating normal from abnormal, the rate of progression of pubertal maturation in deciding how concerned to be about a particular child should be taken into account. For example, in a 7.5-year-old girl with a small amount of breast tissue (Tanner stage 2) on examination and no evidence of a growth spurt, pubertal maturation may progress slowly and often the findings remain the same 6 months later; this girl does not benefit from treatment to suppress puberty (see later). On the other hand, an 8.25-year-old girl who is at Tanner 3 for breast development and has grown 3–4 inches in the past year is clearly progressing more rapidly and needs prompt evaluation. In addition, pediatricians should be more concerned about girls with early and progressive breast development with or without pubic hair than girls who only have pubic hair because girls in the latter group rarely have a condition requiring intervention.

ARE BOYS MATURING EARLIER THAN IN THE PAST AND WHEN SHOULD THEY BE REFERRED?

For many years, the definition of precocious puberty in boys has been signs of maturation starting before the age of 9 years, but there have been relatively few studies on whether the mean age at the onset of puberty in boys has decreased over the past 30 to 40 years. One report based on the NHANES III study seemed to indicate that stage 2 genital growth, a more reliable sign of puberty in boys than pubic hair, was occurring much earlier than earlier studies had found, with a mean age of about 10 years [12]. However, the accuracy of sexual maturation ratings in this survey has been questioned. A study of male puberty in the United States undertaken by the PROS network is nearing completion, and these data should be available in the near future. In the Copenhagen Puberty Study, it was recently reported that compared with the period from 1991 to 1993, boys examined during 2006 to 2008 had slightly earlier attainment of testicular volume of greater than 3 cm^3, which correlated with an increase in BMI [13]. Unlike the situation for girls, it is generally agreed that endocrinologists have observed no increase in the past 40 years in the number of boys referred for true precocious puberty. At present there is no reason to change the age at which pubertal development in boys is considered precocious, which should remain 9 years.

WHAT CAN WE SAY ABOUT WHY GIRLS ARE STARTING PUBERTY EARLIER?

This topic was discussed at length in the author's article in 2004 for this series, and in this section, the author mainly highlights recent articles that bear on the subject. The relationship between increased body fat (typically measured as elevated BMI for age) and earlier puberty has been summarized in a recent review [14]. Multiple studies have documented that higher BMI (which is a good surrogate measure of increased body fat) is correlated with earlier onset of breast development, pubic hair, and menarche. Although the precise cause of this relationship is not known, one possibility is that higher levels of the fat cell–derived protein leptin, seen in children with increased body fat, allow puberty to start earlier. Leptin is required for normal gonadotropin secretion because mice and humans lacking the ability to produce or respond to leptin fail to make LH and FSH, and providing leptin to leptin-deficient mice results in the onset of puberty. One area of debate is whether earlier puberty itself is the cause of the increase in body fat or if an increase in body fat precedes and causes the earlier appearance of breast development. A recent article by Lee and colleagues [15] presented findings that favor the latter interpretation. The study included 354 girls from the National Institute of Child Health and Human Development Study of Early Child Care and Youth Development for whom there was longitudinal data on BMI at ages 36 and 54 months and grades 1, 4, 5, and 6, with pubertal assessments by physical examination in grades 4 to 6. The investigators found that elevated BMI standard deviation scores at ages 36 and 54 months and in grade 1 and the rate of change in BMI from 36 months to grade 1 were associated with increased odds of earlier puberty (defined as Tanner $\geq$2 breasts in grade 4 or Tanner $\geq$3 breasts in grade 6). This finding suggests that well before the onset of puberty, as early as 3 years of age, the presence of increased BMI is an important factor in determining the age of onset of puberty in girls in the United States. It is curious that the same relationship between increased BMI and the timing of puberty has not consistently been found in boys. A recent study from the same group found that boys who were in the highest BMI trajectory through 11.5 years had a significantly higher chance of remaining prepubertal than boys in the lowest BMI trajectory [16], suggesting that increased body fat does not promote earlier puberty in boys, at least in the United States; this contrasts with the recent findings in Danish boys.

Many clinicians and investigators have proposed that chemicals in the environment with weak estrogenlike properties, including certain pesticides, phthalates, bisphenol A, and plant-derived phytoestrogens, or low levels of estrogens itself in the food supply are driving the trend toward earlier puberty in girls [17,18]. The investigators of one review pointed out that prepubertal girls are extremely sensitive to low levels of exogenous estrogens and that exposures previously thought to be safe based on less-sensitive measures of estradiol levels in young children may in fact have important effects on growth and pubertal development, even at levels below the detection limits of most assays [17]. However, except in a few isolated cases, evidence for specific exposures linked to earlier onset of puberty has been difficult to come by. Research on such exposures in girls with earlier pubertal development is ongoing, but it is recognized that examining blood or urine levels of these chemicals in a 7- to 8-year-old girl may miss a potentially higher level of exposure to one or more of these chemicals in the critical perinatal period.

COMMON VARIATIONS OF PUBERTAL DEVELOPMENT

Pediatricians confronted with a child with early breast development or pubic hair need to know how to distinguish the common benign normal variations from children who need prompt referral for possibly treatable conditions, as well as the limited usefulness of hormone testing and radiography in evaluating such children.

Premature adrenarche

PA is the most common cause of referrals for precocious puberty in many US centers. Table 1 suggests why this entity is so common, especially in black girls, and why it may represent, at least in 6- to 8-year old girls, the lower end of the normal range for pubic hair development. At the author's institution, which serves the DC region, over a 2-year period, 430 boys and girls between the ages of 5 and 9 years were referred for signs of early puberty, and 62% were diagnosed as having PA. Of these, 82% were girls. In other parts of the world, the proportion of puberty referrals with PA seems to be much lower. For example, in Israel, of a group of 453 children seen for early puberty over a 5-year period, only 22.2% were diagnosed with PA, whereas 34.4% had CPP [19]. This finding may be at least in part because in certain regions in the United States, there is a high proportion of black children who, as noted in Table 1, are 2 to 3 times more likely than white girls to have early appearance of pubic hair.

The typical features of PA are pubic and/or axillary hair, often accompanied by an adult-type axillary odor, without breast development in girls or penile or testicular enlargement in boys. The amount of pubic hair increases slowly over time, and in many cases, there may be growth acceleration in the year or two before referral, so that most such children are taller than average. The hormonal basis of PA is a precocious increase in secretion of weak androgens of adrenal origin (referred to as adrenarche), primarily DHEA, which is converted to an easily measured storage form, DHEA sulfate (DHEA-S). The cause of this increase is not clear, but it does not seem to be because of an increase in pituitary adrenocorticotropic hormone (ACTH) levels because cortisol levels, which increase when the ACTH level is elevated, are not increased. Several studies have identified obesity as a risk factor for earlier appearance of pubic hair [20,21], but not all children with PA are obese. Another risk factor is having low birth weight. A recent study from Barcelona, Spain found that girls with PA are twice as likely to reach menarche before age 12 years compared with control girls, and among the subset of girls with PA who had low birth weight, menarche before age 12 years was 3-fold more prevalent and adult height was less compared with those in girls who did not have low birth weight [22].

Many pediatricians worry that the appearance of early pubic hair is associated with pathologic conditions often enough that hormonal testing is recommended before referral, as well as radiography of the hand for bone age. In PA, the only hormone level elevated for age is DHEA-S, typically in the range of 30 to 150 μg/dL (DHEA levels are elevated as well but vary much more by time of day than DHEA-S levels and are not clinically useful). The differential diagnosis of early pubic hair development includes adrenal and gonadal androgen-secreting tumors in which DHEA-S levels, testosterone levels, or both are extremely elevated, but those rare cases are generally not difficult to detect because there is enlargement of the clitoris or penis and marked growth acceleration. More difficult to detect clinically but far less worrisome are cases of late-onset or nonclassical congenital adrenal hyperplasia (CAH) due to partial 21-hydroxylase deficiency, the only manifestation of which may be early pubic hair. Studies in which ACTH stimulation testing (the gold standard for diagnosis) has been done in a series of children with PA to check for an exaggerated increase in 17-hydroxyprogesterone (17-OHP) levels have found that between 2% and 8% of children have hormonal findings compatible with nonclassical CAH. A recent study from Paris found nonclassical CAH in 4% of 238 children presenting with early pubic hair, and all had basal 17-OHP levels greater than 200 ng/dL (normal levels in prepubertal children are generally <100 ng/dL) [23].

Testosterone levels may be mildly elevated (20–30 ng/dL) in girls and boys with PA when the tests are run in laboratories which use a traditional radioimmunoassay that is not specific enough for young children. When tested by a more accurate method, liquid chromatography/tandem mass spectrometry, levels are virtually always less than 15 ng/dL. Determination of LH, FSH, and estradiol levels are often recommended in girls with PA but are not helpful because when there is no breast development, there is no need to look for evidence of activation of the pituitary-gonadal axis. In general, it is best to leave the decision as to which tests to order the endocrinologist who will be seeing the child.

The value of a bone age as a screening test to identify pathologic causes of early pubic hair is questionable. The author has seen many cases in which, as a result of finding a bone age advanced by 2 or more years, a large number of tests were recommended, including multiple hormone levels; adrenal and/or pelvic ultrasonography; and, in some cases, brain magnetic resonance imaging (MRI), which did not add anything to the diagnosis. Of the 121 children with PA seen in our department who had a bone age x-ray, 30% had a bone age advanced by 2 or more years [24]. The main difference between these children and those with normal bone ages was that they had greater height and BMI standard deviation scores (ie, they were taller and more likely to be obese). Because bone age advancement is common in PA, is a poor predictor of pathology, and generates considerable anxiety on the part of referring physicians and parents, it is suggested that the decision to order a bone age X-ray be left to the endocrinologist who examines the child.

Several studies have found that girls with PA have an increased risk for polycystic ovary syndrome in the teenage years, particularly for those girls who are born small for gestational age and who are obese [25]. Thus, counseling families of girls with PA on the need to maintain normal body weight is important, and referring those who experience very irregular periods in adolescence to pediatric endocrinologists is advised.

Premature thelarche

Another scenario often encountered is the girl who develops breast tissue, which during a period of observation does not progress. A recent review of 139 cases of premature thelarche (PT) seen at a single center in Israel over a 10-year period indicated that in 42% breast tissue appeared at birth, in 43% between 1 and 24 months, and in only 15% between ages 2 and 8 years [26]. Breast development was bilateral in 78% but had reached stage 3 in only 11%. In most such cases, there is no growth acceleration; pubic hair is occasionally also present but is typically absent. The Israeli study reported that during follow-up, PT regressed in 51%, persisted in 36%, and progressed in only 3%, and 10% had a cyclic course [26]. Therefore, parents should not be counseled to expect resolution of breast tissue. Some investigators have suggested that progression to true precocious puberty occurs often enough that children with this condition need to be monitored for prolonged periods, but the author has never seen this occur in a child with PT starting at less than 3 years of age. Because true precocious puberty starting before age 3 years is uncommon [27], the best approach is reassurance and periodic monitoring of the size of the breasts and the rate of growth, which can be done by the primary care pediatrician after an initial consultation. Laboratory testing is not very helpful in classic cases because LH, FSH, and estradiol levels are invariably in the prepubertal range; pelvic ultrasonography is also not indicated. Bone age may be slightly advanced by 6 to 12 months, but advance of 2 or more years is rare, and ordering a bone age x-ray should be left to the discretion of the endocrinologist.

Genital hair appearing in infancy

Appearance of fine hairs in the genital area in the first year of life (typically along the labia in girls and on the scrotum in boys) seems unusual enough to raise suspicion of an underlying gonadal or adrenal disorder. Typically, the phallus is not enlarged, and there is no evidence of growth acceleration. A recent report of 11 infants seen at a mean age of 8 months found resolution in all cases that returned for follow-up [28], whereas the author's series of 12 such infants found that the genital hair persisted in most. Multiple hormone levels in this series were measured by liquid chromatography/tandem mass spectrometry [29]; in half, there was a slight elevation compared with age-matched controls in DHEA-S levels, suggesting this may be a variant form of PA. In no case was 17-OHP levels elevated, but 1 girl, who had had exposure to testosterone because the father was using a topical androgen (Androgel), had a mild elevation of serum testosterone. As for PA and PT, this entity seems to be a benign normal variation, and routine hormonal and imaging studies are not recommended.

Premature menarche

A puzzling situation that can be easily confused with precocious puberty is the onset of vaginal bleeding in a girl who has not yet started to develop breast tissue, referred to as premature menarche. This occurrence may be described as either intermittent light bleeding or daily spotting continuing for many weeks or episodes of heavier bleeding lasting several days and separated by 3 to 4 weeks. Although these episodes are quite worrisome for the family, they almost always resolve over a period of 1 to 4 months. The differential diagnosis includes such potentially serious conditions as tumors, foreign body inserted into the vagina (which would likely result in a more foul-smelling than bloody vaginal discharge), and sexual abuse. However, in the more than 30 cases seen by the author, the physical examination has invariably been normal, the girls have not acted fearful or withdrawn, and none of these worrisome diagnoses have been found. Pelvic ultrasonographic results are normal but may be useful in reassuring the parents if the bleeding persists for more than a month or two. Hormone testing has not in the author's experience been helpful. The mystery of premature menarche is that one needs estrogen action on the uterus to build up enough endometrium to cause bleeding, but such estrogen exposure should lead to progressive breast enlargement, which is conspicuously absent. There has not been any satisfactory hormonal explanation for this paradox, and nothing new has been published on the subject since the early 1990s.

Central precocious puberty

The diagnosis of CPP should be entertained in girls younger than 8 years who have shown a progressive enlargement in breasts over a period of 4 to 6 months, particularly if accompanied by acceleration of linear growth. It is important to assess breast development by not only inspection but also careful palpation because many chubby girls seem to have breasts while sitting up, but when examined lying down, it is apparent that all or nearly all the tissue under the nipple and areola is adipose. In questionable cases, it is helpful to reexamine the girl in 4 to 6 months to see if the breasts are in fact enlarging because many girls with early breast development have been found to have a nonprogressive or slowly progressive form of precocious puberty, which requires no treatment [11].

Hormonal testing in girls with clearly progressive breast enlargement should be kept simple and may include determining LH, FSH, and estradiol levels, but the LH test is the most reliable for diagnosing CPP. In the past, an increase in LH levels to more than 5 to 8 U/L during stimulation test with gonadotropin-releasing hormone (GnRH) or a synthetic analog of GnRH such as leuprolide was thought to be necessary to confirm the diagnosis of CPP. However, assays for gonadotropins are now more sensitive and specific, and according to a recent study, a single unstimulated LH level of 0.4 U/L or more is sufficient to diagnose CPP in most girls [30]. Prepubertal girls and girls with PT usually have random LH levels less than 0.2 U/L, but some girls with CPP also have low random LH levels, and if the clinical findings are suggestive of CPP, the endocrinologist may perform a GnRH stimulation test. An estradiol level of more than 20 pg/mL is supportive of a diagnosis of CPP, but lower values are sometimes seen in girls who by other criteria clearly are in puberty. Bone age advanced by 2 or more years favors the diagnosis of progressive CPP, but less-advanced bone ages may be seen in patients with CPP of very recent onset.

In boys, the diagnosis of CPP based on physical findings is simpler than in girls, because one will see enlargement of the testes ($\geq$3 cm in diameter or $\geq$6 mL in volume), reflecting increased gonadotropin secretion, as well as growth of the stretched penis to more than 8 cm in length because of increased testosterone levels, generally more than 50 ng/dL, can be seen. If the testes are prepubertal and pubic hair is the main finding, the diagnosis is likely to be PA, which does not require any intervention.

Which children with CPP benefit from treatment?

In November 2007, representatives of the Lawson Wilkins Pediatric Endocrine Society and the European Society for Pediatric Endocrinology met to develop consensus guidelines for the use of GnRH analogs (GnRHas) in children, which were published in *Pediatrics* in 2009 [31]. One key point was that progressive pubertal development and growth acceleration should be documented over a 3- to 6-month period before starting GnRHa therapy, unless a girl is already at Tanner 3 or greater for breast development, in which case an observation period may not be necessary. There was also consensus that the most compelling reason to treat CPP was to prevent compromise of adult stature because of early closure of the epiphyses; however, it has been found that many girls with the slowly progressive form of CPP achieve a normal adult height without treatment [11]. Long-term follow-up studies have shown that the greatest gain in adult height versus that predicted at the time of diagnosis (average of 9–10 cm with much variation among different studies) is seen in girls with onset of puberty before age 6 years, who make up only a small proportion of girls evaluated for precocious puberty. Some girls with onset of puberty between ages 6 and 8 years achieve a modest improvement in adult height with treatment, but an Israeli study found that treatment of girls whose puberty started at ages 8 to 9 years did not improve adult height compared with that predicted based on bone age [32]. At diagnosis, many girls with CPP are quite tall, so that even though the bone age is advanced and growth will be completed at an earlier than normal age, adult height will usually be within the normal range. Thus, parents of a tall girl with early puberty should not be advised that treatment is needed to prevent their child ending up abnormally short.

The greatest concern of many parents of girls with CPP is the potential psychological effect of early menses. The consensus statement points out that using GnRHas solely to delay menses or to alleviate the consequences of a girl being more physically developed than her peers has not been convincingly shown to improve psychological outcomes [31], although controlled studies addressing this issue are lacking. Girls who start puberty at age 8 years or later rarely reach menarche before age 10 years, and according to the author's experience, few experience severe stress, particularly if a parent has discussed this with them ahead of time. Girls with developmental delay sometimes have more difficulties in this area and may benefit from treatment to delay menses, although the use of inexpensive alternatives, such as extended use of combined oral contraceptive, which can be interrupted every 3 months to allow less-frequent periods, or medroxyprogesterone acetate (Depo-Provera) given intramuscularly every 3 months, should be considered before using GnRHas [33]. For girls starting puberty before age 7 years, which progresses rapidly, there is a good chance that menarche will occur by age 9 years, which is often very stressful for both the child and mother, and many parents opt for treatment to delay menses. For girls in whom puberty starts between age 7 and 8 years and progresses, advising the parents on how to prepare the child for early menarche sometimes results in a lower stress level than undertaking a course of treatment to suppress puberty with its frequent injections and follow-up visits.

Most cases of CPP are idiopathic and many seem to be inherited. In an Israeli study that included 156 children (mostly girls) with CPP, 27.5% were thought to have a genetic basis, with most inherited in an autosomal dominant fashion with incomplete penetrance [19]. The proportion of patients with CPP because of a central nervous system (CNS) lesion is low but varies a lot from study to study. The question of whether all girls with CPP require a brain MRI to rule out CNS lesions (astrocytomas, gliomas, hamartomas, or cysts in the area of the pituitary or hypothalamus) is controversial. One study from Paris found abnormal brain imaging in 19% of girls with onset of CPP before age of 6 years but in only 2% of those with onset between the ages of 6 and 8 years [27]. Although many endocrinologists in the United States do not routinely perform MRIs in all 6- to 8-year-old girls with CPP, European endocrinologists are more likely to do so. The consensus conference on the use of GnRHas concluded that all boys with CPP (in whom the incidence of CNS lesions is higher) and girls with onset of puberty before age 6 years require an MRI of the head, whereas for older girls, those with neurologic findings (eg, severe headaches) and those with very rapid progression are more likely to have intracranial pathology [31].

How is CPP treated?

GnRHas acutely stimulate LH and FSH secretion, but when given chronically, these hormones shut off pituitary gonadotropin and estradiol production because the gonadotrophs are programmed to respond to pulses of GnRH secreted by the hypothalamus every 1 to 2 hours and are desensitized by continuous exposure. The most widely used preparation in the United States is Lupron Depot, a slow release form of leuprolide, which is administered by intramuscular injection every 28 days. The typical starting dose is 7.5 mg, with a current average retail price of $9500 per year. Some patients require larger doses or more frequent administration for complete gonadotropin suppression; for the higher 11.25-mg dose given every 4 weeks, the cost comes to about $18,000 per year. There have been pediatric studies of 3-month formulations of Lupron Depot, approved for women with endometriosis and men with advanced prostate cancer. One study suggested that the 11.25-mg dose works as well in most patients as the 7.5-mg monthly preparation for clinical suppression of pubertal development [34]. Suppression of stimulated gonadotropin levels was not as complete, but there was no difference in sex steroid levels in patients on the 2 different regimens. Although the medication itself is very safe, up to 5% of patients develop painful swelling at the site of the injection. Girls who have started menstruating sometimes have 1 additional period before they stop, after which menses do not resume until at least 6 months after the medication is discontinued. In most cases, there is a decrease in the amount of glandular breast tissue within a few months, but slowing of the rapid growth rate may take a few months longer. Treatment is typically stopped at 10 to 11 years of age.

There is now another therapeutic option for girls with CPP, which is a subcutaneous implant of the GnRHa histrelin, called Supprelin, which slowly releases active medication for 12 months [35]. Clinical trials have shown it to be at least as effective as the injectable formulations, with the main disadvantage being the need to have the implants placed (and a year later removed) by a surgeon, typically under localized or light general anesthesia.

Long-term follow-up studies, summarized in the consensus statement, indicate that treatment with GnRHas have no consequences on reproductive function [31]. The time from end of treatment to onset of menses is quite variable and averages about 16 months. Regular cycles occur in the same proportion as in the general population, and no increase in the rate of infertility has been reported. Bone mineral density has been found in some studies to be decreased during treatment, which is expected because of the loss of estrogen effect on bone mass accrual, but after cessation of therapy, bone density normalizes and there is no long-term effect on peak bone mass achieved.

Gonadotropin-independent precocious puberty

A small proportion of boys and girls presenting with signs of progressive pubertal development have conditions in which the production of sex steroids is independent of increasing gonadotropin secretion. All these conditions are rare, and so individually they do not merit detailed discussion. This section focuses on the red flags that might point to one of these conditions, which can then be promptly referred to a subspecialist for further evaluation.

Girls

Estrogen-producing ovarian tumors are characterized by rapid progression of breast development and growth acceleration, accompanied by very high levels of estradiol (often >100 pg/mL) and suppressed levels of LH and FSH. The same scenario can be seen in McCune-Albright syndrome, which may be suspected on the basis of cystic bone lesions (polyostotic fibrous dysplasia) and irregular café-au-lait areas of skin pigmentation. In some cases, vaginal bleeding may precede breast development but usually before 3 years of age, younger than in most patients with premature menarche. Young girls with virilization, the most obvious sign of which is clitoral enlargement (often more impressive than the amount of pubic hair), need prompt evaluation to rule out the rare androgen-producing adrenal or ovarian tumor or nonclassical CAH. On the other hand, isolated stable clitoral enlargement without pubic hair or growth acceleration is usually a normal variation. In many cases, it is the skin of the clitoral hood, and not the clitoris itself, which is prominent and gives the impression of clitoromegaly. The appropriate screening laboratory test results for girls with an enlarged clitoris and evidence of growth acceleration are testosterone, 17-OHP, and DHEA-S levels. Imaging studies of the adrenal gland or ovaries may be ordered by the endocrinologist after review of the physical and hormonal findings.

Boys

Rapid and/or very early growth of the penis and pubic in a young boy without significant testicular enlargement is the major clue to GIPP. In the days before newborn screening for CAH was widespread, nonsalt-wasting CAH was a relatively common cause of GIPP in boys but is still seen in states and countries that do not perform newborn CAH screening. Leydig cell testicular tumors can also present this way, with the major clue being asymmetry on the testicular examination. Familial male precocious puberty presents at 2 to 3 years of age with adult levels of testosterone and suppressed gonadotropins; the cause is an activating mutation in the LH receptor. Because this condition is usually inherited in an autosomal dominant manner, family history taking may be very helpful. Testes are slightly enlarged because of Leydig cell hyperplasia, which is also the case when precocious puberty is caused by ectopic tumors (typically CNS germinomas or thymic tumors) secreting human chorionic gonadotrophin, which has LH-like actions on the Leydig cells. In any of these situations, the presence of high testosterone levels (usually >100 ng/dL) with low LH and FSH levels is sufficient evidence to request that the patient be seen promptly by a subspecialist.

Environmental exposures to sex steroids

In the past 10 years, there have been a modest number of case reports and small case series describing young boys and girls who develop either rapid genital enlargement with pubic hair or breast development as a result of skin contact with a parent using topical androgens (Androgel) [36] or estrogen creams, so asking about the use of these preparations is important. Testosterone or estradiol levels are variably elevated (with prepubertal LH and FSH), depending on the timing of the most recent exposure.

SUMMARY

Children who present with signs of early puberty require a careful history taking and physical examination and review of the growth chart looking for evidence of recent growth acceleration. The benign normal variations reviewed in this article are significantly more common than CPP, at least in the United States. Why there seems to be large differences in the incidence of PA between the United States and the other parts of the world should be the subject of further research looking for environmental and/or genetic factors. Ordering multiple hormone tests and radiography before having the child evaluated by a subspecialist should be resisted, unless there is clear evidence of rapid progression of findings over the previous 6 months (eg, a girl who presents before age 8 years with Tanner stage 3 breast development or a boy younger than 9 years with penis and/or testicular enlargement). Even girls diagnosed with CPP often do not require treatment because many have the slowly progressive form that does not result in early menarche and compromise of adult stature. In addition, studies suggest that the benefit of treatment in terms of preservation of normal adult stature is clearest for the minority of patients who have onset of CPP before age 6 years, and those girls whose onset of puberty is early but at age 8 years or more do not benefit from treatment with an increase in adult stature.

References

[1] Kaplowitz P. Precocious puberty: update on secular trends, definitions, diagnosis, and treatment. Adv Pediatr 2004;51:37–62.
[2] Susman EJ, Houts RM, Steinberg L, et al. Longitudinal development of secondary sexual characteristics in girls and boys between ages 91/2 and 151/2 years. Arch Pediatr Adolesc Med 2010;164(2):164–73.
[3] Marshall WA, Tanner JW. Variations in pattern of pubertal changes in girls. Arch Dis Child 1969;44(235):291–303.
[4] Herman-Giddens ME, Slora EJ, Wasserman RC, et al. Secondary sexual characteristics and menses in young girls seen in office practice: a study from the Pediatric Research in Office Settings network. Pediatrics 1997;99(4):505–12.
[5] Kaplowitz PB, Oberfield SE. Reexamination of the age limit for defining when puberty is precocious in girls in the United States: implications for evaluation and treatment. Pediatrics 1999;104(4):936–41.
[6] Wu T, Mendola P, Buck GM. Ethnic differences in the presence of secondary sex characteristics and menarche among US girls: the Third National Health and Nutrition Examination Survey, 1988–1994. Pediatrics 2002;110(4):752–7.
[7] Biro FM, Galvez MP, Greenspan LC, et al. Pubertal assessment method and baseline characteristics in a mixed longitudinal study of girls. Pediatrics 2010;126(3):e583–90.
[8] Aksglaede L, Sørensen K, Petersen JH, et al. Recent decline in age at breast development: the Copenhagen Puberty Study. Pediatrics 2009;123(5):e932–9.
[9] Ma H, Du M, Luo X-P, et al. Onset of breast and pubic hair development and menses in urban Chinese girls. Pediatrics 2009;124(2):e269–77.
[10] McDowell MA, Brody DJ, Hughes JP. Has age at menarche changed? Results from the National Health and Nutrition Examination Survey (NHANES) 1999–2004. J Adolesc Health 2007;40:227–31.
[11] Palmert MR, Malin HV, Boepple PA. Unsustained or slowly progressive puberty in young girls: initial presentation and long-term follow-up of 20 untreated patients. J Clin Endocrinol Metab 1999;84(2):415–23.
[12] Herman-Giddens ME, Wang L, Koch G. Secondary sexual characteristics in boys: estimates from the national health and nutrition examination survey III, 1988–1994. Arch Pediatr Adolesc Med 2001;155(9):988–9.
[13] Sørensen K, Aksglaede L, Petersen JH, et al. Recent changes in pubertal timing in healthy Danish boys: associations with body mass index. J Clin Endocrinol Metab 2010;95(1):263–70.
[14] Kaplowitz PB. Link between body fat and the timing of puberty. Pediatrics 2008;121(Suppl 3):S208–17.
[15] Lee JM, Appugliese D, Kaciroti N, et al. Weight status in young girls and the onset of puberty. Pediatrics 2007;119(3):e624–30.
[16] Lee JM, Kaciroti N, Appugliese D, et al. Body mass index and timing of pubertal initiation in boys. Arch Pediatr Adolesc Med 2010;164(2):139–44.
[17] Aksglaede L, Juul A, Leffers H, et al. The sensitivity of the child to sex steroids: possible impact of exogenous estrogens. Hum Reprod Update 2006;12(4):341–9.
[18] Nebesio TD, Pescovitz OH. Historical perspectives: endocrine disruptors and the timing of puberty. Endocrinologist 2005;15(1):44–8.
[19] deVries L, Kauschansky A, Shohat M, et al. Familial central precocious puberty suggests autosomal dominant inheritance. J Clin Endocrinol Metab 2004;89(4):1794–800.
[20] Rosenfield RL, Lipton RB, Drum ML. Thelarche, pubarche, and menarche attainment in children with normal and elevated body mass index. Pediatrics 2009;123(1):84–8.
[21] Kaplowitz PB. Clinical characteristics of 104 children referred for evaluation of precocious puberty. J Clin Endocrinol Metab 2004;89(8):3644–50.
[22] Ibanez L, Jiminez R, de Zegher F. Early puberty-menarche after precocious pubarche: relation to prenatal growth. Pediatrics 2006;117(1):117–21.

[23] Armengaud JB, Charkaluk ML, Trivin C, et al. Precocious pubarche: distinguishing late-onset congenital adrenal hyperplasia from premature adrenarche. J Clin Endocrinol Metab 2009;94(8):2835–40.
[24] Desalvo D, Mehra R, Vaidyanathan P, et al. In patients with premature adrenarche, bone age advancement by 2 or more years is relatively common and generally benign. Presented at the Annual Meeting of the Pediatric Academic Societies. Denver (CO), April 30–May 3, 2011.
[25] Van Weissenbruch MM. Premature adrenarche, polycystic ovary syndrome and intrauterine growth retardation: does a relationship exist? Curr Opin Endocrinol Diabetes Obes 2007;14(1):35–40.
[26] De Vries L, Guz-Mark A, Lazar L, et al. Premature thelarche: age at presentation affects clinical course but not clinical characteristics or risk to progress to precocious puberty. J Pediatr 2010;156(3):466–71.
[27] Chalumeau M, Chemaitilly W, Trivin C, et al. Central precocious puberty in girls: an evidence-based diagnosis tree to predict central nervous system abnormalities. Pediatrics 2002;109(1):139–41.
[28] Nebesio TD, Eugster EA. Pubic hair of infancy: endocrinopathy or enigma? Pediatrics 2006;117(3):951–4.
[29] Kaplowitz P, Soldin S. Steroid profiles in serum by liquid chromatography-tandem mass spectrometry in infants with genital hair. J Pediatr Endocrinol Metab 2007;20(5):597–605.
[30] Houk CP, Kunselman AR, Lee PA. Adequacy of a single unstimulated luteinizing hormone level to diagnose central precocious puberty in girls. Pediatrics 2009;123(6):e1059–63.
[31] Carel J-C, Eugster E, Rogol A, et al. Consensus statement on the use of gonadotropin-releasing hormone analogs in children. Pediatrics 2009;123(4):e752–62.
[32] Lazar L, Kauli R, Pertzelan A, et al. Gonadotropin-suppressive therapy in girls with early and fast puberty affects the pace of puberty but not total pubertal growth or final height. J Clin Endocrinol Metab 2002;87(5):2090–4.
[33] Albanese A, Hopper NW. Suppression of menstruation in adolescents with severe learning disabilities. Arch Dis Child 2007;92(7):629–32.
[34] Badaru A, Wilson DM, Bachrach LK, et al. Sequential comparisons of one-month and three-month depot leuprolide regimens in central precocious puberty. J Clin Endocrinol Metab 2006;91(5):1862–7.
[35] Eugster EA, Clarke W, Kletter GB, et al. Efficacy and safety of histrelin subdermal implant in children with central precocious puberty: a multicenter trial. J Clin Endocrinol Metab 2007;92(5):1697–704.
[36] Kunz GJ, Klein KO, Clemons RD, et al. Virilization of young children after topical androgen use by their parents. Pediatrics 2004;114(1):282–4.

Advances in Pediatrics 58 (2011) 259–276

ADVANCES IN PEDIATRICS

Update on Pediatric Epilepsy

Agnes H. Chen, MD

Division of Pediatric Neurology, Los Angeles County-Harbor-UCLA Medical Center, David Geffen School of Medicine at University of California Los Angeles, Box 468, 1000 West Carson Street, Torrance, CA 90502-2004, USA

The understanding of seizures and epilepsy has grown tremendously in the past decade, and many more treatment options have become available. Yet, pediatric epilepsy still remains a great challenge for clinicians to manage. This article describes how seizures and epilepsy are understood and classified today and how to approach the management of patients with seizures and updates the pediatrician on the newest approaches to epilepsy treatment.

CLASSIFICATION OF SEIZURES AND EPILEPSY

The International League Against Epilepsy (ILAE) defines a seizure as "a transient occurrence of signs and/or symptoms due to abnormal excessive or synchronous neuronal activity in the brain" [1]. Diagnosis of seizures and epilepsy largely depends on being able to identify a seizure clinically. However, most seizures are not witnessed by medical professionals, and the diagnosis depends on a caregiver's description.

Most seizures are characterized by unresponsiveness and eye opening. In fact, eye closure during a seizure is a sensitive indicator of pseudoseizure [2]. In addition, most patients who are having a seizure are unresponsive to painful stimuli. Parents of children with staring spells often say that the child does not respond to his or her name being called. This can be the case even with daydreaming. Parents are often asked to shake the child on the shoulder to see if they can abort the staring. If they cannot, it is more likely to be a seizure.

The ILAE has been working on a revision to the organization of seizures and epilepsy for many years. Their recent report has simplified the classification of seizures (Box 1) [3].

It is to be noted that the term "focal" is used instead of "partial." Focal seizures are no longer broken down into "complex partial" and "simple partial". This terminology was thought to be confusing and misused. It is also to be noted that the use of simple and complex in terms of febrile seizures is completely unrelated to simple and complex partial seizures. Nevertheless, the commission recognizes that it is important to describe any alteration of consciousness as part of a seizure [3].

E-mail address: ahchen@ucla.edu

0065-3101/11/$ – see front matter
doi:10.1016/j.yapd.2011.03.001

Box 1: Classification of seizures

- Generalized seizures
    - Tonic-clonic
    - Absence
        - Typical
        - Atypical
        - Absence with special features
            - Myoclonic absence
            - Eyelid myoclonia
    - Myoclonic
        - Myoclonic
        - Myoclonic atonic
        - Myoclonic tonic
    - Clonic
    - Tonic
    - Atonic
- Focal seizures
- Unknown
    - Epileptic spasms

Data from Revised terminology and concepts for organization of seizures and epilepsies: report of the ILAE commission on classification and terminology, 2005–2009. Epilepsia 2010;51(4):676–85.

Absence seizures have been subcategorized further. A typical absence seizure involves an abrupt staring spell often accompanied by eyelid blinking and an abrupt return to responsiveness. There is no prodrome, no loss of tone, and no postictal phase. Often the children will be talking, then stop talking to stare into space for a few seconds, and then resume talking where they last left off. Atypical absence seizures are less abrupt; they last longer and can have postictal confusion. Myoclonic absence is an absence seizure with myoclonic jerks of the head, shoulders, and arms. Prominent eyelid myoclonus followed by absence seizure is also recognized as an absence subtype.

Myoclonic seizures are characterized by brief contractions of the whole body, or isolated parts of the body. A myoclonic jerk followed by the sudden loss of tone of the whole body is known as a myoclonic atonic seizure. Myoclonic atonic and myoclonic tonic seizures while a patient is standing can result in falls and injury.

Clonic seizure consists of rhythmic jerking of the body that can be asymmetric, even in a generalized clonic seizure. Tonic seizures involve sustained muscle contraction, and patients can appear to be in a decerebrate posture. A tonic-clonic seizure usually consists of a tonic phase in which the patient loses consciousness, falls to the ground, and is stiff for less than 30 seconds and then, a clonic phase in which the patient jerks all limbs for longer than 30 seconds, sometimes minutes. Tonic-clonic seizures have a postictal phase in which patients are lethargic and confused for up to an hour, or longer if sedative medications are given.

Focal seizures can consist of myoclonic jerks or can have tonic or clonic components. What distinguishes focal seizures is that they are thought to arise from one hemisphere. Sometimes this origin can be difficult to tell clinically. Also, focal seizures can just have sensory changes, or cognitive changes such as confusion, hallucinations, and staring. Both focal seizures and absence seizures can be described as staring spells, and it can be difficult to distinguish between them.

Infantile spasms are categorized as an "epileptic spasm." It is unclear whether this type of seizure is focal or generalized, therefore, it has been categorized as "unknown."

CLASSIFICATION OF EPILEPSY

The epilepsies have a separate classification from seizures. For example, a patient has to have an absence seizure to have absence epilepsy, but patients with childhood absence epilepsy can have other types of seizures as well. Epilepsy describes a propensity for seizures because of an "enduring alteration in the brain" [1]. This alteration can be because of a known underlying structural cause, such as a remote encephalitis, or it can be because of a known epilepsy syndrome. The 1989 international classification of epilepsies categorized epilepsy syndromes as "idiopathic," "symptomatic," and "crytogenic" [4]. These terms have been abandoned because of their inaccuracy and inconsistency with new genetic and neuroscience knowledge. The commission now recognizes epilepsies called "electroclinical syndromes" (Box 2). These are a cluster of clinical symptoms and electroencephalographic (EEG) characteristics that appear at certain ages. In addition, there are "distinctive constellations," which are also recognizable clusters of clinical symptoms but do not have the strong developmental component of the electroclinical syndromes.

It is beyond the scope of this article to describe every electroclinical syndrome, but the author describes a few of the syndromes in the other sections of this article.

APPROACH TO SEIZURES AND EPILEPSY

Evaluation of a child with a seizure should always begin with an assessment of the cardiopulmonary status, including airway, breathing, and circulation. It is common during generalized tonic-clonic seizures for the patient to have increased secretions from the mouth, therefore it is recommended that unconscious seizure patients be placed lying on their side to allow secretions to escape and to prevent aspiration. Although it is not uncommon for parents of a child with seizures to request oxygen tanks to have at home, clinically significant hypoxia during a seizure is rare. Suctioning of the mouth can be helpful,

Box 2: Electroclinical syndromes and other epilepsies (abbreviated)

Electroclinical syndromes arranged by age at onset

- Neonatal period
  - Benign familial neonatal epilepsy
  - Ohtahara syndrome
- Infancy
  - West syndrome
  - Myoclonic epilepsy in infancy
  - Benign infantile epilepsy
  - Benign familial infantile epilepsy
  - Dravet syndrome
- Childhood
  - Febrile seizures plus
  - Panayiotopoulos syndrome
  - Epilepsy with myoclonic atonic seizures
  - Benign epilepsy with centrotemporal spikes
  - Autosomal dominant nocturnal frontal lobe epilepsy
  - Epilepsy with myoclonic absences
  - Lennox-Gastaut syndrome
  - Epileptic encephalopathy with continuous spike and wave during sleep
  - Landau-Kleffner syndrome
  - Childhood absence epilepsy
- Adolescence-Adult
  - Juvenile absence epilepsy
  - Juvenile myoclonic epilepsy
  - Progressive myoclonus epilepsies
- Distinctive constellations
  - Mesial temporal lobe epilepsy with hippocampal sclerosis
  - Rasmussen syndrome
  - Gelastic seizures with hypothalamic hamartoma
- Epilepsies attributed to and organized by structural-metabolic causes
  - Malformations of cortical development, neurocutaneous syndrome, tumor, infection, trauma, angioma, perinatal insults, stroke, etc.
- Epilepsies of unknown cause
- Conditions with epileptic seizures that are traditionally not diagnosed as a form of epilepsy per se
  - Benign neonatal seizures
  - Febrile seizures

Data from Revised terminology and concepts for organization of seizures and epilepsies: report of the ILAE commission on classification and terminology, 2005–2009. Epilepsia 2010;51(4):676–85.

especially in the hospital setting. The blood glucose level is frequently measured by paramedics in the field.

Besides an increase in respiratory secretions, other autonomic changes are frequently noted during a seizure. Most patients with complex partial seizure or generalized tonic-clonic seizures have tachycardia and hypertension. Changes in respiratory rate in either direction are frequent as well. In most seizure patients who have not been given antiepileptic medication, the cardiopulmonary changes are not severe enough to require resuscitation and mechanical ventilatory support. Other autonomic changes during a seizure can include flushing, pallor, sweating, bilateral pupillary dilation, abdominal pain, vomiting, and urinary incontinence [5].

Once it is established that the patient has stable cardiopulmonary status, the patient's mental status should be assessed. Commonly, the patient is in a postictal state. If the patient had a generalized tonic-clonic seizure, the postictal state is characterized by the ceasing of limb movement, stupor or coma, and normalizing of the heart rate, blood pressure, and respiration. The length of the postictal period is related to the length of the seizure. Generalized tonic-clonic seizures lasting less than a few minutes are usually followed by a postictal stupor or coma of 5 to 30 minutes. The patient can remain depressed for longer, especially if given benzodiazepines to treat the seizure.

In rare cases, a patient who seems to be in the postictal state may be having nonconvulsive seizure activity. This situation is more likely if the original convulsive seizure was prolonged, meeting the definition for status epilepticus. The patient should be observed for normalization of vital signs and for gradual return of responsiveness. An EEG should be considered for patients who remain comatose. Status epilepticus is discussed in a separate section later.

After the patient is stabilized, a complete history and physical examination can be obtained. Questions and examination should be directed in an attempt to determine the cause of the seizure. Table 1 lists the common causes of seizures and the studies that can be done to help confirm the diagnosis.

With an accurate history and physical examination, few to none of the studies in Table 1 will need to be performed acutely. Conversely, children with known epilepsy should still have investigations into the secondary causes of seizure, such as infection and trauma, if clinically warranted. The main piece of clinical information to obtain is to determine whether the child has returned to his or her baseline neurologic status. These children are only likely to need further studies on an outpatient basis. Children who remain lethargic after an appropriate postictal period need continued monitoring, possible admission, and further studies, such as lumbar puncture for viral encephalitis or subarachnoid hemorrhage or computed tomography of the head for subdural hematoma or hydrocephalus.

All children with a first-time afebrile seizure without an obvious secondary cause such as trauma should have an EEG [6]. EEG can be done as an outpatient if the patient is at the baseline neurologic status when presenting after the seizure. Antiepileptic drug therapy is generally not recommended after a first

Table 1
Common causes of seizures

Cause of Seizure	Suggested Studies
Metabolic abnormalities: hypoglycemia or hyperglycemia, hyponatremia or hypernatremia, hypocalcemia or hypercalcemia, hypomagnesemia, uremia, liver failure, hyperammonemia	Basic chemistries, calcium and magnesium levels, liver function tests, ammonia levels
Infection: meningoencephalitis, sepsis, neurocysticercosis	Lumbar puncture, send cerebrospinal fluid for appropriate infectious titers/PCR, sepsis evaluation, head CT, MRI with gadolinium
Neoplasm, vascular malformation	Head CT, MRI with gadolinium
Trauma	Head CT
Inherited neurodegenerative disorder	Appropriate genetic testing
Toxic causes, drug withdrawal	Urine toxicology screen, ethanol levels, other specific drug tests
Perinatal stroke/asphyxia	Head CT, MRI
Congenital brain malformation	Head CT, MRI
Febrile seizure	Lumbar puncture in selected cases
Epilepsy	EEG, antiepileptic drug levels (to check for compliance)

Abbreviations: CT, computed tomography; MRI, magnetic resonance imaging; PCR, polymerase chain reaction.

seizure, but this decision should be individualized [7]. There is no evidence that treating after the second seizure, as opposed to the first seizure, changes the long-term course or prognosis of the patient's epilepsy.

ANTIEPILEPTIC DRUGS

Medications are first line in the treatment of epilepsy. Once it is determined that a child has recurrent seizures, that is, epilepsy, initiating a daily medication in an attempt to prevent seizures is recommended. The choice of medication depends on many factors, including seizure type and syndrome, side effect profiles, forms of administration, drug interactions, underlying medical conditions, and cost.

There are many antiepileptic medications available in the United States. Tables 2 and 3 list the commonly used medications, the year they were made available in the United States, and a recommended dosing range. With the exception of bromide salts, many of the earliest seizure medications, such as phenobarbital and phenytoin, are still in clinical use today. Phenytoin was the first anticonvulsant to be screened through an animal model of epilepsy. Also called the electroshock model, the animal (a cat in the original experiment) was hooked up to mouth and scalp electrodes and given gradually increased electric current until a seizure occurred. The level of current was the cat's seizure threshold. Then, the cat was premedicated with a test drug. If the drug increased the seizure threshold by an amount comparable to phenobarbital, it was considered for further testing as an anticonvulsant [8]. Drugs undergoing testing at present

Table 2
Traditional antiepileptic medications

Medication	Available in the United States	Recommended Dosing Ranges
Bromide	19th century	Not currently used for seizures in the United States
Phenobarbital	1912	3–5 mg/kg/d, qd to bid
Phenytoin	1938	3–9 mg/kg/d, qd to bid
Acetazolamide	1953	500–1000 mg/d, bid
Primidone	1954	Start 50 mg q hour, titrate slowly to 10–25 mg/kg/d tid, maximum 2 g/d
Ethosuximide	1960	20 mg/kg/d to a maximum of 1.5 g/d, bid
Diazepam	1963	Recommended for status epilepticus, not daily prophylaxis
Carbamazepine	1974	Start 10 mg/kg/d, increase to 20–30 mg/kg/d, bid to tid
Clonazepam	1975	0.05–0.2 mg/kg/d, bid
Valproic acid	1978	Start 10 mg/kg/d, increase to 20–60 mg/kg/d, bid

are screened with rodents through the "maximal electroshock model," which uses principles similar to the original electroshock experiments in cats [9].

In the early 1970s, the National Institutes for Neurologic Disorders and Stroke started the Anticonvulsant Drug Development program in an effort to screen many more drugs for potential anticonvulsant activity. Thousands of drugs have been screened through the maximal electroshock model as well as other animal models of epilepsy, such as the subcutaneous pentylenetetrazol

Table 3
Newer antiepileptic medications

Medication	Available in the United States	Recommended Dosing Ranges
Felbamate	1993	15–45 mg/kg/d, tid
Lamotrigine	1994	Start 0.3 mg/kg/d, increase to 5–8 mg/kg/d, bid, lower if concurrent valproic acid
Fosphenytoin	1996	Same as phenytoin
Topiramate	1996	1–9 mg/kg/d, bid
Levetiracetam	1999	20–60 mg/kg/d, bid
Oxcarbazepine	2000	Start 15 mg/kg/d, increase to 30–60 mg/kg/d, bid
Zonisamide	2000	100–600 mg/d, bid
Pregabalin	2004	150–600 mg/d, bid
Rufinamide	2008	Start 10–15 mg/kg/d to a maximum of 50–60 mg/kg/d, bid
Vigabatrin	2009	50–150 mg/kg/d, bid
Lacosamide	2009	Start 50 mg bid, increase to 100–200 mg bid

and kindling models [8]. Drugs developed for the treatment of epilepsy by mass screening through animal models are not designed with a particular mechanism of action in mind. This is partly because not all the mechanisms of epilepsy are known. However, in examining the potential mechanisms of these drugs and potential mechanisms of the animal models in causing seizures and in studying the brains of people with epilepsy, our understanding of the development of epilepsy and the potential targets is rapidly growing.

In a prospective study comparing a traditional antiepileptic drug with a newer antiepileptic drug, there was no significant difference in the seizure remission rate after either drug was given in subjects who completed the study [10]. There are not many trials of head-to-head comparisons between seizure medications, but generally, increased efficacy has not been seen with the newer agents. Always, one-third of patients do not respond to one or more seizure drugs, and these patients are labeled refractory. Generally, however, the newer antiepileptics have a more tolerable side-effect profile.

Medication choice based on seizure type and syndrome

After phenytoin became widely used, it was noted that it did not prevent petit mal seizures very well. Since then, further evidence has demonstrated that phenytoin and carbamazepine, as well as several other drugs, seem to worsen seizures in patients who have an idiopathic generalized epilepsy [11]. These drugs, considered narrow spectrum (Box 3), should be reserved for patients with focal and/or secondarily generalized seizures. They should be avoided in patients with idiopathic or primary generalized epilepsy, which are age-related epilepsy syndromes characterized by generalized spike-and-wave discharges on the EEG, such as childhood absence epilepsy and juvenile myoclonic epilepsy (JME).

Conversely, most of the other antiepileptic drugs as listed in Tables 2 and 3 are considered broad spectrum and therefore have been shown to work against a variety of seizure types. Some exceptions include ethosuximide, which is regarded as first-line treatment for typical absence seizures, but not enough evidence exists to use it for partial seizures.

Box 3: Narrow-spectrum antiepileptic drugs

- Phenytoin
- Carbamazepine
- Oxcarbazepine
- Pregabalin
- Gabapentin
- Vigabatrin
- Tiagabine

Medication choice based on potential toxicity

There are many different antiepileptic medications that have the potential to be effective for any particular patient. Often, choices are narrowed down to avoid certain toxicities. For example, many neurologists would not use valproic acid in women of childbearing age because of the association of valproic acid with polycystic ovary disease, obesity, and hyperandrogenism [12].

Box 4 lists some prominent and unique side effects and toxicities of the antiepileptic drugs. The author has not listed headache, dizziness, nausea, abdominal pain, or sedation because these side effects have been reported for every anticonvulsant.

Box 4: Unique side effects and toxicities of antiepileptic medications

- Phenytoin
  - Gingival hyperplasia, hirsutism, rash, osteopenia
- Carbamazepine
  - Hyponatremia, blood dyscrasias, allele HLA-B*1502 is associated with toxic epidermal necrolysis and Stevens-Johnson syndrome
- Felbamate
  - Liver failure, aplastic anemia
- Lamotrigine
  - Serious rash, worse with concurrent valproate
- Levtiracetam
  - Behavior or personality change
- Oxcarbazepine
  - Similar to carbamazepine
- Phenobarbital
  - Hyperactivity, aggressiveness, and insomnia in children, lowering of IQ, osteopenia
- Primidone
  - Similar to phenobarbital, more acute early toxicity that is transient
- Topiramate
  - Cognitive impairment, weight loss, paresthesias, kidney stones, metabolic acidosis, oligohidrosis
- Valproic cid
  - Hepatic toxicity, weight gain, tremor, polycystic ovaries, thrombocytopenia, tremor, hair loss
- Vigabatrin
  - Irreversible visual field defects, intramyelinic edema
- Zonisamide
  - Similar to topiramate, also do not use in sulfa-allergic patients

THE NEWEST ANTIEPILEPTICS

The newest antiepileptics to be approved by the US Food and Drug Administration (FDA) are rufinamide, lacosamide, and vigabatrin. Vigabatrin is discussed in the section on "Infantile Spasms."

Rufinamide, like many other antiepileptics, affects sodium channels, and in in vitro studies of cultured neurons, this drug has prolonged the inactivated state of the channel. In a randomized, double-blind, placebo-controlled study for Lennox-Gastaut syndrome (LGS), adjunct therapy with rufinamide was found to reduce the number of drop attacks (which can be the most disabling seizure type in LGS) by 42.5% [13]. In the same study, rufinamide also demonstrated a 32.7% decrease in the total seizure frequency over 28 days compared with the 11.7% decrease for placebo. These results are comparable to those of clinical trials for other drugs tried for LGS, namely topiramate, lamotrigine, and felbamate [14]. Based on these results, the FDA approved rufinamide in November 2008 for the treatment of LGS in patients aged 4 years or older. Rufinamide has also been tried in older children and adults with partial-onset seizures showing modest efficacy [14].

Patients who are taking rufinamide are often on other antiepileptics and may have failed several antiepileptics previously. Rufinamide has minimal drug-drug interactions, but, like many other drugs, its level can be decreased by cytochrome P450 inducing seizure medications such as phenobarbital, carbamazepine, and phenytoin. The concurrent administration of valproic acid can increase levels of rufinamide; therefore, caution should be taken when starting rufinamide on patients who are already taking valproic acid. Generally, the starting dose should be lowered and the titration much slower.

The main side effect in the author's experience has been somnolence, and this is alleviated by a slower titration. In addition, one can consider lowering the dose of other sedating antiepileptics such as topiramate. The author recommends starting rufinamide at 10 to 15 mg/kg/d divided twice daily. The dose is doubled after one week to 20 to 30 mg/kg/d. If there is no improvement, the dose is further increased by 10 to 15 mg/kg/d weekly until a maximum of 50 to 60 mg/kg/d.

At present, rufinamide is available in 200-mg and 400-mg tablets, which are scored and can be cut in half. In addition, the tablets can be crushed for administration through gastrostomy tubes. The manufacturer has applied to the FDA for approval of an oral suspension 40 mg/mL in the summer of 2010.

In 2009, lacosamide was approved for the adjunctive treatment of partial seizures in adults. In a double-blind placebo-controlled trial in which patients were randomized to 4 arms of different dosing (200 mg, 400 mg, 600 mg, and placebo), there was a median reduction of 40% in the 400-mg and 600-mg groups compared with 10% in the placebo group [15]. There were dose-related adverse events that included dizziness, nausea, fatigue, ataxia, headache, diplopia, and nystagmus. Because of these side effects, the clinical recommendation is to start at 50 mg twice daily and increase the dose weekly by 100 mg to a target dose of 200 to 400 mg. The author reports that an even slower titration, 50 mg per week, is better tolerated.

There are not enough data on the efficacy of lacosamide in younger populations. It is approved for patients aged 17 years and older. As with other antiepileptics, it will likely find a place in the treatment of pediatric epilepsy. Advantages of lacosamide include low drug-drug interactions and an intravenous (IV) formulation, with a 1:1 oral to IV substitution.

INFANTILE SPASMS

Infantile spasms were first described in the medical literature in 1941 by Dr William James West, whose infant son had a peculiar seizure disorder consisting of rapid flexor jerks [16]. It has since been learned that infantile spasms are associated with a specific EEG pattern called hypsarrhythmia and that infantile spasms can occur in older children. The new ILAE revised terminology has categorized infantile spasms under the term epileptic spasms, and it is unknown whether these seizures are generalized or focal [3].

The triad of infantile spasms, developmental regression or arrest, and hypsarrhythmia is now known as the West syndrome. The possible underlying cause should be searched when an infant presents with this triad of symptoms. Secondary causes of seizures as described in Table 1 should be investigated. A thorough physical examination looking for neurocutaneous and other genetic syndromes should be done. A brain magnetic resonance imaging (MRI) is helpful to look for cerebral malformations, evidence of prior hypoxic-ischemic injury, trauma, or infection. An underlying cause is found in about two-thirds of patients with West syndrome.

The treatment of infantile spasms has been controversial, but adrenocorticotropin and oral steroids showed particularly efficacy when they were tried in the midtwentieth century. Recently, the Infantile Spasms Working Group established recommended guidelines for the treatment of infantile spasms in the United States [17]. Adrenocorticotropic hormone (ACTH) is recommended as first-line treatment based on prospective randomized controlled trials. However, the optimal dose and duration of the treatment is unclear. The side effects of ACTH are severe and worse at high doses. Patients need to be carefully monitored for signs of infection, hyperglycemia, cardiomyopathy, electrolyte abnormalities, and hypertension. There are published protocols for a high-dose and a low-dose ACTH regimen. The high-dose regimen starts at 150 IU/m^2 per day in 2 divided doses for 1 week and a careful taper over 10 weeks total. The lower-dose schedule starts at 40 IU/d total, and increases to 60 to 80 IU/d if there is no response after 2 weeks at 40 IU. Because response to ACTH is generally seen after 1 to 2 weeks, it is recommended to taper the dosage after 2 weeks if it has not been effective [18].

Vigabatrin has also been found to be effective for infantile spasms. There is evidence that it works better in patients who have infantile spasms secondary to tuberous sclerosis [19]. As with ACTH, the optimal dose of vigabatrin is not known, although most recommend starting at 50 mg/kg/d, divided twice daily, and titrating up to 100 to 150 mg/kg/d. The use of vigabatrin has been limited because of 2 serious adverse effects: intramyelinic edema and irreversible visual field defects. Edema in the myelin sheaths has been observed in rats given vigabatrin, but not in primates. In infants given vigabatrin for infantile spasm, MRI T2 signal abnormalities have appeared that seem to be dose related and have resolved after treatment is discontinued [20]. It is unclear whether these transient MRI changes are related to intramyelinic edema seen in rats.

Visual field defects were first reported in 1997 [21]. Usually the defects are bilateral and concentric. Further studies have demonstrated retinal injury in the cone system [20]. The pathophysiology of retinal injury is unclear, but up to 40% of patients who have taken vigabatrin are affected, with adults being more affected than children. Because of this adverse effect, the use of vigabatrin is restricted only to physicians who have registered with a program that includes frequent ophthalmologic screening for patients prescribed vigabatrin.

EXAMPLE CASE IN THE MANAGEMENT OF PEDIATRIC EPILEPSY

Henry is a healthy 13-year-old boy who presents in the pediatric emergency department with a generalized seizure. He had just woken up and was getting dressed when his mother heard a loud bang. She ran into his room and found him lying on his bedroom floor shaking. His eyes were rolled back in his head, and he was unresponsive when she called his name. Paramedics were called, and Henry stopped shaking by the time they arrived. A rapid glucose test showed glucose levels of 120 mg/dL. Henry was groggy but responsive to pain. He woke up further in the ambulance and was awake by the time he was in the pediatric emergency department.

On examination, Henry is afebrile with stable vital signs. He has a scalp hematoma on the back of his head. Henry remembers riding in the ambulance and waking up in his room, but nothing in between. The result of neurologic examination is normal.

On further questioning, Henry and his parents state that over the past few months he has been having brief body jerks. The jerks usually occur in the morning, and he has dropped things from his hands before.

Discussion

As with all acute seizure presentations, once the child is stabilized, an investigation into the cause of the seizure is begun. Because Henry is a previously healthy boy who is neurologically normal and is on no medications, a metabolic condition is not suspected. A urine toxicology screen is sent, and the result is negative. There is minimal suspicion for drug exposure. Because Henry is at his baseline mental status and afebrile, suspicion for meningitis or encephalitis is low. There are no focal neurologic signs, so emergent neuroimaging is not required.

This seems to be a first unprovoked seizure; however, the history of brief body jerks is concerning for myoclonic type seizure. Henry's age and presentation could fit the electroclinical syndrome of JME. An EEG is recommended to look for 4- to 6-Hz spike and polyspike and wave discharges that are bilateral and symmetric, and classic, for JME. JME is considered a primary generalized epilepsy, therefore the patient should not be placed on narrow-spectrum antiepileptic medications such as phenytoin or carbamazepine. Valproic acid is considered the drug of choice for JME, although if Henry was a girl, another drug might be considered because of the possible increased risk of polycystic ovarian syndrome associated with valproic acid.

If one were confident that the body jerks were seizures, then it would be reasonable to start Henry on valproic acid right away. If Henry weighs 50 kg, the reasonable starting dose of valproic acid is 250 mg administered orally twice daily. It would also be reasonable to wait until the EEG is performed before starting medication.

STATUS EPILEPTICUS

The author has emphasized that the child should be stabilized before investigations are made into the cause of the seizure; however, in status epilepticus, treatment of the seizure, determination of the precipitating cause, and treatment of the cause (if possible) should be done simultaneously. The Epilepsy Foundation of America Working Group on Status Epilepticus has defined status epilepticus as longer than 30 minutes of either continuous seizure activity or 2 or more sequential seizures without full recovery of consciousness between the seizures [22]; however, any continuous seizure should be treated as status epilepticus because there is evidence that the more prolonged a seizure the more difficult it is to control [23].

As stated earlier, seizure management first includes management of the airway. Because metabolic derangements can be rapidly treated, and because seizures caused by metabolic abnormalities are resistant to antiepileptic medication, the level of glucose and electrolytes should be measured right away. An IV line should be placed, but if this proves difficult, medication can be given via the rectum.

Treatment of status epilepticus begins with a benzodiazepine, such as lorazepam, 0.1 mg/kg of which is given via a slow IV push (0.75 mg/min). The drug should be given a few minutes to take effect. If the seizure does not stop, another dose should be given. If there is no IV access, diazepam, 0.3 mg/kg, can be given intrarectally.

If the patient is still having a seizure, fosphenytoin (or phenytoin) is recommended at 20 mg/kg [24]. At this point, the seizure has been continuing for 20 minutes or more. The recommended drugs vary by institution. If the patient is known to be taking valproic acid, a 20-mg/kg load of valproic acid can be given. Another 10 mg/kg of fosphenytoin can be given. Phenobarbital, 10 to 20 mg/kg, can be given, but caution must be taken to observe for respiratory compromise. Often, patients require intubation and mechanical ventilation at this point because they are no longer protecting their airway. Once patients are intubated, IV anesthesia can be administered with a midazolam or propofol drip [24].

NONMEDICATION EPILEPSY TREATMENT OPTIONS

Nonmedication epilepsy treatment options include the ketogenic diet, vagus nerve stimulation (VNS), and epilepsy surgery.

The ketogenic diet

The ketogenic diet, which was reviewed in the previous issue of this journal, is a high-fat low-carbohydrate diet used to treat epilepsy. The goal of the diet is to mimic the metabolic changes of starvation because fasting has been noted since biblical times to reduce the number of seizures in epileptics. The ketogenic diet was developed in the 1920s, but its use decreased as phenytoin and other antiepileptic medications were developed and marketed. In the past 15 years, however, due in part to the efforts of patients and families for whom the standard antiepileptic drugs have not been effective, awareness and use of the ketogenic diet has been increasing.

The classic ketogenic diet has a 4:1 ratio of grams of fats to grams of protein and carbohydrate. For the diet to be effective, a dietician must work with the family to carefully calculate everything that the child ingests. Other diets, such as the modified Atkins diet and the low glycemic index treatment, which are less strict because they have higher amounts of protein and carbohydrate, have been tried and show results similar to the ketogenic diet in small uncontrolled trials [25].

The ketogenic diet is generally started in conjunction with the antiepileptic medications that the child is already taking. There are a few inherited metabolic conditions in which the ketogenic diet would be started as first-line therapy, including glucose transporter 1 (GLUT-1) deficiency and pyruvate dehydrogenase deficiency, and a few conditions in which the ketogenic diet would be absolutely contraindicated, such as primary carnitine deficiency, fatty acid oxidation disorders, and pyruvate carboxylase deficiency. Screening for these conditions should be done before initiating the diet [26].

There are several cohort studies, mostly retrospective, showing efficacy of the ketogenic diet in patients who were already refractory to multiple medication regimens [27]. In a combined analysis of the outcome data in 2000, more than half of the patients had a greater than 50% reduction in seizure frequency, which is a frequently used outcome measure in medication trials [27]. In 2008, the first randomized controlled trial of the ketogenic diet was published [28]. In this study, 145 children were randomized to the diet or no diet for 3 months. On intention-to-treat analysis, 38% of the diet group had a greater than 50% reduction in seizures compared with 6% of the control group ($P < .001$). Around 7% of the diet group had a greater than 90% reduction in seizures compared with none in the control group ($P < .05$).

Patients who are on the ketogenic diet need to be closely monitored, both for compliance as well as for side effects. Effectiveness does depend on ketone production, so parents are taught to monitor urine ketone levels. Constipation is the most common side effect of the ketogenic diet, and this can be managed with the usual fiber, stool softeners, and increased fluid regimen. Also, the addition of medium chain triglyceride oil to improve ketosis can help with the constipation because of its laxative properties [29]. Other side effects include vitamin and mineral deficiencies (supplementation is required), kidney stones, and lipid elevation [30].

An international consensus guideline recommends that patients remain on the ketogenic diet for at least 3.5 months before tapering because of inefficacy [31]. If the diet does result in a significant reduction in the seizure frequency, the recommendation is to remain on the diet for 2 years [31]. There is limited information about the long-term use of the ketogenic diet. In a retrospective study of almost 600 children, 12% became seizure free after 2 years on the diet and most of these patients were medication free. However, 13% of these patients eventually had seizure recurrence at a median of 2.4 years after discontinuing the diet. Most of the patients were able to regain seizure control after resuming the diet [32].

Vagus nerve stimulator

VNS was approved by the FDA in 1997 as adjunctive treatment or partial epilepsy in patients aged 12 years and older. It was also approved in 2005 for treatment-resistant depression and is currently undergoing clinical trials for chronic pain, migraine, and even Alzheimer disease.

It is unclear how the vagus nerve stimulator works, but its wide applicability as listed earlier, reinforces the fact that connections from the vagus nerve project widely to the forebrain. Studies in dogs demonstrated attenuation of experimentally induced seizures [33]. Based on these animal studies, a VNS therapy system was developed using a pacemakerlike pulse generator.

The generator is implanted subcutaneously in the upper left part of the chest, and bipolar leads are tunneled up the neck and attached to the left vagus nerve. The left vagus nerve is used because it has fewer sinoatrial fibers than the right vagus nerve. The generator provides intermittent electric stimulation at programmable preset intervals. For example, the device can be set to 30 seconds of "on time" and 5 minutes of "off time." During the 30 seconds of on time, electric current is delivered at a certain preset frequency and pulse width. The VNS runs continuously 24 hours, 7 days a week, turning on every 5 minutes until the settings are changed or until the battery runs out. At typical stimulation settings, the battery lasts 7 to 10 years [34].

The VNS system also comes with a small strong magnet that can be worn on the patient's wrist. The magnet activates the stimulator and provides a current that is usually set higher and longer than the baseline current that is given around the clock. This on-demand stimulus is meant to interrupt or shorten an ongoing seizure. Usually, the magnet is used by a caregiver because the patient does not have the capacity to use it during a seizure.

Physicians can check the device and change the settings with a programming wand that is connected to a hand-held computer. The wand is placed over the generator on the patient's chest and can detect signals through clothing. The physician can set the proportion of on time to off time (known as the duty cycle) as well as change the current, frequency, and pulse width. The device does not allow high-enough settings that could lead to severe pain and nerve damage [35].

The vagus nerve stimulator was tested in 2 double-blind clinical trials in which patients were randomized to receive high-stimulation versus low-stimulation parameters. Both studies showed a reduction in seizure frequency by half in about 30% of subjects in the high-stimulation group [36,37]. Patients on VNS followed up for 12 months continued to show improvements, with additional patients demonstrating a significant reduction in seizure frequency [38].

Similar to the ketogenic diet, vagus nerve stimulator therapy is recommended for patients who have failed traditional antiepileptic medication treatments (usually at least two drugs). Contraindications for VNS implantation include prior left cervical vagotomy and underlying cardiac or pulmonary disease. Side effects include changes in voice, cough, and dyspnea. These side effects are generally mild, well tolerated, and stimulation dependent. Therefore, the settings can be lowered if the side effects are intolerable. Surgical problems such as wound infections, fluid accumulation at the generator site, and unilateral vocal cord paralysis are very rare.

Epilepsy surgery

A detailed discussion of epilepsy surgery is beyond the scope of this article. Generally, referrals for surgery are made after it is determined that a child has a focal epilepsy and is not responding to antiepileptic medications. Also, it is recommended that patients who have a resectable epileptogenic lesion should be referred to surgery before VNS or ketogenic diet therapy [31,39]. Medical centers with expertise in epilepsy surgery have the capability with prolonged video EEG monitoring and PET scanning to detect small epileptogenic foci, such as cortical dysplasias, that may be amenable for surgical removal.

SUMMARY

Seizures and epilepsy in children remain challenging to manage. Newer classification reflects the more sophisticated understanding of the genetic, anatomic, and neurophysiologic bases of seizures and epilepsy syndromes. Seizure management includes knowledge of emergency procedures and awareness of a broad differential diagnosis. Epilepsy management requires knowledge of the numerous electroclinical syndromes and high familiarity with the many drugs that are available. Although many patients remain refractory, with rapid advances in elucidating the animal models of epilepsy, it is to be hoped that drug mechanisms and nonmedication treatment options will free more patients from their seizures.

References

[1] Fisher RS, van Emde Boas W, Blume W, et al. Epileptic seizures and epilepsy: definitions proposed by the International League Against Epilepsy (ILAE) and the International Bureau for Epilepsy (IBE). Epilepsia 2005;46(4):470–2.
[2] Chung SS, Gerber P, Kirlin KA. Ictal eye closure is a reliable indicator for psychogenic nonepileptic seizures. Neurology 2006;66(11):1730–1.
[3] Berg AT, Berkovic SF, Brodie MJ, et al. Revised terminology and concepts for organization of seizures and epilepsies: report of the ILAE Commission on Classification and Terminology, 2005–2009. Epilepsia 2010;51(4):676–85.
[4] Proposal for revised classification of epilepsies and epileptic syndromes. Commission on Classification and Terminology of the International League Against Epilepsy. Epilepsia 1989;30(4):389–99.
[5] Devinsky O. Effects of seizures on autonomic and cardiovascular function. Epilepsy Curr 2004;4(2):43–6.
[6] Freeman JH. Practice parameter: evaluating a first nonfebrile seizure in children: report of the quality standards subcommittee of the American academy of neurology, the child neurology society, and the American epilepsy society. Neurology 2001;56(4):574.
[7] Hirtz D, Berg A, Bettis D, et al. Practice parameter: treatment of the child with a first unprovoked seizure: report of the quality standards subcommittee of the American Academy of Neurology and the Practice Committee of the Child Neurology Society. Neurology 2003;60(2):166–75.
[8] Arzimanoglou A, Ben-Menachem E, Cramer J, et al. The evolution of antiepileptic drug development and regulation. Epileptic Disord 2010;12(1):3–15.
[9] Bialer M, White HS. Key factors in the discovery and development of new antiepileptic drugs. Nat Rev Drug Discov 2010;9(1):68–82.
[10] Kwan P, Brodie MJ. Early identification of refractory epilepsy. N Engl J Med 2000;342(5): 314–9.
[11] Benbadis SR, WO Tatum, Gieron M. Idiopathic generalized epilepsy and choice of antiepileptic drugs. Neurology 2003;61(12):1793–5.
[12] Bilo L, Meo R. Polycystic ovary syndrome in women using valproate: a review. Gynecol Endocrinol 2008;24(10):562–70.
[13] Glauser T, Kluger G, Sachdeo R, et al. Rufinamide for generalized seizures associated with Lennox-Gastaut syndrome. Neurology 2008;70(21):1950–8.
[14] Wheless JW, Vazquez B. Rufinamide: a novel broad-spectrum antiepileptic drug. Epilepsy Curr 2010;10(1):1–6.
[15] Ben-Menachem E, Biton V, Jatuzis D, et al. Efficacy and safety of oral lacosamide as adjunctive therapy in adults with partial-onset seizures. Epilepsia 2007;48(7):1308–17.
[16] Eling P, Renier WO, Pomper J, et al. The mystery of the Doctor's son, or the riddle of West syndrome. Neurology 2002;58(6):953–5.
[17] Pellock JM, Hrachovy R, Shinnar S, et al. Infantile spasms: a U.S. consensus report. Epilepsia 2010;51(10):2175–89.
[18] Go CY, Snead OC. Adrenocorticotropin and steroids. In: Wyllie E, editor. Wyllie's treatment of epilepsy: principles and practice. Philadelphia (PA): Lippincott Williams and Wilkins; 2010. p. 763–70.
[19] Chiron C, Dumas C, Jambaque I, et al. Randomized trial comparing vigabatrin and hydrocortisone in infantile spasms due to tuberous sclerosis. Epilepsy Res 1997;26(2): 389–95.
[20] Lerner JT, Salamon N, Sankar R. Clinical profile of vigabatrin as monotherapy for treatment of infantile spasms. Neuropsychiatr Dis Treat 2010;6:731–40.
[21] Eke T, Talbot JF, Lawden MC. Severe persistent visual field constriction associated with vigabatrin. BMJ 1997;314(7075):180–1.
[22] Treatment of convulsive status epilepticus. Recommendations of the Epilepsy Foundation of America's Working Group on Status Epilepticus. JAMA 1993;270(7):854–9.

[23] Shinnar S, Hesdorffer DC, Nordli DR Jr, et al. Phenomenology of prolonged febrile seizures: results of the FEBSTAT study. Neurology 2008;71(3):170–6.
[24] Lowenstein DH. The management of refractory status epilepticus: an update. Epilepsia 2006;47(Suppl 1):35–40.
[25] Kossoff EH, Zupec-Kania BA, Rho JM. Ketogenic diets: an update for child neurologists. J Child Neurol 2009;24(8):979–88.
[26] Cross JH, McLellan A, Neal EG, et al. The ketogenic diet in childhood epilepsy: where are we now? Arch Dis Child 2010;95(7):550–3.
[27] Lefevre F, Aronson N. Ketogenic diet for the treatment of refractory epilepsy in children: a systematic review of efficacy. Pediatrics 2000;105(4):E46.
[28] Neal EG, Chaffe H, Schwartz RH, et al. The ketogenic diet for the treatment of childhood epilepsy: a randomised controlled trial. Lancet Neurol 2008;7(6):500–6.
[29] Zupec-Kania BA, Spellman E. An overview of the ketogenic diet for pediatric epilepsy. Nutr Clin Pract 2008 Dec–2009 Jan;23(6):589–96.
[30] Freeman JM, Kossoff EH. Ketosis and the ketogenic diet, 2010: advances in treating epilepsy and other disorders. Adv Pediatr 2010;57(1):315–29.
[31] Kossoff EH, Zupec-Kania BA, Amark PE, et al. Optimal clinical management of children receiving the ketogenic diet: recommendations of the International Ketogenic diet study group. Epilepsia 2009;50(2):304–17.
[32] Martinez CC, Pyzik PL, Kossoff EH. Discontinuing the ketogenic diet in seizure-free children: recurrence and risk factors. Epilepsia 2007;48(1):187–90.
[33] Zabara J. Inhibition of experimental seizures in canines by repetitive vagal stimulation. Epilepsia 1992;33(6):1005–12.
[34] Wheless J. Vagus nerve stimulation therapy. In: Wyllie E, editor. Wyllie's treatment of epilepsy: principles and practice. Lippincott Williams and Wilkins; 2010. p. 797–808.
[35] Naritoku D. Vagus Nerve Stimulation. In: Rho J, Sankar R, Cavazos J, editors. Epilepsy: Scientific Foundations of Clinical Practice. New York (NY): Marcel Dekker, Inc; 2004. p. 285–98.
[36] Handforth A, DeGiorgio CM, Schachter SC, et al. Vagus nerve stimulation therapy for partial-onset seizures: a randomized active-control trial. Neurology 1998;51(1):48–55.
[37] Ben-Menachem E, Manon-Espaillat R, Ristanovic R, et al. Vagus nerve stimulation for treatment of partial seizures: 1. A controlled study of effect on seizures. First International Vagus Nerve Stimulation Study Group. Epilepsia 1994;35(3):616–26.
[38] DeGiorgio CM, Schachter SC, Handforth A, et al. Prospective long-term study of vagus nerve stimulation for the treatment of refractory seizures. Epilepsia 2000;41(9):1195–200.
[39] Fisher RS, Handforth A. Reassessment: vagus nerve stimulation for epilepsy: a report of the therapeutics and technology assessment subcommittee of the American academy of neurology. Neurology 1999;53(4):666–9.

Advances in Pediatrics 58 (2011) 277–296
ADVANCES IN PEDIATRICS

Hearing Loss and Cochlear Implantation in Children

Patricia J. Yoon, MD

Department of Otolaryngology-Head & Neck Surgery, University of Colorado School of Medicine, The Bill Daniels Center for Children's Hearing, The Children's Hospital, 13123 East 16th Avenue, B455, Aurora, CO 80045, USA

Hearing loss is the most common congenital sensory impairment, with an incidence of 2 to 3 per 1000 live births. Approximately half of these newborns have severe-profound loss. Hearing loss can significantly hinder a child's expressive and receptive communication and, as a result, be detrimental to cognitive, educational, and psychosocial development. Fortunately, with the advent of universal newborn hearing screening, which is now mandated in most states, hearing loss is usually discovered very early in life. This screening provides the opportunity to intervene in the nascent stages of childhood development. Early intervention has far-reaching impact not only in terms of furthering a child's communication abilities, but also in its potential to change the direction of a child's life.

Cochlear implantation has become a very successful treatment option for some children with severe-profound hearing loss. Over the past several decades, significant advances in implant technology, coupled with increased understanding of auditory development, have enabled many hearing impaired children to successfully become a part of the "hearing world."

TYPES OF HEARING IMPAIRMENT

To understand the role of cochlear implantation, the different types of hearing impairment must first be understood. Hearing loss is primarily characterized as conductive or sensorineural in nature. Mixed hearing loss is a combination of the two. Another category of hearing impairment is auditory neuropathy spectrum disorder (ANSD).

Conductive hearing loss occurs when sound transmission is physically blocked between the opening of the external ear and the cochlear hair (receptor) cells. The most common cause of conductive hearing loss in children is otitis media and related conditions, such as middle ear effusion and Eustachian tube dysfunction. Conductive loss has numerous other causes, including cerumen

E-mail address: yoon.patricia@tchden.org

0065-3101/11/$ – see front matter
doi:10.1016/j.yapd.2011.03.013

impaction, tympanic membrane perforation, and ossicular fixation or disruption. In a conductive loss, no dysfunction of the cochlear hair cells or auditory nerve is present. Cochlear implantation is not used to treat conductive hearing losses.

A sensorineural hearing loss (SNHL) is caused by a neural defect in the transmission of sound at the level of the cochlea, which is where the receptor cells for sound, known as *hair cells*, are found. SNHL may be congenital or acquired, and both congenital and acquired losses may be hereditary (genetic) or nonhereditary in nature. Approximately 30% of hereditary hearing loss is considered syndromic. More than 400 genetic syndromes that include hearing loss have been described. The other 70% are nonsyndromic, or not associated with any visible abnormalities or medical problems. Well-recognized risk factors for SNHL in infants and children include family history of childhood SNHL, birth weight less than 1500 g, low Apgar scores, craniofacial anomalies, hypoxia, in utero infections (eg, TORCH), and history of mechanical ventilation for more than 5 days.

SNHL is also characterized as being prelingual or postlingual. Prelingual hearing loss is present before speech develops and is very often congenital; postlingual hearing loss occurs after the development of normal speech.

Auditory neuropathy was first recognized as an entity in the 1990s, and was renamed ANSD in 2008 [1]. It is diagnosed when there is a discrepancy between cochlear and neural function. In ANSD, the outer hair cells function normally, but sound is not properly transmitted from the outer hair cells to the auditory cortex. This dysfunction is thought to be caused by desynchronized action potentials in the auditory nerve. Presentation varies widely. Children with ANSD may have hearing thresholds that range from normal to profound levels on audiometric testing; however, they usually exhibit disproportionately poor speech perception abilities for their degree of hearing loss. Some patients with ANSD have only very mild impairment, whereas others present as functionally deaf. Some have impairment that fluctuates in severity. Children with ANSD typically have difficulty hearing in noise. ANSD children may hear words but have difficulty understanding what is being said.

ANSD may not be detected on newborn hearing screening if otoacoustic emissions (OAE) testing is used, because this modality only tests the function of the cochlear outer hair cells, and not the auditory nerve. Auditory brainstem response (ABR) is either absent or grossly abnormal on testing. ANSD accounts for a relatively small percentage of hearing impairment. Risk factors include prematurity, severe jaundice, low birth weight, and hypoxia. It is genetic in some cases. Some children with ANSD actually have deficient or absent cochlear nerves, whereas others have global neuropathies, such as seen in Charcot-Marie-Tooth disease or Friedreich ataxia.

Cochlear implantation is an option for some children with severe-profound sensorineural hearing loss or significant impairment caused by ANSD.

THE COCHLEAR IMPLANT

The U.S. Food and Drug Administration (FDA) approved the modern, multichannel cochlear implant in 1985 for use in adults. The FDA approved the device in 1990 for children down to the age of 2 years, and in 2002 down to the age of 12 months.

A cochlear implant is not a hearing aid. Hearing aids merely amplify sound. A cochlear implant bypasses the cochlear hair cells and directly electrically stimulates the auditory nerve. It does not restore normal hearing, but rather allows for the perception of sound sensation.

The device has internal and external parts (Figs. 1 and 2). The external parts include a microphone, speech processor, and transmitter. The microphone picks up sounds from the environment. The speech processor digitizes the sounds and then these signals are sent via the transmitter to the internal portion of the device, which is surgically implanted. The receiver, which is under the scalp, picks up the signals and delivers them to the electrode array that is

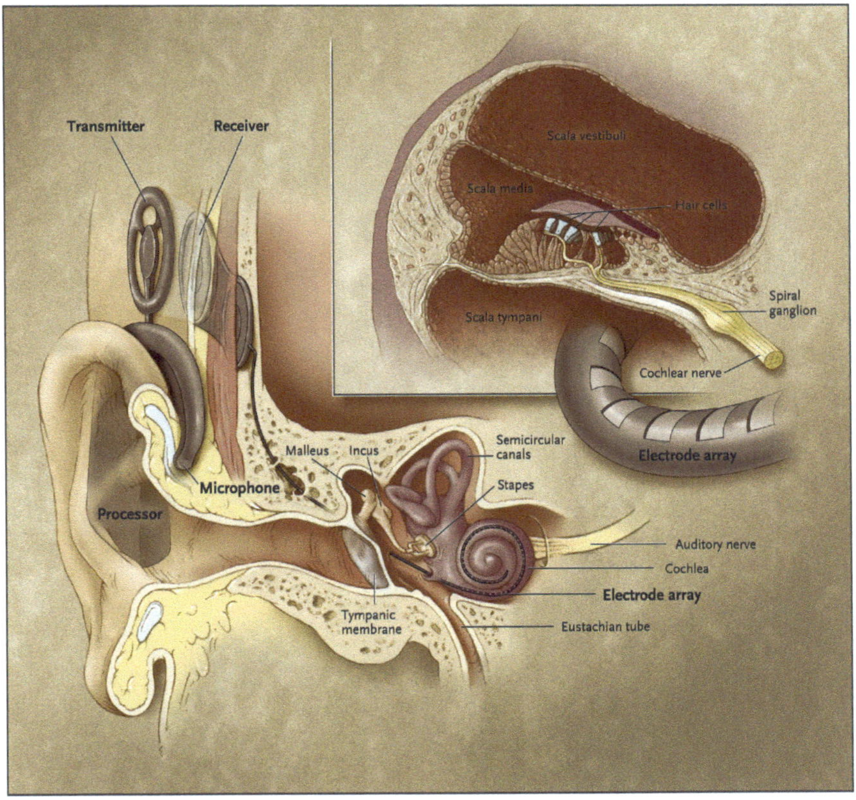

Fig. 1. This diagram shows how the internal and external portions of a cochlear implant are positioned. The microphone, which is worn on the ear, picks up sounds which are then digitized by the speech processor. The transmitter sends these signals through the scalp to the receiver, and the impulses are sent into the electrode array which directly stimulates the auditory nerve. (*Reprinted from* Papsin BC, Gordon KA. Cochlear implants for children with severe-to-profound hearing loss. N Engl J Med 2007;357:2380–7; with permission.)

inserted into the cochlea. The electrodes along the array directly stimulate the auditory nerve. The cochlea is tonotopically organized: high frequencies are picked up at the base of the cochlea, and low frequencies are detected at the apex of the snail-shaped organ.

Currently available cochlear implants have up to 24 electrodes along the array. The speech processor contains software that transforms sounds into electrical signals. The software contains speech-encoding algorithms designed to optimize the conveyance of speech information. Different manufacturers use different processing strategies and no one strategy has consistently produced better overall results than the others. As of this writing, there are three major manufacturers in the world.

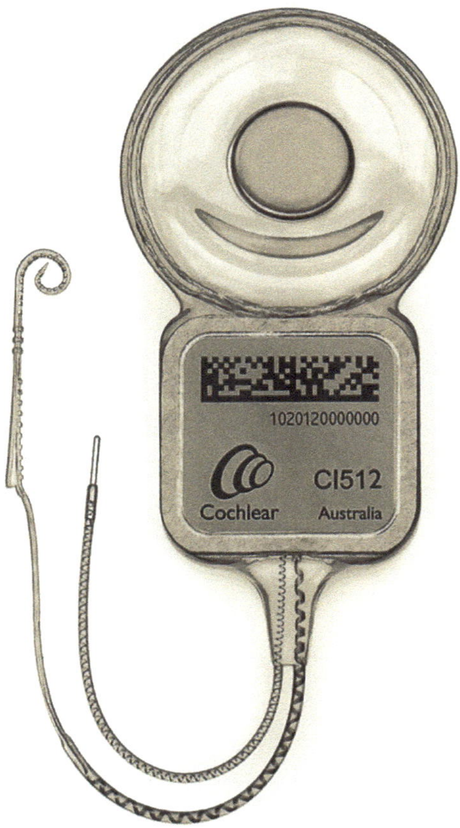

Fig. 2. The internal portion of a cochlear implant. The receiver is surgically implanted under the scalp, and has a ground electrode and a curved electrode array which is placed in the cochlea. (Photo provided *Courtesy of* Cochlear Americas, 2009 Cochlear Americas; with permission.)

CANDIDACY FOR IMPLANTATION

Before any discussion regarding candidacy for implantation, it is important to note that not all people desire cochlear implants or wish to be a part of the "hearing world." Some view deafness not as a disability, but rather a different human experience. For this population, Deafness is a cultural identity, much like an ethnic identity, and the capital "D" is used to signify use of the term as a cultural label. American Sign Language (ASL) forms the linguistic basis for their identity. The Deaf population prides itself on being a close-knit, supportive community, with its own language and rich heritage. Thus, cochlear implantation, and the view that hearing-impaired children must be brought into an oral-hearing world, are antithetical to the Deaf identity, and have been the topic of many contentious debates. Both sides of this debate share the common goal of promoting language development in and bettering the life of deaf children. Both sides have pros and cons.

The decision of whether to implant a child is pivotal, and one of lifelong consequence, because it can profoundly influence the future direction of a child's life. It is a complex decision based on many factors in addition to hearing status, such as available educational options and support systems. The surgical placement of the device alone does not result in improved hearing and, in fact, is only the beginning of a long and involved learning process. Success depends on motivation and a long-term commitment to therapy and education. For this reason, in many centers a team approach is used to evaluate candidates, with the involvement of otolaryngologists, audiologists, speech–language pathologists, social workers, psychologists, and educational specialists.

From a medical standpoint, a candidate must be healthy enough to withstand general anesthesia and surgery, and must have a cochlea and an auditory nerve. Rarely, deafness is the result of an absent auditory nerve or cochlear agenesis. Other cochlear and inner ear malformations are not usually contraindications to surgery but must be evaluated on a case-by-case basis.

Obtaining an accurate assessment of an infant or child's hearing status is necessary to determine candidacy. Previously, the belief was that only children with bilateral profound (pure-tone averages >90 dB) sensorineural hearing loss, receiving little to no benefit from hearing aids, should be considered for implantation. However, as understanding of auditory development and outcomes has evolved, the criteria have broadened to include patients with greater degrees of residual hearing. The trend has been toward a more functional assessment of a candidate's hearing, with a focus on language acquisition abilities, instead of reliance on pure-tone averages alone.

All cochlear implant candidates should receive a trial of binaural amplification, fit appropriately, according to American Academy of Audiology pediatric hearing aid fitting guidelines. A 3- to 6-month trial of hearing aid use, in conjunction with intensive therapy, is typically necessary to evaluate benefit. To determine whether the hearing aids are providing enough useful auditory input to allow for communication and language acquisition, open-set aided speech recognition testing is performed in older children. In younger children, closed-set speech recognition tests may provide useful information. The FDA criteria vary slightly for different manufacturers' devices, but speech discrimination scores of 50% to 60% or below with optimal amplification are currently required for candidacy. Receiving benefit from amplification no longer disqualifies one from receiving a cochlear implant, because most patients who are able to recognize approximately 50% of words using hearing aids have now been shown to generally have even higher speech recognition scores postimplantation, compared with their best preoperative scores [2,3]. For children with asymmetric hearing loss, the literature supports continued use of a hearing aid in the better-hearing, nonimplanted ear, with implantation of the worse-hearing ear. Greater residual hearing at implantation and shorter duration of deafness seem to be associated with improved language outcomes; conversely, poorer outcomes seem to be associated with prolonged use of hearing aids before implantation [4,5].

For infants and very young children who cannot undergo speech perception testing, the assessment relies heavily on a team approach. Audiometric testing and appropriately fit hearing aids are the first requirement, and then evidence of benefit, or lack thereof, is based on regular audiologic evaluations, results of outcome questionnaires, and reports from parents and early intervention providers. A speech-language pathologist who is familiar with this population works collaboratively with the implant audiologist to assess progress in auditory skills. Because the evaluation of infants is not straightforward, a hearing aid trial of at least 6 months, with appropriate early intervention and speech-language services, is usually desired before making a decision regarding implantation.

A situation in which the decision to implant is often expedited is when deafness occurs secondary to bacterial meningitis, particularly if *Streptococcus pneumoniae* is the pathogen. In these cases, because of the powerful inflammatory response triggered by the pneumococcal cell wall, rapid fibrosis and ossification of the cochlea may occur, often beginning within several weeks of the infection [6]. Ossification can lead to a more difficult surgery, incomplete electrode insertion, and poorer outcomes. For this reason, many advocate a more aggressive time line for surgery, including implantation under the age of 12 months if necessary. This recommendation is a matter of some debate, because hearing recovery in post-meningitic patients has been reported; for advocates of the watchful waiting approach, serial MRI scanning is performed, with urgent cochlear implantation for signs of ossification.

The age of implantation continues to decrease. Understanding of auditory development and brain plasticity has given physicians the impetus to implant children at a younger age, and earlier implantation has been correlated with improved communication outcomes [4,7–12]. A narrow window of time exists during development, known as a *sensitive period*, within which the central auditory cortex must be stimulated by sound if it is to develop normally. If the auditory cortex is deprived of stimulus during this period, it will reorganize to be used for other purposes. For example, studies using functional MRI have shown that in deaf individuals, areas of the auditory cortex were activated by visual stimuli; this was not seen in normal hearing controls [13]. Because of this reallocation of brain function, once the sensitive period has passed, auditory development becomes much more challenging.

Sharma and colleagues [13–15] looked to assess the effect of age at cochlear implantation on auditory development and found that the brain is maximally plastic for the first 3.5 years, and that the optimal time for implantation is within this period. Plasticity then declined, but was found to remain in varying degrees until approximately 7 years of age, which marked the end of the sensitive period. Some studies have shown that different language skills may have different sensitive periods. For example, one study concluded that there might be an earlier sensitive period for vocabulary-building skills than for speech perception skills [7].

Research has been directed toward further narrowing down the optimal age for implantation. No consensus has been reached, but most literature supports that younger is better [7,10,16]. The FDA currently approves cochlear implantation down to 12 months of age, but some centers have been implanting even younger infants.

As understanding of ANSD has grown, cochlear implants have also become recognized as a viable option for some children with this disorder. One might question the efficacy of a cochlear implant in patients with abnormal auditory nerve conduction, but it is postulated that the discrete electrical signals produced by a cochlear implant may be more effective at eliciting a synchronous neural response than acoustic stimuli. Several studies report that children with ANSD derive benefit from cochlear implantation, and some report outcomes comparable to those of implanted children with SNHL [17–20]. In 2008, a consensus panel recommended that cochlear implants should be considered in children with ANSD, regardless of audiometric threshold, if progress is not being made in language development, despite appropriate amplification.

However, children with ANSD are a heterogeneous group, and not all patients with ANSD should be implanted. Research has shown that for individuals with a cochlear nerve deficiency or hypoplastic cochlear nerve, outcomes are much poorer [21,22]. This does not mean that this group should automatically be excluded from consideration, but they should be carefully assessed for any auditory sensation, and expectations should be tempered.

There is also a chance that auditory function may improve in ANSD. This has been documented in several studies. In a 2002 study, 50% of children with ANSD and evidence of severe SNHL spontaneously improved, with a mean improvement time of 5.8 months. The children whose ANSD was attributed to hyperbilirubinemia had a greater tendency to improve. These children achieved a stable audiogram at a mean age of 18 months [23]. Thus, caution must be exercised before proceeding with implantation in infants and very young children who carry this diagnosis.

Cochlear implant programs in the past tended to exclude deaf children with other handicaps, but the number of children with other disabilities being implanted is increasing rapidly, and accounts for a large percentage of implant recipients at some centers. For most children, the goal of implantation is spoken language. For children with developmental delays or other disabilities, the goals of implantation may be different. Speech and language outcomes may be limited by cognitive deficits, but these children may still derive benefit from improved use of language, as well as sound awareness, and increased environmental and social connectedness. Communication by nonverbal modalities may still be supported by sound. Mere sound awareness can be useful in terms of social attachment, attention, and safety. Thus, these children should not automatically be excluded from implant candidacy [24,25].

In addition to audiometric, speech, language, and medical considerations, candidacy evaluation must also include assessments of a child's support systems, psychosocial situation, and educational environment. The importance of these aspects cannot be underestimated. A cochlear implant recipient must have access to appropriate therapy and educational services to learn to understand speech and develop spoken language. This may be difficult in some rural areas or in areas with a low population of deaf or implanted children. Efforts must be made to line up these services during the candidacy process. The potential recipient must be motivated and have adequate family/caregiver support to participate in intensive therapy and education. A psychological evaluation may be needed to assess whether a child has met general and cognitive developmental targets and whether he/she will be able to use the device effectively. It may also identify behavioral issues or other areas of concern that may affect candidacy.

It is critical that potential implant recipients and their families have realistic expectations regarding the implant and outcomes, and that they be willing to revise their expectations throughout the process. While a cochlear implant may allow a child to "hear" sounds, there are always limitations, and there is no guarantee that a child will be able to function as a hearing child. Numerous factors, some intrinsic and others extrinsic to the child, will influence outcome. A cochlear implant does not cure deafness, and the recipient and family must understand that hearing with a cochlear implant is different from how most people perceive sound. Perhaps most important is the understanding that language comprehension and the ability to speak will not develop without intensive, long-term therapy and education, and significant effort on both the part of the recipient, his/her family, and the educational system.

The Children's Implant Profile, often referred to as ChIP, was devised in 1991 as a systematic method for determining implant candidacy, and has been widely used around the world. ChIP examines 11 factors that contribute to successful implantation and rates them on a 3-point scale. These include age, duration of deafness, medical or radiologic anomalies, secondary handicaps, functional hearing level, speech-language abilities, family support, expectations, educational environment, availability of support services to monitor implant use, and cognitive learning style [26]. Several modifications of the protocol have been made since then [27,28].

SURGICAL AND MEDICAL CONSIDERATIONS

The surgeon assesses the candidate in terms of medical risk and surgical feasibility. Comorbid medical conditions, cognitive status, and otologic history are all taken into account. The patient must be stable enough to undergo general anesthesia and withstand surgery and the potential, realistic benefit for that individual must outweigh the risks.

All cochlear implant candidates must be evaluated with radiographic imaging. High resolution computed tomography (CT) scanning of the temporal bone is obtained to evaluate any anatomic abnormalities of the inner ear structures, such as a dysplastic cochlea or enlarged vestibular aqueduct. Use of magnetic resonance imaging (MRI) is becoming more widespread for preoperative evaluation because of its superior ability to reveal soft tissue abnormalities of the inner ear, such as cochlear nerve hypoplasia or agenesis, cochlear fibrosis, or dilated endolymphatic sac [29]. Findings such as a cochlear nerve asymmetry or cochlear obstruction might influence the decision to implant one side over the other. In all cases of ANSD, MRI should be obtained to evaluate for cochlear nerve hypoplasia or absence. Lack of a cochlear nerve would be a contraindication to surgery. MRI of the inner ear and brain should also be obtained in children with other neurologic pathologies, at least as a baseline, since an MRI cannot easily be obtained once a child has been implanted due to potential damage to the device and compromise of the image due to artifact.

All cochlear implant recipients are at increased risk for bacterial meningitis. An opening is created in the cochlea during surgery to accommodate insertion of the electrode. Although the opening is plugged with soft tissue, it remains a potential route through which bacteria, such as those causing acute otitis media, may enter the inner ear and cerebrospinal fluid. Some inner ear malformations associated with hearing loss also inherently place patients at increased meningitis risk. Therefore, all cochlear implant candidates and recipients should receive all age-appropriate doses of pneumococcal conjugate and *Haemophilus influenza* type b conjugate vaccines, in addition to an annual influenza vaccination. At age 24 months, the 23-valent pneumococcal polysaccharide vaccine should also be administered. The tetravalent meningococcal vaccine should be considered, but there is no evidence that individuals with cochlear implants are at any increased risk for meningitis caused by *N. meningitidis*. Because of the meningitis risk, acute otitis media at the time of planned implant surgery is a contraindication to proceeding. Tympanostomy tube placement should be considered before implantation in patients with recurrent acute otitis media or chronic middle ear effusions [30].

With large numbers of children being implanted during their most otitis-prone years, primary care providers are becoming more likely to encounter children with cochlear implants and acute otitis media. Acute otitis media must be treated aggressively in this population, without delay. The risk of complications from acute otitis media may be higher in the first few months after implantation. Empiric treatment with an oral antibiotic such as high-dose amoxicillin or amoxicillin-clavulanate is appropriate if the patient is at least 2-months post-implant surgery, he/she does not have an inner ear malformation, he/she does not appear severely ill, and the cochlear implant does not have a spacer/positioner. (This was found in an implant model which was available from 1999 through 2002, when it was voluntarily recalled from the market.) For patients who do not meet these criteria, parenteral antibiotics, such as ceftriaxone or cefotaxime, are recommended as initial treatment. Referral to an otolaryngologist is appropriate if symptoms worsen despite 24 hours of antibiotic therapy [30].

Concerns have been raised about the safety of implanting very young infants. Issues unique to this population, from a surgical standpoint, include thinner and more delicate tissues, lower circulating blood volume, large amounts of calvarial bone marrow, decreased pneumatization of the temporal bone, and more superficial position of the facial nerve. However, studies support the safety and efficacy of the procedure, and preliminary data seem to indicate language growth rates comparable to normal hearing children [31,32].

THE IMPLANT PROCEDURE

The typical cochlear implantation procedure is described here. The surgery is performed in the supine position under general anesthesia. Paralytic agents are not used, as intraoperative facial nerve monitoring is performed. (The facial nerve traverses the surgical area and is therefore at some risk.) Perioperative intravenous antibiotics are administered to cover normal skin flora. The facial nerve monitor electrodes are placed, the postauricular area is injected with local anesthetic with epinephrine, and then the patient is prepped and draped in sterile fashion. A skin incision is created in the postauricular area and carried down to expose the mastoid area and cranium. Posterior and superior to the ear, most surgeons drill a depression or well in the skull in which the implant receiver will sit. Next, a mastoidectomy is performed: the mastoid bone, immediately behind the ear, is opened using a surgical drill, down to a depth where the lateral semicircular canal and incus can be seen; the middle ear space is accessed from here (Fig. 3). An opening called the facial recess is created, and through this, one can see the bone overlying the cochlea. A cochleostomy, or hole, is created into the scala tympani of the cochlea through which the implant electrode will be threaded (Fig. 4). A trough is drilled to connect the well with the mastoidectomy, providing a channel for the electrode. The cochlear implant is then positioned and secured in the well, the electrode array is threaded into the cochlea, and the cochleostomy is plugged with small pieces of soft tissue such as temporalis muscle or fascia (Figs. 5 and 6). The incision is then closed in layers and a head-wrap dressing is applied. After the implant has been placed, many centers perform intraoperative testing to measure implant electrode impedances and to verify and record neural responses to electrical stimuli. Plain films or fluoroscopy may also verify electrode placement. Cochlear implantation is frequently performed in an ambulatory surgery setting.

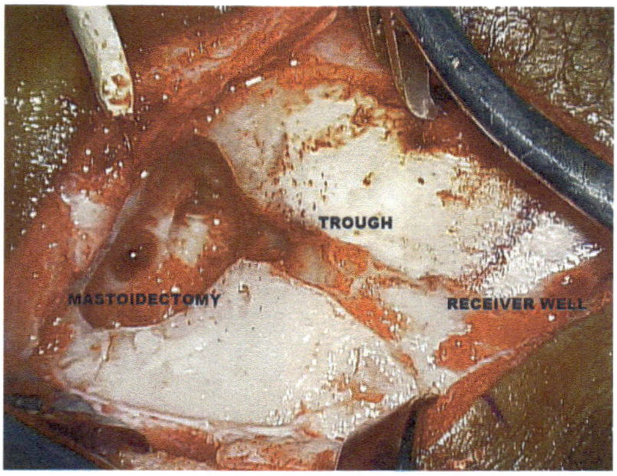

Fig. 3. This photograph shows the temporal bone in the postauricular area after the receiver well, mastoid, and trough have been drilled. This is a left ear.

The cochlear implant surgical procedure has evolved over time. In the past, generous areas of hair were shaved as part of the surgical preparation, large incisions and scalp flaps were created, and large wells were drilled in the skull to accommodate the receiver, often exposing dura. Holes were drilled in the skull through which sutures were passed to tie down the implant. As with many other surgeries, the trend has been toward making cochlear implantation minimally invasive. The implants themselves have become smaller over time, making possible some recent changes in technique. Cochlear implants are now being placed through significantly smaller skin incisions, often without any hair being shaved. Some surgeons do not drill a well, but rather just create a pocket under the pericranium to hold the receiver. Some do not secure the implants with sutures. Others feel that without one or both of these steps, the device is at significantly increased risk for displacement.

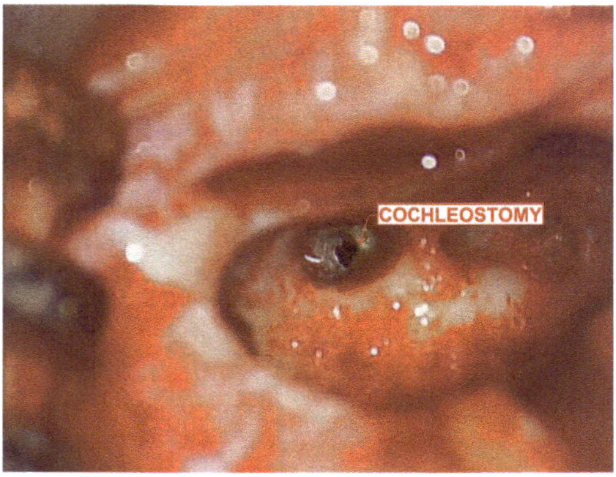

Fig. 4. The cochleostomy.

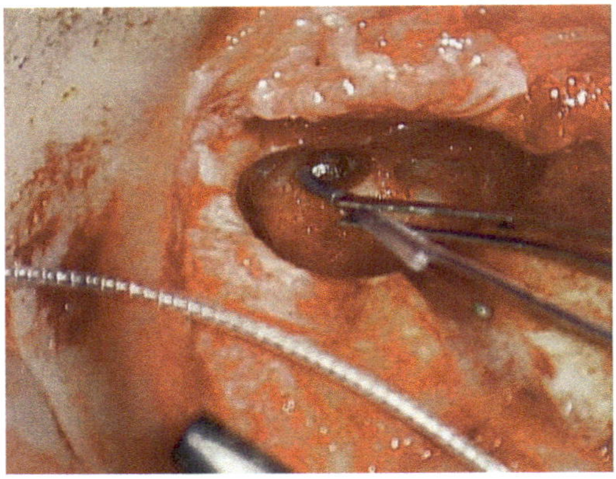

Fig. 5. Insertion of the electrode array into the cochleostomy.

The potential major and minor risks of cochlear implant surgery which are typically stated on a surgical consent form include the following: facial nerve injury, meningitis, cerebrospinal fluid leak, perilymphatic fluid leak, vertigo, hematoma, seroma, wound infection, tinnitus, taste disturbance, ear numbness, and device failure. The published data on rates of complications in cochlear implant surgery is somewhat limited, but the overall rate of major perioperative complications in the pediatric population is low and compares favorably with that of the adult population [33]. The revision surgery rate in the pediatric population, however, is higher than is seen in adults, with a quoted rate of 8–13%, as compared with 5.4–6.9% in adults [34–36]. Cited reasons for revision implantation surgery included internal device failure ("hard failure"), scalp flap complications, device migration, infection, electrode extrusion, technology upgrade, unexplained deterioration of performance ("soft failure"), and facial

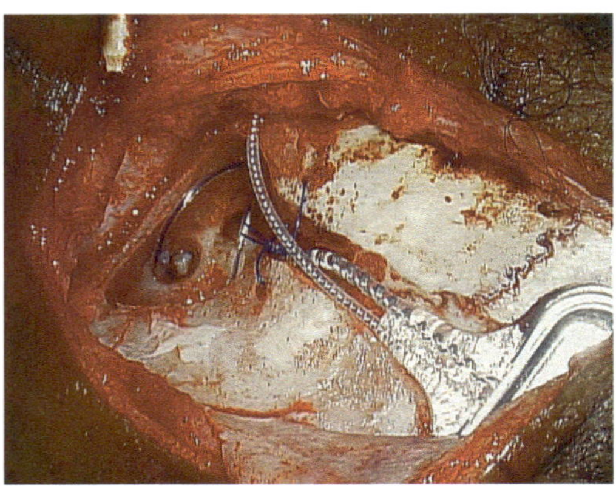

Fig. 6. The internal device in place.

nerve stimulation. In all articles reviewed, "hard failure" of the device accounted for the most revision surgeries. Head trauma was noted to precede almost half of the pediatric hard failures in one study [37]. For this reason, some implant centers discourage participation in contact sports among recipients. Fortunately, studies report excellent outcomes for reimplantation surgery, with equal or improved performance in most cases [38].

AFTER COCHLEAR IMPLANT SURGERY

After cochlear implant surgery, most centers will wait approximately 2–4 weeks before activating the device to allow time for healing. There is no ability to hear with the implant during this period. At the time of activation, the audiologist will place the external device (transmitter) directly over the receiver which is implanted under the scalp; this is held in place by a magnet. The internal portion of the cochlear implant is then checked by computer to ensure that it is working properly; communication between the external and internal devices is checked, along with each individual electrode. The speech processor is then programmed or "mapped." Each electrode is turned on and a current is delivered until the patient hears a tone; this is the threshold. The loudness is then increased until a comfortable listening level is achieved. After each electrode has been mapped, this information is downloaded into the speech processor and the implant is activated. For infants, mapping is primarily based on objective measurement of neural responses to stimulation, but also relies on behavioral responses as observed by the parents and audiologist. The reaction at switch-on is different for each child, but common reactions include crying or a look of bewilderment in infants and toddlers, and excitement, happiness or anxiety in older children. At the beginning, sounds may seem garbled and unfamiliar, as the brain must adapt to processing the new input, but over time, sounds become clearer and gain meaning. As the recipient becomes familiar with and is better able to use the implant, the audiologist will adjust mapping and fine-tune the settings to enhance the quality of sound for the individual.The initial activation visit usually takes several hours and may take place over two visits. Mapping visits occur frequently early-on, and then once a stable map is achieved, typically after about 2 months of use, visits may be spaced out to every 3 months, and then every 6 months to yearly. Stimulation thresholds change over time, so monitoring and adjustments are necessary throughout life. In addition, a typical therapy schedule for infants and young children is twice a week for the first 1–2 years after implantation, and then weekly until school begins, at which point, therapy usually takes place through school.

Once a patient has a cochlear implant, there are some important precautions and restrictions which must be remembered. The external device is not waterproof, so recipients can swim but must first remove the external portion of the device. MRI is contraindicated because the powerful magnetic field created by MRI scanners can damage the implant. Some newer implant models are MRI compatible and can withstand up to 1.5 Tesla, and there are also some models with removable magnets in case MRI scanning should be necessary. A brief surgical procedure is necessary to remove the magnet. Monopolar electrosurgical instruments should not be used in the head or neck of a cochlear implant recipient, as the currents produced could flow through the electrode array and cause damage to the implant or cochlear tissue. A common scenario in which this can be a factor is when a cochlear implant patient requires a tonsillectomy or adenoidectomy. In general, bipolar cautery may be safely used. Ionizing radiation therapy can damage the implant. The sound from a cochlear implant can be distorted when in close proximity to sources of electromagnetic interference which include radio or television transmission towers, airport metal detectors and some types of mobile communications equipment, including some mobile phones. Static electricity can potentially damage the device or, more commonly, erase the speech processor program. Certain activities known to create significant electrostatic discharge, such as sliding down a plastic slide, should either be avoided, or the processor should first be removed.

BILATERAL IMPLANTATION

While unilateral cochlear implant users appreciate significant benefit as compared with severe-to-profoundly deaf patients without an implant, they still experience the problems associated with unilateral deafness, such as difficulty with localization of a sound source and listening in background noise. Some still benefit from hearing aid use in the contralateral ear, but for many this provides no recognizable benefit. In recent years, with the backing of research which has examined auditory outcomes, safety, efficacy and cost-utility, bilateral implantation has become a standard medical practice where clinically appropriate [39,40].

The advantages of bilateral implantation which have been reported in multiple studies include improved speech perception, not only in noisy environments, but also in quiet settings. Bilateral implant users have shown improved abilities in localizing the direction from which a sound originates. Another benefit cited is the fact that with two implants, it is less likely that a recipient will have to spend time "off the air" if the batteries should lose charge, or if one of the devices should fail [39]. There is also evidence of specialization of the auditory cortices in each hemisphere [41]. Thus, it seems reasonable to conclude that input from two implants may complement each other, each providing slightly different information.

Bilateral implantation can be performed simultaneously or sequentially. Advantages of simultaneous implantation include the need for only one surgery and anesthetic, as well as the ability to activate both devices at the same time. Disadvantages include longer operative time on a given day, with greater blood loss and potentially increased anesthetic risk. The blood loss factor may be significant in infants who inherently have a lower circulating blood volume and a marrow-filled temporal bone. If sequential bilateral implantation is chosen, it is recommended that the second implant be placed with minimal delay [41,42]. In a 2009 study, Gordon and Papsin reported better speech perceptions scores for children in whom the inter-implant delay was less than 12 months, as compared with those in whom the delay was more than 2 years. It is postulated that there are sensitive periods for development of binaural hearing, so this may be, at least in part, a function of age. Peters and colleagues [43] found that children younger than age 8 who had received a sequential second implant had a faster rate of improvement and achieved a higher mean speech perception score than children in the 8–13 year age group.

OUTCOMES

The goal of most cochlear implant recipients is to develop age-appropriate expressive and receptive language abilities; however, there is significant variation in performance. In general, the best outcomes are seen in cognitively normal children who were implanted at an early age, who have motivated families and educators, and who are in an environment rich in oral communication. Many children are able to achieve open-set speech recognition within the first year of implantation [44]. A 10-year follow up study out of France reported that with cochlear implants, many profoundly hearing-impaired children are able to develop functional speech perception and production and achieve satisfactory performance in school [9]. In this study, 79% of implant recipients were able to use the telephone, 67% developed intelligible speech, and 78% were able to attend mainstream schools. Recipients averaged 72% open-set word recognition in quiet settings and 45% in noise. These children had more difficulty with receptive language, with 75% scoring below the median value of their normal-hearing peers. A 2005 English study showed similar findings 10–14 years post-implant, with 87% able to understand conversations without visual cues such as lip-reading, 60% able to speak on the telephone with a familiar speaker, and 77% able to produce intelligible speech [45].

Despite the significant benefits seen in word recognition and speech intelligibility, however, many children with cochlear implants still experience difficulties with elements of communication, such as syntax, semantics, and pragmatics [25]. And because of the multifaceted and integrated nature of language and communication development in the brain, deafness affects nonauditory skills, such as attention, reading, and written language. The average 18-to-19 year old deaf student reads at the level of an average normal-hearing 9 year old. Several factors have been identified as contributing to this deficiency, including the fact that most normal-hearing children learn to read by drawing upon their knowledge of spoken vocabulary and grammar. Early implant recipients with normal cognition may have less impairment, but most implanted children still lag behind normal hearing children in reading skills [11,25,46,47].

Several factors influence outcomes in children. Shorter duration of deafness before cochlear implantation was an important positive predictor of better outcome [12]. This generally correlates with younger age at time of implantation. It is also suspected that with a shorter duration of deafness, it is likely that more of the auditory system is intact and better able to process the signals produced by a cochlear implant. This supports the idea of implantation in the setting of residual hearing [5].

As discussed earlier in this article, early implantation minimizes the period of sensory deprivation and takes advantage of sensitive periods in auditory development. Numerous studies correlate younger age at implantation with improved outcome, but as of yet, there is no clear agreement on the optimal age for implantation. In several studies, the best outcomes are seen in recipients age 2 years and under [4,10,48]. Promising results have been reported in children implanted under 12 months of age but other studies have found no significant language outcome advantage in children implanted before 12 months of age as compared with children implanted at 13–24 months [16,32].

The recipient's method of communication and educational environment also influence outcome. Although children using both total communication (oral and sign language) and oral communication make gains in language acquisition after implantation, oral communicators overall outperform total communicators [49–51]. Long-term follow up of a large group of cochlear implant recipients found that those who relied on spoken language early on fared better in speech perception, speech intelligibility, verbal rehearsal skills, and literacy [50].

Other factors noted to influence language outcomes include socioeconomic status and strength of parent-child interactions [4]. Perhaps not surprisingly, one of the strongest influences on outcome, after correcting for other factors, was found to be the recipient's nonverbal intelligence [49,52].

For children with ANSD, studies indicate that cochlear implantation is beneficial and most studies report outcomes that are not significantly different from those seen in non-ANSD implanted children [17,18,20]. The exception was in children who had preoperative MRI evidence of central nervous system pathology and/or cochlear nerve hypoplasia; this group had poorer language-acquisition outcomes [21,22].

Children with inner ear malformations frequently undergo cochlear implant surgery, and despite more frequent intraoperative difficulties such as perilymphatic leaks and aberrant facial nerve anatomy, outcomes are often very successful [53,54]. However, the various types of inner ear malformations have different prognoses. Buchman and colleagues found that children with an incompletely partitioned cochlea, enlarged vestibular aqueduct (EVA) and dilated vestibule (Mondini malformation), as well as children with isolated EVA or partial semicircular canal aplasia had better outcomes in terms of speech perception than children with total semicircular canal aplasia, isolated incomplete partitioning, cochlear hypoplasia or common cavity deformity. Papsin also found poorer performance in children with narrowed internal auditory/cochlear canals, common cavity deformity, and a hypoplastic cochlea. However, both authors noted that these deformities should not automatically preclude a candidate from implantation, and that individual evaluation is necessary.

COST EFFECTIVENESS AND QUALITY OF LIFE

In the current health care environment, with economic pressures discouraging the use of expensive technologies, much attention has turned toward cost-effectiveness studies of new innovations. Cost-effectiveness and quality of life outcomes have been difficult to assess in children, as they often rely on parental reporting, and normative data in this population, with its diverse developmental phases, is scarce [55]. However, available studies support cochlear implantation as a cost-effective intervention with significant societal cost-savings [56,57]. One study estimates the lifetime cost of profound deafness to exceed $1 million, and estimates that cochlear implantation may save $53,198 per child when reduced educational costs and increased earnings are taken into account. The pediatric cochlear implant fares well in terms of cost-utility when compared with several other common medical interventions [40,57].

SUMMARY

In the mid-1980s, it was discovered that birds, unlike humans, have the ability to produce new cochlear hair cells after acoustic trauma or ototoxic drugs had damaged existing hair cells. Since then, research in hair cell regeneration has been one of the most active areas of inquiry in the hearing sciences. Many scientists are working furiously to unlock the key to human hair cell regeneration and to thereby make hearing restoration possible. This, or another breakthrough, may one day render the cochlear implant obsolete. But until that time comes, we work to advance implant technology and to better understand how to get the most out of these devices.

Children have now been receiving cochlear implants for approximately the past two decades. Implantation has become a standard option for many patients with severe-profound hearing loss and has become a possibility for populations who were not previously considered appropriate for this technology. Cochlear implants provide these children with the opportunity to become a part of the hearing world, or at least to allow sound perception to enrich their lives. Studies to date support the idea of sensitive periods of auditory development, and indicate that implantation at a very early age provides recipients with the best language acquisition outcomes, particularly in an environment of oral communication. Bilateral implantation offers the advantages of binaural hearing and should be considered when implantation is being evaluated.

The first pediatric multichannel cochlear implant recipients are just now entering adulthood. Research on these subjects is giving us insight into how this technology can impact recipients across the lifespan, from infancy into later years. We still have much to learn about auditory development, cognition and how these and other factors influence outcome.

Acknowledgments

Thank you to Jennifer Kolb, M.Ed., CCC-A and Susan Dreith, Au.D., CCC-A for their audiologic expertise.

References

[1] Starr A, Picton TW, Sininger Y, et al. Auditory neuropathy. Brain 1996;119:741–53.
[2] Dowell RC, Hollow R, Winton E. Outcomes for cochlear implant users with significant residual hearing. Arch Otolaryngol Head Neck Surg 2004;130:575–81.

[3] Dettman SJ, D'Costa WA, Dowell RC, et al. Cochlear implants for children with significant residual hearing. Arch Otolaryngol Head Neck Surg 2004;130:612–8.
[4] Niparko JK, Tobey EA, Thal DJ, et al. Spoken language development in children following cochlear implantation. JAMA 2010;303(15):1498–506.
[5] Gantz BJ, Rubenstein T, Tyler RS, et al. Long-term results of cochlear implants in children with residual hearing. Ann Otol Rhinol Laryngol Suppl 2000;185:33–6.
[6] Philippon D, Bergeron F, Ferron P, et al. Cochlear implantation in postmeningitic deafness. Otol Neurotol 2010;31:83–7.
[7] Houston DM, Miyamoto RT. Effects of early auditory experience on word learning and speech perception in deaf children with cochlear implants: implications for sensitive periods of language development. Otol Neurotol 2010;31:1248–53.
[8] Nikolopoulos TP, O'Donoghue GM, Archbold S. Age at implantation: its importance in pediatric cochlear implantation. Laryngoscope 1999;109:595–9.
[9] Uziel AS, Sillon M, Vieu A, et al. Ten-year follow-up of a consecutive series of children with multichannel cochlear implants. Otol Neurotol 2007;28:615–28.
[10] DeRaeve L. A longitudinal study on auditory perception and speech intelligibility in deaf children implanted younger than 18 months in comparison to those implanted at later ages. Otol Neurotol 2010;31:1261–7.
[11] Geers AE, Hayes H. Reading, writing, and phonological processing skills of adolescents with 10 or more years or cochlear implant experience. Ear Hear 2011;32:49S–59S.
[12] Geers AE, Sedey AL. Language and verbal reasoning skills in adolescents with 10 or more years of cochlear implant experience. Ear Hear 2011;32:39S–48S.
[13] Sharma A, Gilley PM, Dorman MF, et al. Deprivation-induced cortical reorganization in children with cochlear implants. Int J Audiol 2007;46:494–9.
[14] Sharma A, Dorman MF, Kral A. The influence of a sensitive period on central auditory development in children with unilateral and bilateral cochlear implants. Hear Res 2005;203:134–43.
[15] Sharma A, Dorman MF, Spahr AJ. A sensitive period for the development of the central auditory system in children with cochlear implants: implications for the age of implantation. Ear Hear 2002;23:532–9.
[16] Holt RF, Svirsky MA. An exploratory look at pediatric cochlear implantation: is earliest always best? Ear Hear 2008;29:492–511.
[17] Buss E, Labadie RF, Brown CJ, et al. Outcome of cochlear implantation in pediatric auditory neuropathy. Otol Neurotol 2002;23:328–32.
[18] Gibson WP, Sanli H. Auditory neuropathy: an update. Ear Hear 2007;28:102S–6S.
[19] Rance G, Barker EJ. Speech perception in children with auditory neuropathy/dyssynchrony managed with either hearing aids or cochlear implants. Otol Neurotol 2008;29:179–82.
[20] Madden C, Hilbert L, Rutter M, et al. Pediatric cochlear implantation in auditory neuropathy. Otol Neurotol 2002;23:163–8.
[21] Walton J, Gibson WP, Sanli H. Predicting cochlear implant outcomes in children with auditory neuropathy. Otol Neurotol 2008;29:302–9.
[22] Teagle HF, Roush PA, Woodard JS, et al. Cochlear implantation in children with auditory neuropathy spectrum disorder. Ear Hear 2010;31:325–35.
[23] Madden C, Rutter M, Hilbert L, et al. Clinical and audiological features in auditory neuropathy. Arch Otolaryngol Head Neck Surg 2002;128:1026–30.
[24] Holt RF, Kirk KI. Speech and language development in cognitively delayed children with cochlear implants. Ear Hear 2005;26:132–48.
[25] Kral A, O'Donoghue GM. Profound deafness in childhood. N Engl J Med 2010;363:1438–50.
[26] Niparko JK, Lingua C, Carpenter RM. Assessment of candidacy for cochlear implantation. In: Niparko JK, editor. Cochlear implants: principles and practices. 2nd edition. Philadelphia: Lippincott Williams and Wilkins; 2009. p. 137–46.

[27] Lazaridis E, Therres M, Marsh RR. How is the children's implant profile used in the Cochlear implant candidacy process? Int J Pediatr Otorhinolaryngol 2010;74:412–5.
[28] Edwards L, Thomas F, Rajput K. Use of a revised children's implant profile (GOSHChIP) in candidacy for paediatric cochlear implantation and in predicting outcome. Int J Audiol 2009;48:554–60.
[29] Parry DA, Booth T, Roland PS. Advantages of magnetic resonance imaging over computed tomography in preoperative evaluation of pediatric cochlear implant candidates. Otol Neurotol 2005;26:976–82.
[30] Rubin LG, Papsin B, Committee on Infectious Diseases and Section on Otolaryngology Head and Neck Surgery. Cochlear implants in children: surgical site infections and prevention and treatment of acute otitis media and meningitis. Pediatrics 2010;126:381–91.
[31] Roland JT, Cosetti M, Wang KH, et al. Cochlear implantation in the very young child: long-term safety and efficacy. Laryngoscope 2009;119:2205–10.
[32] Dettman SJ, Pinder D, Briggs RJ, et al. Communication development in children who receive the cochlear implant younger than 12 months: risks versus benefits. Ear Hear 2007;28: 11S–8S.
[33] Tucci DL, Pilkington TM. Medical and surgical aspects of cochlear implantation. In: Niparko JK, editor. Cochlear implants: principles and practices. 2nd edition. Philadelphia: Lippincott Williams and Wilkins; 2009. p. 161–86.
[34] Marlowe AL, Chinnici JE, Rivas A, et al. Revision cochlear implant surgery in children: the Johns Hopkins experience. Otol Neurotol 2009;31:74–82.
[35] Cote M, Ferron P, Bergeron F, et al. Cochlear reimplantation: causes of failure, outcomes, and audiologic performance. Laryngoscope 2007;117:1225–35.
[36] Migirov L, Taitelbaum-Swead R, Hildesheimer M, et al. Revision surgeries in cochlear implant patients: a review of 45 cases. Eur Arch Otorhinolaryngol 2007;264:3–7.
[37] Cullen RD, Fayad JN, Luxford WM, et al. Revision cochlear implant surgery in children. Otol Neurotol 2008;29:214–20.
[38] Roland JT, Huang TC, Cohen NL. Revision cochlear implantation. Otolaryngol Clin North Am 2006;39:833–9.
[39] Basura GJ, Eapen R, Buchman CA. Bilateral cochlear implantation: current concepts, indications, and results. Laryngoscope 2009;119:2395–401.
[40] Bichey BG, Miyamoto RT. Outcomes in bilateral cochlear implantation. Otolaryngol Head Neck Surg 2008;138:655–61.
[41] Gordon KA, Wong DD, Papsin BC. Cortical function in children receiving bilateral cochlear implants simultaneously or after a period of interimplant delay. Otol Neurotol 2010;31: 1293–9.
[42] Gordon KA, Papsin BC. Benefits of short interimplant delays in children receiving bilateral cochlear implants. Otol Neurotol 2009;30:319–31.
[43] Peters BR, Litovsky R, Parkson A, et al. Importance of age and postimplantation experience on speech perception measures in children with sequential bilateral cochlear implants. Otol Neurotol 2007;28:649–57.
[44] Kirk KI, Choi S. Clinical investigations of cochlear implant performance. In: Niparko JK, editor. Cochlear implants: principles and practices. 2nd edition. Philadelphia: Lippincott Williams and Wilkins; 2009. p. 191–222.
[45] Beadle EA, McKinley DJ, Nikolopoulos TP, et al. Long-term functional outcomes and academic-occupational status in implanted children after 10–14 years of cochlear implant use. Otol Neurotol 2005;26:1152–60.
[46] Archbold S, Harris M, O'Donoghue GO, et al. Reading abilities after cochlear implantation: the effect of age at 5 and 7 years after implantation. Int J Pediatr Otorhinolaryngol 2008;72:1471–8.
[47] Schopmeyer B. Reading and deafness. In: Niparko JK, editor. Cochlear implants: principles and practices. 2nd edition. Philadelphia: Lippincott Williams and Wilkins; 2009. p. 263–5.

[48] Hayes H, Geers AE, Treiman R, et al. Receptive vocabulary development in deaf children with cochlear implants: achievement in an intensive auditory-oral educational setting. Ear Hear 2009;30:128–35.
[49] Tobey EA, Geers AE, Brenner C, et al. Factors associated with development of speech production skills in children implanted by age five. Ear Hear 2003;24:36S–45S.
[50] Geers AE, Strube MJ, Tobey EA, et al. Epilogue: factors contributing to long-term outcomes of cochlear implantation in early childhood. Ear Hear 2011;32:84S–92S.
[51] Robbins AM. Rehabilitation after cochlear implantation. In: Niparko JK, editor. Cochlear implants: principles and practices. 2nd edition. Philadelphia: Lippincott Williams and Wilkins; 2009. p. 269–312.
[52] Geers AE, Nicholas JG, Sedey AL. Language skills of children with early cochlear implantation. Ear Hear 2003;24:46S–58S.
[53] Papsin BC. Cochlear implantation in children with anomalous cochleovestibular anatomy. Laryngoscope 2005;115(Suppl):1–26.
[54] Buchman CA, Copeland BJ, Yu KK, et al. Cochlear implantation in children with congenital inner ear malformations. Laryngoscope 2004;114(2):309–16.
[55] Lin FR, Niparko JK, Francis HW. Outcomes in cochlear implantation: assessment of quality-of-life impact and economic evaluation of the benefits of the cochlear implant in relation to costs. In: Niparko JK, editor. Cochlear implants: principles and practices. 2nd edition. Philadelphia: Lippincott Williams and Wilkins; 2009. p. 229–44.
[56] O'Neill C, O'Donghue GM, Archbold SM, et al. A cost-utility analysis of pediatric cochlear implantation. Laryngoscope 2000;110:156–60.
[57] Cheng AK, Rubin HR, Powe NR, et al. Cost-utility analysis of the cochlear implant in children. JAMA 2000;284:850–6.

Advances in Pediatrics 58 (2011) 297–311
ADVANCES IN PEDIATRICS

Neuroblastoma

Nadja C. Colon, MD[a], Dai H. Chung, MD[a,b,*]
[a]Department of Pediatric Surgery, Vanderbilt University Medical Center, 2200 Children's Way, Suite 7100, Nashville, TN 37232, USA
[b]Department of Cancer Biology, Vanderbilt University Medical Center, Nashville, TN 37232, USA

In the discipline of pediatric cancer biology, neuroblastoma signifies an oncologic conundrum given the clinical range with which it presents. Prognosis correlates with age and the degree of differentiation, and thus, outcomes vary from high rates of survival (with possible tumor regression) to recurrence and mortality. Although the standard of treatment is a combination of chemotherapy, radiation, and surgical resection, there is growing evidence that aggressive neuroblastomas are resistant to our therapies. To this end, research has been focused on the molecular mechanisms behind differentiation, cell survival and apoptosis, angiogenesis, and metastasis to elucidate where the process goes awry. The basis of this research has led to the development of novel therapies that are directed toward key targets, some of which are quite promising. While discussing clinical background, this article aims to provide a synopsis of the latest, up-and-coming developments in the field of neuroblastoma.

EPIDEMIOLOGY

Neuroblastoma is the most common extracranial solid tumor in infants and children, representing 8% to 10% of all childhood tumors. It accounts for approximately 15% of all cancer-related deaths in the pediatric population [1]. The incidence of neuroblastoma is 10.2 cases per million children under 15 years of age [2], and nearly 500 new cases are reported annually. Although 90% of cases are diagnosed before 5 years of age, 30% of those are within the first year. The median age of diagnosis is 22 months [3]. Rarely does it present in adolescence and adulthood, but outcomes are much poorer in this age group. There does not appear to be an increased prevalence among races, but there is a slight predilection for boys (1.2:1.0) [1].

This work was supported by grant R01 DK61470 from the National Institute of Health and Rally Foundation for Cancer Research.

*Corresponding author. Department of Pediatric Surgery, Vanderbilt University Medical Center, 2200 Children's Way, Suite 7100, Nashville, TN 37232. *E-mail address*: dai.chung@vanderbilt.edu

0065-3101/11/$ – see front matter
doi:10.1016/j.yapd.2011.03.011

With a family history noted in 1% to 2% of diagnoses, there are reports of autosomal dominant patterns of inheritance [3]. In such pedigrees, patients are frequently diagnosed at an earlier age (median age of 9 months) than those with sporadic disease and are more likely to have multiple associated primary cancers. Neuroblastoma has also been diagnosed in conjunction with other congenital conditions, such as Hirschsprung disease, congenital hypoventilation disorder, and neurofibromatosis type 1 [1]. There was early interest in the co-occurrence of neuroblastoma and neurofibromatosis, as they are both disorders of neural crest cells. However, this may represent coincidence rather than a true association [4].

Outcomes in patients with neuroblastoma have improved steadily over the last 30 years with 5-year survival rates rising from 52% to 74% [2]. The improvement is likely secondary to improved cure rates in the low-risk group, who have survival rates of up to 92%. It is estimated that 50% to 60% of patients in the high-risk group experience relapse [2], and as such, they have only seen a modest decrease in mortality. In a study by the International Neuroblastoma Risk Group, the median time to relapse was 13.2 months, and 73% of those who relapsed were aged 18 months or older. Taken together, their overall survival rates remain quite abysmal (~20% at 5 years) despite more aggressive therapies [5].

CLINICAL PRESENTATION

Multiple factors play into a patient's clinical presentation because it depends largely on tumor location, size, degree of invasion, effects from catecholamine secretion, and symptoms caused by paraneoplastic syndromes. Nearly 65% of tumors arise in the abdomen with half of those localized to the medulla of the adrenal gland. However, they can occur in the neck (5%), chest (20%), or pelvis (5%), and 1% of patients have no detectable primary [1,6]. Many patients are asymptomatic, yet some may present with constitutional symptoms (malaise, fevers, and weight loss), an enlarging mass, pain, abdominal distension, lymphadenopathy, or respiratory distress secondary to compression or hepatomegaly. Pelvic masses may cause constipation or difficulty with urination, whereas thoracic involvement can cause dysphagia, dyspnea, or rarely thoracic outlet syndrome [7]. For cervical tumors, a patient may develop Horner syndrome, and in up to 15% of patients, epidural extension may result in neurologic deficits, such as progressive paralysis [1].

At the time of diagnosis, 50% of patients present with localized disease, whereas 35% already have regional lymph node spread [1]. Metastasis can occur by hematogenous or lymphatic route, seeding bone marrow, liver, and bone. Commonly, the orbits are involved, which manifests as periorbital swelling and proptosis (raccoon eyes). When dissemination occurs to the skin, patients develop blue subcutaneous nodules known as blueberry muffin syndrome. Surprisingly, this is associated with a favorable prognosis with likely spontaneous tumor regression.

Because of its neuroendocrine properties, neuroblastoma has the potential to secrete catecholamines, which results in early-onset hypertension and tachycardia. Patients may also experience paraneoplastic syndromes. Examples include intractable diarrhea with electrolyte disturbances caused by release of vasoactive intestinal peptide (VIP), encephalomyelitis, or sensory neuropathy. There have been reports of the development of opsoclonus-myoclonus syndrome (OMS), which occurs when antibodies cross-react with cerebellar tissue [8]. The characteristic symptoms and signs of OMS include rapid, conjugate eye nystagmus with involuntary spasms of the limbs. Interestingly, the patients with intractable diarrhea caused by VIP secretion or OMS generally tend to present with less aggressive neuroblastomas. Nonetheless, symptomatic paraneoplastic syndromes are quite rare and are estimated to occur in less than 0.01% of *all* cancers [9].

CLASSIFICATION AND STAGING

Neuroblastoma belongs to a group collectively known as peripheral neuroblastic tumors, which also includes intermixed ganglioneuroblastoma, ganglioneuroma, and nodular ganglioneuroblastoma. Neuroblastoma can further be divided based on the degree of neuroblastic differentiation (undifferentiated, poorly differentiated, and differentiating) and the mitosis-karyorrhexis index (MKI; low, intermediate, or high) [10]. Histologically, it has limited Schwannian cell production, is stroma-poor, and has abundant neuroblasts [8].

The International Neuroblastoma Pathology Classification has been used to predict prognosis based on the histopathology of the tumor and age of patients. This system takes into account the degree of cell differentiation, MKI, and the presence of Schwann cells. Following these guidelines, the unfavorable group encompasses patients with any tumor more than 60 months; undifferentiated tumors with a high MKI at any age; and undifferentiated or poorly differentiated tumors with intermediate or high MKI in children older than 18 months [11].

Staging is dictated by the International Neuroblastoma Staging System (INSS) (Box 1). The Children's Oncology Group currently stratifies patients into low-, intermediate-, or high-risk categories based on patients' age at diagnosis, INSS stage, tumor histopathology, DNA index, and *MYCN* amplification status (Table 1) [12]. Because the INSS is based on tumor resection, a new system, called the International Neuroblastoma Risk Group Staging System, was introduced in hopes of better stratifying pretreatment patient risk based on clinical criteria and image-defined risk factors (Fig. 1). This staging system classifies neuroblastoma into L1 (localized disease that does not involve vital structures and is confined to one body compartment); L2 (localized disease with image-defined risk factors); M (distant metastatic disease); and MS (metastatic disease confined to the skin, liver or bone marrow in children younger than18 months) [13]. Based on this, patients can be sorted into pretreatment very low-, low-, intermediate-, and high-risk groups [14]. This classification has implications as to what treatment algorithm is recommended.

Box 1: The International Neuroblastoma Staging System

Stage 1

Localized tumor with complete gross excision with or without microscopic residual disease; ipsilateral and contralateral lymph nodes (LN) negative for tumor microscopically

Stage 2A

Unilateral tumor with incomplete gross resection; ipsilateral and contralateral LN negative for tumor microscopically

Stage 2B

Unilateral tumor with or without complete gross excision with ipsilateral LN positive for tumor; contralateral LN negative microscopically

Stage 3

Tumor infiltrating across the midline with or without regional LN involvement, localized unilateral tumor with contralateral regional LN involvement, or midline tumor with bilateral extension by infiltration (unresectable) or by LN involvement

Stage 4

Any primary tumor with dissemination to distant LN, bone, bone marrow, liver, skin, or other organs (except as defined for stage 4S)

Stage 4S

Localized primary tumor (as defined for stage 1 or 2) with dissemination limited to skin, liver, or bone marrow (limited to infants younger than 1 year)

Table 1
Children's oncology group risk stratification

INSS	Age (y)	*MYCN* status	Shimada	DNA index	Risk group
1	0–21	Any	Any	Any	Low
2A/2B	<1	Any	Any	Any	Low
	≥1–21	Normal	Any	—	Low
	≥1–21	Amplified	Favorable	—	Low
	≥1–21	Amplified	Unfavorable	—	High
3	<1	Normal	Any	Any	Intermediate
	<1	Amplified	Any	Any	High
	≥1–21	Normal	Favorable	—	Intermediate
	≥1–21	Normal	Unfavorable	—	High
	≥1–21	Amplified	Any	—	High
4	<1	Normal	Any	Any	Intermediate
	<1	Amplified	Any	Any	High
	≥1–21	Any	Any	—	High
4S	<1	Normal	Favorable	>1	Low
	<1	Normal	Any	=1	Intermediate
	<1	Normal	Unfavorable	Any	Intermediate
	<1	Amplified	Any	Any	High

INRG Stage	Age (months)	Histologic Category	Grade of Tumor Differentiation	*MYCN*	11q Aberration	Ploidy	Pretreatment Risk Group
L1/L2		GN maturing; GNB intermixed					A Very low
L1		Any, except GN maturing or GNB intermixed		NA			B Very low
				Amp			K High
L2	< 18	Any, except GN maturing or GNB intermixed		NA	No		D Low
					Yes		G Intermediate
	≥ 18	GNB nodular; neuroblastoma	Differentiating	NA	No		E Low
					Yes		H Intermediate
			Poorly differentiated or undifferentiated	NA			
				Amp			N High
M	< 18			NA		Hyperdiploid	F Low
	< 12			NA		Diploid	I Intermediate
	12 to < 18			NA		Diploid	J Intermediate
	< 18			Amp			O High
	≥ 18						P High
MS	< 18			NA	No		C Very low
					Yes		Q High
				Amp			R High

Fig. 1. International Neuroblastoma Risk Group Classification. EFS, event-free survival; L1, localized tumor confined to one body compartment and with absence of image-defined risk factors (IDRFs); L2, locoregional tumor with presence of one or more IDRFs; M, distant metastatic disease (except stage MS); MS, metastatic disease confined to skin, liver, or bone marrow in children younger than18 months; NA, not applicable. (*From* Cohn SL, Pearson AD, London WB, et al. The International Neuroblastoma Risk Group [INRG] Classification System: An INRG Task Force Report. J Clin Oncol 2009;27(2):295, Fig. 2; with permission.)

GENOMICS

From a genomic standpoint, neuroblastoma occurs in the setting of chromosomal losses and gains. DNA mutations can fall into 2 prognostic categories: whole-chromosome gains and segmental chromosomal aberrations. The former results in hyperdiploidy that is associated with a favorable prognosis, whereas the latter is characterized by *MYCN* amplification and regional gains or losses that tend to be associated with worse outcomes.

It has been shown that deletion of the chromosome 1p36 region occurs in 70% of tumors and may correlate with an increased risk of relapse in patients with localized tumors [15,16]. Interestingly, a promising candidate suppressor gene in the 1p36 region is *CHD5*, which is expressed in the nervous system and controls cellular proliferation, senescence, and apoptosis. Studies have confirmed that *CHD5* expression is low in neuroblastoma tumors that have a chromosome 1p deletion, and when these cells were transfected with *CHD5,* clonogenicity and tumor growth were decreased [17]. Whether this has any prognostic significance is unknown, but it does appear to play a role in neuroblastoma tumorigenesis.

Gain of chromosome 17q occurs in approximately 80% of neuroblastomas, making it the most common genetic aberration. Although whole-chromosome 17 gain is associated with a good prognosis [16], unbalanced translocations of chromosome 17q with either 1p or 11q have been reported to be an independent poor prognostic factor. Likewise, deletions of chromosome 11q have been identified in 15% to 22% of neuroblastomas and are also associated with unfavorable patient outcomes and a lessened time of progression-free survival [8]. Chromosome 11q and 3p deletions are often found together and occur in high-stage tumors without *MYCN* amplification that is typical of aggressive neuroblastoma [16]. With 3p deletions frequently noted in patients who are older at the time of diagnosis (median age of 60.5 months), some speculate that 3p loss is an event that occurs later in oncogenesis [18].

In instances of familial neuroblastoma, recent evidence points to mutations of the anaplastic lymphoma kinase (*ALK*) oncogene as the putative cause. *ALK* is a tyrosine kinase receptor whose expression is important in neural differentiation, proliferation, and survival. Its malignant transformation is thought to arise from missense mutations that are linked to chromosomal region 2p23–24 and result in constitutive kinase activity. However, *ALK* can also be mutated at specific hotspots, such as R1275Q and F1174L, in up to 12% of sporadic cases, with the latter mutation being the most common [19]. Currently, efforts are being made to determine the pathways by which *ALK* exerts its effects and whether inhibitors of *ALK* would be feasible therapeutically.

Lastly, the *MYCN* oncogene, which is amplified at chromosome 2p24 in 25% of cases, is used as a biomarker for disease stratification. *MYCN* amplification is defined as greater than or equal to 10 gene copies per nuclei because tumors with fewer than this do not behave as aggressively [20]. *MYCN* amplification is found in 30% to 40% of stage 3 and 4 neuroblastomas, but only in 5% of localized or stage 4S neuroblastomas. It encodes for multiple transcription factors that, when overexpressed, lead to deregulated growth and proliferation [4]. Several *MYCN* downstream targets have been identified, including p53, Aurora A kinase, and MDM2 [21]. However, the exact mechanisms remain unknown.

DIAGNOSIS

Based on clinical presentation, the index of suspicion must be high. Initial diagnostic testing should include basic blood work (complete blood count, serum electrolytes, liver function tests) and a chest radiograph, which may reveal calcifications or a posterior mediastinal mass. Additional diagnostic findings will include increased levels of urine or serum catecholamines or catecholamine metabolites (dopamine, vanillylmandelic acid, and homovanillic acid). Patients may have elevated levels of nonspecific biomarkers, such as lactate dehydrogenase (>1500 U/mL), ferritin (>142 ng/mL), and neuron-specific enolase (>100 ng/mL), which may be associated with advanced stage or relapse [15].

For diagnostic imaging, a computed tomography scan of the neck, chest, or abdomen is the gold standard, as it can simultaneously localize the tumor and determine the degree of involvement (see Fig. 1). Ultrasound may be used initially to characterize the mass. A magnetic resonance imaging may be useful if there is concern for spinal extension, and imaging of the brain is only necessary in the setting of neurologic symptoms. Although not routinely used, a $^{123/131}$iodine-meta-iodobenzylguanidine (MIBG) scan is valuable in both the detection of primary tumor and metastases because metaiodobenzylguanidine, a norepinephrine analog, is selectively concentrated in sympathetic tissue. It has also proven to be practical in surveillance of treatment response and recurrence. The role of fluorodeoxyglucose positive emission tomography (FDG-PET) remains controversial, but a small retrospective study has suggested that although MIBG is generally more sensitive for the detection of lesions, FDG-PET may be better at localizing soft-tissue metastases [22].

Despite advances in diagnostic medicine, the diagnosis of neuroblastoma can only be confirmed pathologically with tissue obtained from tumor or bone marrow. Specimens can be obtained either during resection of the primary tumor or as an open biopsy for unresectable disease. Bilateral posterior iliac crest marrow aspirates are required to exclude metastatic disease. Molecular studies, such as fluorescent in situ hybridization, can be performed on tissue samples to note ploidy, *MYCN* amplification, and the presence of other chromosomal aberrations.

TREATMENT

The mainstay of treatment consists of chemotherapy, surgical resection, or radiotherapy. However, many aggressive neuroblastomas have developed resistance to chemotherapeutic agents, making the likelihood of relapse quite high. Treatment can be hindered by aggressive neuroblastomas that exhibit drug resistance, and this may be related to the selection of clones that express multidrug resistant-associated protein (*MRP1*) [23]. The treatment algorithm is dependent on the patients' stage and risk stratification. The goal of induction chemotherapy is to achieve remission by reducing the tumor burden, which then allows for a more complete resection when indicated. Induction chemotherapy consists of some combination of cyclophosphamide, doxorubicin, cisplatin, melphalan, carboplatin, etoposide, topotecan, ifosfamide, and vincristine. After induction, treatment is consolidated with one or more courses of high-dose chemotherapy to induce bone marrow ablation, which necessitates autologous hematopoietic stem cell support. Rescue is not without complication as it can lead to growth failure, endocrinopathy, and the occurrence of secondary malignancies [24].

For high-risk patients, radiotherapy is needed for local and metastatic control. It is indicated when there is minimal residual disease post-induction chemotherapy and resection. Current radiation protocols use a dose of 2100 cGy, and based on the practices at the Memorial Sloan-Kettering Cancer Center, the combination of chemotherapy, surgery, and radiation therapy has resulted in a local relapse rate of less than 10% [20]. Radiation is contraindicated for intraspinal tumors because it can lead to vertebral damage, growth arrest, and scoliosis. Yet, it may be necessary for palliation in the setting of pain or acute neurologic symptoms caused by cord compression [8].

Surgery is recommended based on the ability to obtain complete resection, which is itself dependent on location and invasiveness of the tumor. In preoperative planning, important considerations include tumor size, extent of adherence or extension into adjacent structures, and the likelihood of surgical cure. Resection is correlated with a reduced risk of local recurrence, especially in combination with induction chemotherapy and local radiotherapy. Thus, surgical resection should be pursued only after adjuvant therapy because it both increases the degree of complete excision and decreases morbidity. For stage 1–2B tumors, resection is recommended. For more advanced-stage neuroblastoma (stages 3 and 4), surgical intervention is limited to an open biopsy. For those infants who are stage 4S, surgical resection is not recommended because these tumors tend to spontaneously differentiate and regress.

Presently, patients receive 6 courses of 13-*cis*-retinoic acid (CRA) to eradicate residual disease that may still be present despite meeting imaging criteria for complete remission. This treatment is based on the finding that high-dose therapy with 13-*cis*-retinoic acid given after chemoradiation significantly improved event-free survival in high-risk neuroblastoma. Side effects, such as skin dryness and cheilitis, are the dose-limiting factor and, consequently, CRA therapy consists of 2-week courses alternating with 2 weeks for mucocutaneous recovery [25].

Trials involving myeloablative chemotherapy and ^{131}I-MIBG have been underway in an effort to minimize adverse side effects by making therapies more targeted. Previous studies have shown that ^{131}I-MIBG exhibits activity against refractory neuroblastoma with response rates ranging from 10% to 50% [26]. In a phase I trial of ^{131}I-MIBG therapy for relapsed neuroblastoma, myelosuppression was the most significant toxicity at doses greater than 15 mCi/kg, as nearly half of the patients enrolled required hematopoietic cell transfusion. Despite this, the response rate (36%), event-free survival (18% at 1 year), and overall survival (49% at 1 year; 29% at 2 years) were found to be significantly higher in patients older than 12 years and who had fewer than 3 prior treatment regimens [27]. Subsequently, a phase I dose-escalation study of ^{131}I-MIBG with myeloablative chemotherapy and stem cell rescue showed a significant response rate of 25% in patients with primary refractory disease. Given these findings, ^{131}I-MIBG may prove to be useful in conjunction with other treatment modalities.

The total length of therapy averages nearly 1 year, and most treatment failures are caused by minimal residual disease that was not eradicated following high-dose chemotherapy. Although the aim of further treatment is remission, prolonged disease stabilization is usually the reality because most patients who relapse eventually die of disease progression. Even patients who achieve a cure with initial therapy remain at risk for developing long-term complications related to treatment, including hearing loss, infertility, and second malignancies [28].

CURRENT RESEARCH MILESTONES AND PROPOSED NOVEL THERAPIES

Retinoic acid

Retinoids are vitamin A derivatives that can cause arrest of cell growth and induce differentiation of human neuroblastoma cells. Although 13-*cis*-retinoic acid is being used clinically for this purpose, fenretinide (4-HPR) is another retinoid derivative currently in phase I trials which has been reported to inhibit growth in vitro in a dose-dependent manner. At the higher end of the dose spectrum, it also seems to be active against retinoic acid-resistant neuroblastoma cell lines that harbor mutations in the retinoic acid receptor (RAR). Unlike all-trans and 13-*cis* retinoic acids, 4-HPR does not induce differentiation, but is actually cytotoxic and pro-apoptotic and may do so in a receptor-independent manner [25,29]. So far, it appears that 4-HPR is minimally toxic with no evidence of myelosuppression; the most common side effect reported is decreased night vision.

mTOR inhibitors

One promising target is the mammalian target of rapamycin (mTOR), which is a serine/threonine protein kinase that regulates cell growth, proliferation, motility, metabolism, and survival. It can exert its effects through several different signaling pathways, notably the phosphatidylinositol-3 kinase (PI3K)-AKT pathway. Rapamycin, a bacterial byproduct, is the classically cited mTOR inhibitor, and it does so by complexing with the intracellular receptor FKBP12 to bind directly to the FKBP12-rapamycin binding (FRB) domain on mTOR [30]. This process leads to activation of downstream effectors, such as cyclin D1, p21, and HIF1α/β. Treatment with mTOR inhibitors leads to downregulation of *MYCN* and vascular endothelial growth factor (VEGF).

Temsirolimus, a rapamycin analog, is being investigated in phase II trials in patients with relapsed neuroblastoma. One study showed that treatment with an insulin-like growth factor (IGF)-1 receptor inhibitor and temsirolimus in vitro was more effective at inducing cell death than either agent alone [31]. Known side effects include skin rashes, stomatitis, and hyperglycemia.

Aurora A kinase

Aurora A kinase is a serine/threonine kinase important in regulating progression through the cell cycle, particularly during the G_2 to M phase transition. Aurora A kinase has an important role in centrosome maturation, spindle assembly, meiotic maturation, and spindle orientation. Selective inhibition of Aurora A kinase results in inhibition of autophosphorylation and p53 phosphorylation, monopolar spindles, and G_2-M arrest [32]. MLN8237, a reversible Aurora A kinase inhibitor, is being investigated in phase I clinical trials by the COG for patients who have experienced relapse. In vitro and in vivo studies with MLN8237 have shown that in addition to inducing apoptosis, it upregulates p53 and the tumor suppressor genes p21 and p27 [33]. Dose-escalation and combination therapy studies are currently underway.

TrkB inhibitors

The Trk family is a group of tropomyosin kinases that are known to modulate neuronal differentiation and survival. There are 3 isoforms (TrkA, TrkB, and TrkC) that each has an affinity for a specific ligand (NGF, BDNF, and NT-3, respectively). Ligand binding causes receptor homodimerization, which leads to autophosphorylation, docking of downstream effectors, and activation of PI3K/AKT, phospholipid C (PLC) $\gamma 1$, and Ras/mitogen-activated protein kinase (Ras-MAPK) signaling [34]. Their ligands can similarly bind p75, a nonselective and low-affinity death receptor, to induce apoptosis via the c-Jun amino terminal kinase (JNK) pathway [35]. Although TrkA expression is associated with favorable prognosis, TrkB has been found to correlate with *MYCN* amplification and clinically aggressive neuroblastoma. In studies, neuroblastoma tumor cells treated with brain-derived nerve factor (BDNF) appear to be less sensitive to cytotoxic drugs, survive in a less than optimal microenvironment, are more invasive, and produce increased levels of VEGF. Furthermore, inhibitors were found to slow growth and induce apoptosis. Thus, the Trk inhibitor CEP-701 is presently being used as an oral phase I agent with the premise that it will be most effective in conjunction with conventional chemotherapeutic agents.

Immunotherapy

The ganglioside GD2 is expressed in the surface of tumors of neuroectodermal origin, including neuroblastoma. Anti-GD2 monoclonal antibodies have been developed because they are specific, high affinity, and fairly nontoxic. They kill tumor cells through both complement and cell-mediated lysis. The antibody 3F8 is a murine IgG_3 monoclonal antibody that has been shown to activate complement on malignant neuroblastomas with ensuing lysis. Moreover, it is thought that granulocyte-macrophage colony-stimulating factor (GM-CSF) can potentially amplify 3F8 antitumor activity by increasing granulocytes [36]. However, its clinical use has been complicated by the formation of human anti-mouse antibodies. To circumvent this, chimeric mouse-human antibodies, such as Ch14.18 (a monoclonal antibody against the tumor-associated GD2), have been generated. Although they were thought to be less immunogenic, 28% of patients reportedly still developed antibodies in a phase I trial [37]. In other studies, beta-glucan has been found to enhance anti-GD2 antibody antitumor effects through increasing iC3b-mediated cytotoxicity. An ongoing phase I trial is comparing the efficacy of 3F8 when given with oral beta-glucan. Other trials are focused on using Ch14.18 in conjunction with other agents, such as interleukin-2 and GM-CSF, after high-dose chemotherapy with stem-cell rescue. A recent study demonstrated that immunotherapy with Ch14.18, GM-CSF, and interleukin-2 was found to be associated with significantly improved overall outcome when compared with standard therapy in high-risk group patients with neuroblastoma [38].

Angiogenesis inhibitors

VEGF has been established as an important growth factor that promotes tumor angiogenesis by inducing endothelial cell proliferation. It has been found to play a significant role in tumorigenesis because in hypoxic environments, such as those in rapidly growing tumors, hypoxia-inducing factor (HIF) stimulates VEGF production. This process results in downstream activation of several signaling pathways, including PI3K/AKT (increased vascular permeability) and MAPK/ERK (endothelial cell proliferation). In neuroblastoma murine models, VEGF inhibitors were found to decrease cell proliferation [39]. Bevacizumab, a human-derived VEGF monoclonal antibody, is approved by the Food and Drug Administration for the treatment of colorectal, breast, and lung cancer, and it is now being used in phase II studies in neuroblastoma, as it has not previously been used in children.

MDM2 and ODC1 as a *MYCN* targets

Mutations of the gene p53 are rare in neuroblastoma and several studies have shown that it appears to be functional because it is capable of activating downstream apoptotic effectors in response to DNA damage [40]. MDM2 is a negative regulator of p53, being a key player in its ubiquitination. It has been suggested that deregulated MDM2 expression may explain aberrant p53 function. Notably, MDM2 is transactivated by *MYCN*, and downregulation of *MYCN* leads to decreased MDM2 expression, p53 stabilization, and cell death. Therefore, dysregulation of MDM2 is thought to decrease p53 activity, and in vitro studies with the MDM2 inhibitor nutlin showed that it could stabilize p53 and induce G_1 cell cycle arrest and apoptosis [41,42]. Further investigations are needed, but this class of agents may represent an untapped resource.

Recently, *ODC1*, an oncogene that encodes for an enzyme needed in polyamine biosynthesis, was tagged as a potential therapeutic candidate. Polyamines enhance transcription, translation, and replication and are, therefore, essential for cell survival as depletion leads to growth arrest and apoptosis. *MYCN* functions as a transcription factor that dimerizes with another factor known as MAX to form a complex that can then activate *ODC1* transcription [43]. *MYCN*-amplified tumors have elevated levels of ODC1 and exhibit deregulated polyamine synthesis. In mouse models, studies revealed that treatment with cyclophosphamide and α-difluoromethylornithine (DFMO), an ODC inhibitor, led to an increased overall survival (80% vs 20% at 3 months) than with cyclophosphamide alone [44]. It is now being piloted in phase I clinical trials with and without etoposide administration.

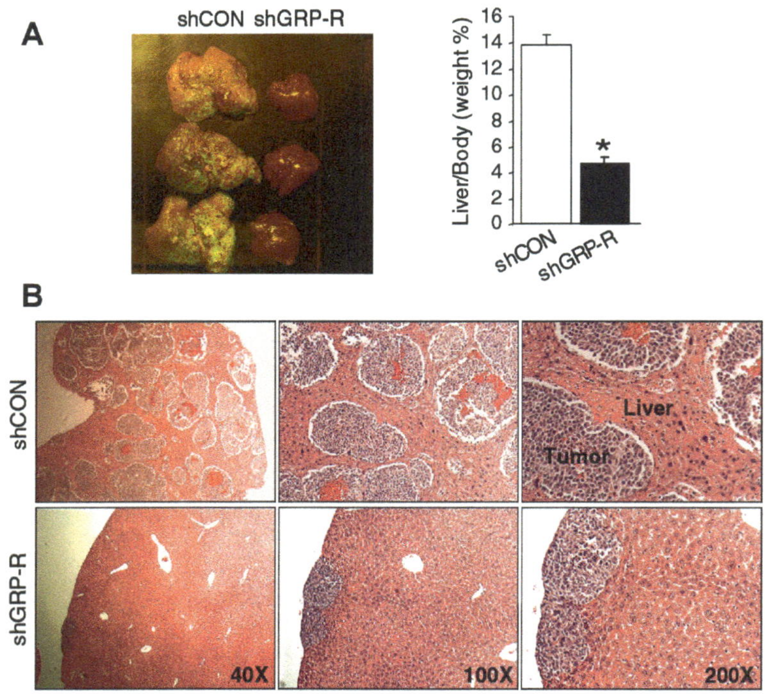

Fig. 2. Effects of GRP-receptor knockdown on neuroblastoma metastasis in vivo. Spleen injection liver metastasis murine model was used using human neuroblastoma BE(2)-C cells transfected with pEGFP/shGRP-R (silenced GRP receptors) or pEGFP/shCON (controls). (*A*) Livers from mice injected with BE(2)-C/GFP/shGRP-R (short-hairpin silenced GRP-receptors) and control cells (shCON). Silencing of GRP-receptors (shGRP-R; *right column*) attenuated liver metastasis of BE(2)-C tumors. Quantitative analysis of liver weight relative to body weight (* $P<.05$ vs shCON) shows significantly less weight in GRP-R silenced group. (*B*) Representative hematoxylin-eosin–stained sections of livers from mice injected with BE(2)-C/GFP/shCON (controls; *upper*) and BE(2)-C/GFP/shGRP-R (GRP receptor silenced; *lower*) cells. Extensive liver metastases are seen in mice from constitutive GRP-receptor expressing BE(2)-C cells (*upper*). (*Adapted from* Qiao J, Kang J, Ishola TA, et al. Gastrin-releasing peptide receptor silencing suppresses the tumorigenesis and metastatic potential of neuroblastoma. Proc Natl Acad Sci USA 2008;105(35):12895, Fig. 6; with permission.)

GRP receptor

Gastrin-releasing peptide (GRP) receptors, a member of G-protein coupled receptor family, are abundantly expressed in undifferentiated neuroblastomas. As in other well-characterized cell surface tyrosine kinase receptor's function in cancers (eg, epidermal growth factor receptor), GRP receptor may also be an important therapeutic cell membrane target in neuroblastomas. GRP ligand is produced and secreted by neuroblastomas to stimulate its tumor growth, and hence, it functions as an autocrine growth factor [45]. GRP binds to GRP receptors to activate the PI3K/AKT pathway in promoting tumorigenesis in neuroblastomas [46]. Targeted silencing of GPR receptors in neuroblastoma cells showed significantly attenuated xenograft growth as well as liver metastases when compared with controls with constitutive expression of GRP receptors [47]. Knockdown of GRP receptors demonstrated inhibition of tumor metastasis to liver in vivo (Fig. 2) [47].

SUMMARY

In spite of the knowledge provided within, neuroblastoma remains a therapeutic enigma. As we are driven to improve outcomes and survival, the ideal therapy also remains elusive. However, there are many fronts on which to attack and it seems unquestionable that the cure will require a multimodal approach. Part of the solution is to effectively eradicate minimal residual disease, as this appears to put patients at highest risk for relapse and progression. Until then, we remain vulnerable to a cancer that continues to evolve.

Acknowledgments

The authors thank Karen Martin for manuscript preparation.

References

[1] Park JR, Eggert A, Caron H. Neuroblastoma: biology, prognosis, and treatment. Hematol Oncol Clin North Am 2010;24:65–86.
[2] Maris JM. Recent advances in neuroblastoma. N Engl J Med 2010;362:2202–11.
[3] Esiashvili N, Anderson C, Katzenstein HM. Neuroblastoma. Curr Probl Cancer 2009;33:333–60.
[4] Brodeur GM. Neuroblastoma: biological insights into a clinical enigma. Nat Rev Cancer 2003;3:203–16.
[5] London WB, Matthay KK, Ambros PF, et al. Clinical and biological features predictive of survival after relapse of neuroblastoma: a study from the International Neuroblastoma (NB) Risk Group (INRG) Database. J Clin Oncol 2010;28:9518.
[6] Kushner BH. Neuroblastoma: a disease requiring a multitude of imaging studies. J Nucl Med 2004;45:1172–88.
[7] Haase GM, LaQuaglia MP. Neuroblastoma. In: Ziegler MM, Azizkhan RG, Weber TR, editors. Operative pediatric surgery. New York: McGraw-Hill; 2003. p. 1181–92.
[8] Ishola TA, Chung DH. Neuroblastoma. Surg Oncol 2007;16:149–56.
[9] Darnell RB, Posner JB. Paraneoplastic syndromes involving the nervous system. N Engl J Med 2003;349:1543–54.
[10] Goto S, Umehara S, Gerbing RB, et al. Histopathology (International Neuroblastoma Pathology Classification) and MYCN status in patients with peripheral neuroblastic tumors: a report from the Children's Cancer Group. Cancer 2001;92:2699–708.

[11] Janoueix-Lerosey I, Schleiermacher G, Delattre O. Molecular pathogenesis of peripheral neuroblastic tumors. Oncogene 2010;29:1566–79.
[12] Maris JM. The biologic basis for neuroblastoma heterogeneity and risk stratification. Curr Opin Pediatr 2005;17:7–13.
[13] Monclair T, Brodeur GM, Ambros PF, et al. The International Neuroblastoma Risk Group (INRG) staging system: an INRG Task Force report. J Clin Oncol 2009;27:298–303.
[14] Cohn SL, Pearson AD, London WB, et al. The International Neuroblastoma Risk Group (INRG) classification system: an INRG Task Force report. J Clin Oncol 2009;27: 289–97.
[15] Kim S, Chung DH. Pediatric solid malignancies: neuroblastoma and Wilms' tumor. Surg Clin North Am 2006;86:469–87, xi.
[16] Van Roy N, De Preter K, Hoebeeck J, et al. The emerging molecular pathogenesis of neuroblastoma: implications for improved risk assessment and targeted therapy. Genome Med 2009;1:74.
[17] Fujita T, Igarashi J, Okawa ER, et al. CHD5, a tumor suppressor gene deleted from 1p36.31 in neuroblastomas. J Natl Cancer Inst 2008;100:940–9.
[18] Vandesompele J, Baudis M, De Preter K, et al. Unequivocal delineation of clinicogenetic subgroups and development of a new model for improved outcome prediction in neuroblastoma. J Clin Oncol 2005;23:2280–99.
[19] Kelleher FC, McDermott R. The emerging pathogenic and therapeutic importance of the anaplastic lymphoma kinase gene. Eur J Cancer 2010;46:2357–68.
[20] Modak S, Cheung NK. Neuroblastoma: therapeutic strategies for a clinical enigma. Cancer Treat Rev 2010;36:307–17.
[21] Bell E, Chen L, Liu T, et al. MYCN oncoprotein targets and their therapeutic potential. Cancer Lett 2010;293:144–57.
[22] Taggart DR, Han MM, Quach A, et al. Comparison of iodine-123 metaiodobenzylguanidine (MIBG) scan and [18F]fluorodeoxyglucose positron emission tomography to evaluate response after iodine-131 MIBG therapy for relapsed neuroblastoma. J Clin Oncol 2009;27:5343–9.
[23] Peaston AE, Gardaneh M, Franco AV, et al. MRP1 gene expression level regulates the death and differentiation response of neuroblastoma cells. Br J Cancer 2001;85:1564–71.
[24] Yalcin B, Kremer LC, Caron HN, et al. High-dose chemotherapy and autologous haematopoietic stem cell rescue for children with high-risk neuroblastoma. Cochrane Database Syst Rev 2010;5:CD006301.
[25] Reynolds CP, Matthay KK, Villablanca JG, et al. Retinoid therapy of high-risk neuroblastoma. Cancer Lett 2003;197:185–92.
[26] Kang TI, Brophy P, Hickeson M, et al. Targeted radiotherapy with submyeloablative doses of 131I-MIBG is effective for disease palliation in highly refractory neuroblastoma. J Pediatr Hematol Oncol 2003;25:769–73.
[27] Matthay KK, Yanik G, Messina J, et al. Phase II study on the effect of disease sites, age, and prior therapy on response to iodine-131-metaiodobenzylguanidine therapy in refractory neuroblastoma. J Clin Oncol 2007;25:1054–60.
[28] Wagner LM, Danks MK. New therapeutic targets for the treatment of high-risk neuroblastoma. J Cell Biochem 2009;107:46–57.
[29] Wu JM, DiPietrantonio AM, Hsieh TC. Mechanism of fenretinide (4-HPR)-induced cell death. Apoptosis 2001;6:377–88.
[30] Yip CK, Murata K, Walz T, et al. Structure of the human mTOR complex I and its implications for rapamycin inhibition. Mol Cell 2010;38:768–74.
[31] Coulter DW, Blatt J, D'Ercole AJ, et al. IGF-I receptor inhibition combined with rapamycin or temsirolimus inhibits neuroblastoma cell growth. Anticancer Res 2008;28:1509–16.
[32] Moore AS, Blagg J, Linardopoulos S, et al. Aurora kinase inhibitors: novel small molecules with promising activity in acute myeloid and Philadelphia-positive leukemias. Leukemia 2010;24:671–8.

[33] Gorgun G, Calabrese E, Hideshima T, et al. A novel Aurora-A kinase inhibitor MLN8237 induces cytotoxicity and cell-cycle arrest in multiple myeloma. Blood 2010;115:5202–13.
[34] Brodeur GM, Minturn JE, Ho R, et al. Trk receptor expression and inhibition in neuroblastomas. Clin Cancer Res 2009;15:3244–50.
[35] Thiele CJ, Li Z, McKee AE. On Trk–the TrkB signal transduction pathway is an increasingly important target in cancer biology. Clin Cancer Res 2009;15:5962–7.
[36] Kushner BH, Kramer K, Cheung NK. Phase II trial of the anti-G(D2) monoclonal antibody 3F8 and granulocyte-macrophage colony-stimulating factor for neuroblastoma. J Clin Oncol 2001;19:4189–94.
[37] Ozkaynak MF, Sondel PM, Krailo MD, et al. Phase I study of chimeric human/murine anti-ganglioside G(D2) monoclonal antibody (ch14.18) with granulocyte-macrophage colony-stimulating factor in children with neuroblastoma immediately after hematopoietic stem-cell transplantation: a Children's Cancer Group Study. J Clin Oncol 2000;18:4077–85.
[38] Yu AL, Gilman AL, Ozkaynak MF, et al. Anti-GD2 antibody with GM-CSF, interleukin-2, and isotretinoin for neuroblastoma. N Engl J Med 2010;363:1324–34.
[39] Shusterman S, Grupp SA, Barr R, et al. The angiogenesis inhibitor tnp-470 effectively inhibits human neuroblastoma xenograft growth, especially in the setting of subclinical disease. Clin Cancer Res 2001;7:977–84.
[40] Barbieri E, Mehta P, Chen Z, et al. MDM2 inhibition sensitizes neuroblastoma to chemotherapy-induced apoptotic cell death. Mol Cancer Ther 2006;5:2358–65.
[41] Slack A, Lozano G, Shohet JM. MDM2 as MYCN transcriptional target: implications for neuroblastoma pathogenesis. Cancer Lett 2005;228:21–7.
[42] Van Maerken T, Speleman F, Vermeulen J, et al. Small-molecule MDM2 antagonists as a new therapy concept for neuroblastoma. Cancer Res 2006;66:9646–55.
[43] Casero RA Jr, Marton LJ. Targeting polyamine metabolism and function in cancer and other hyperproliferative diseases. Nat Rev Drug Discov 2007;6:373–90.
[44] Hogarty MD, Norris MD, Davis K, et al. ODC1 is a critical determinant of MYCN oncogenesis and a therapeutic target in neuroblastoma. Cancer Res 2008;68:9735–45.
[45] Kim S, Hu W, Kelly DR, et al. Gastrin-releasing peptide is a growth factor for human neuroblastomas. Ann Surg 2002;235:621–9 [discussion: 629–30].
[46] Kang J, Ishola TA, Baregamian N, et al. Bombesin induces angiogenesis and neuroblastoma growth. Cancer Lett 2007;253:273–81.
[47] Qiao J, Kang J, Ishola TA, et al. Gastrin-releasing peptide receptor silencing suppresses the tumorigenesis and metastatic potential of neuroblastoma. Proc Natl Acad Sci U S A 2008;105:12891–6.

Advances in Pediatrics 58 (2011) 313–317

ADVANCES IN PEDIATRICS

INDEX

Note: Page numbers of article titles are in **boldface** type.

0065-3101/11/$ – see front matter
doi:10.1016/S0065-3101(11)00027-2

Kolibri 360 GmbH
Ferdinand-Jühlke-Straße 7
99095 Erfurt, Deutschland
produktsicherheit@kolibri360.de